# Ethical Decisions in Medicine

# Ethical Decisions in Medicine

# Howard Brody

Department of Human Development,
Michigan State University College of
Human Medicine, East Lansing

Foreword by
Joseph F. Fletcher, S.T.D., D.Litt.
Visiting Professor of Medical Ethics,
University of Virginia School of Medicine, Charlottesville,
and Visiting Professor, The University of Texas
Health Science Center at Houston Medical School

First Edition

Second Printing

Library of Congress catalog card No. 75-30279

ISBN 0-316-10898-7

Printed in the United States of America

Little, Brown and Company   Boston

# Foreword

Medical ethics has come a long way. The A.M.A. code of 1847 proposed that a physician should "unite condescension with authority"—a quaint paternalism by current standards. In the first part of this century medical ethics had shifted its emphasis to the problems of obligation between doctors and patients but was still fairly limited to clinical situations. When I published *Morals and Medicine* in 1954, medical ethics still meant for the most part medical manners—deportment, guild rules, propriety. Should the doctor sit on the bed? Should he "smell" of tobacco?

Now we have reached a third stage, which combines problems in patient care with what "ought" to be done about the value choices posed in a broad range of social-policy issues along the biological front: allocation of medical resources (not just clinical triage), elective death or "euthanasia" for certain defective newborns and for patients in terminal illness, quality of life weighed against quantity, limits for tissue and organ transplants, rules for animal and human experimentation, resuscitation, artificial modes of human reproduction, psychosurgery, fetal interventions, dangerous viral and bacterial innovations in molecular biology—the list is long. At this stage of "biomedical ethics" we must look at the life sciences in social as well as clinical terms.

Howard Brody is in an excellent position to discuss with authority these rapidly developing areas of medical ethics. A student both of medicine and of ethics, he is young enough and close enough to those who are encountering this complex field for the first time to be aware of the needs of those who will be using this book. He is also humble enough to call up the recognized experts and careful enough to have already tested his ideas thoroughly in the classrooms of a first-class medical school. Although he is admirably candid about his own personal positions, the book is realistic: it has not been tied to any arcane metaphysics or easy moralistic and loftier-than-thou injunctions. It is the first survey of this field tailored specifically to the needs and questions of medical students of all faiths and backgrounds. And it makes intriguing use of both real and hypothetical case illustrations.

Our thanks go to the author for two things especially. First, he makes it clear that medical ethics is a branch of ethics, not of medicine. Second, he deals with his subject without being limited by any rigid "system" of beliefs. The book's virtue is that it is not an answer manual. Books can stimulate thinking and offer suggestions; only people can make decisions.

Joseph Fletcher

# Preface

This book is a self-instructional unit in that it is designed to be used by the student, if need be, independent of any formal course or lectures—although group discussion enhances the consideration of the cases. It may also be termed a "programmed text" in that it uses some programmed features. In some places, the reader may skip ahead without loss of continuity. In other places, the reader is asked to choose among two or more answers to a question, and is then directed to proceed to one of several discussions depending on his choice. Wherever possible, the reader is directed back to relevant sections, so that he may refresh his memory on parts of the text that he had forgotten or had not fully understood before.

Because the physician or health professional must put ethical knowledge to work in the clinical setting, this book relies on many sample cases to illustrate major points. Each case concludes with a question. As you read the text, you can treat these as rhetorical questions, but you will get much more out of the unit if you pause and arrive at your own reasoned answer before continuing your reading.

This book requires some basic college-level understanding of biology, especially elementary genetics for Chapters 14 and 15, but does not assume any specifically medical knowledge beyond recourse to a medical dictionary. It is aimed at about the level of a first-year medical student or a junior nursing student. Instructors in more philosophically oriented medical ethics courses may find this book useful as a topic outline and collection of discussion cases, while assigning additional reading to cover points on ethical methodology not included here.

Since medical ethics is such a complex field, and since the literature on the subject has accumulated immensely over the past several years, a book of this size can serve only as an introduction. On completing this book, the reader should have a sort of road map to the subject matter rather than an in-depth knowledge of medical ethics. However, if you read in addition a good number of the suggested materials listed in the back of this book, you will be able to achieve a high degree of familiarity with current discussion of ethical issues in medicine.

If your time for reading this book is limited, first read Chapters 1 through 8, then Chapters 17 and 18. You can then go back to cover the specific topics in Chapters 9 through 16 as you have the opportunity.

H.B.

# Acknowledgments

Drs. William B. Weil, Jr., James E. Trosko, and Thomas A. Helmrath of the Department of Human Development, and Dr. Bruce Miller of the Department of Philosophy, Michigan State University, reviewed portions of the manuscript of this book and made many helpful recommendations.

Among the many others from whose comments I have benefited are: Dr. Arthur F. Kohrman, Department of Human Development; Dr. Scott N. Swisher and Dr. Anthony Bowdler, Department of Medicine; Dr. Edward D. Coppola, Department of Surgery; Steven Posar, medical student; Drs. Martin Benjamin, Harold T. Walsh, and Donald Koch, Department of Philosophy; and Dr. June Goodfield, College of Human Medicine, Michigan State University. I am also indebted to Dr. Robert Baker, formerly of the Department of Philosophy, Wayne State University.

I received special benefit from the Institute of Society, Ethics, and the Life Sciences in attending their workshop on teaching medical ethics in Berkeley, California, July 1973. Dr. Robert M. Veatch has been most generous in providing case material which was adapted for this text.

I was assisted in revising the original book, following comments from students and faculty, by a teaching assistantship at the Institute of Medical Humanities, University of Texas Medical Branch at Galveston, with special assistance from Dr. H. Tristram Engelhardt, Jr., Dr. Chester R. Burns, and Mr. George Agich.

The design and production of the book was the work of Mr. Harry Andrews and the staff of the Biomedical Communications Center of Michigan State University.

I have modified most of my source material to suit the needs of this book, so that except where identified by direct quotations, none of the above individuals are responsible for any errors or oversimplifications that might appear.

# Contents

# Contents

# List of Cases for Discussion

# Key to Symbols

26 ↓

The text is continued in Frame 26. (If no number, the text is continued in the next frame below.)

UNCLEAR *43

If this statement is unclear, go to Frame 43 for more discussion.

LEGAL
IMPLICATIONS? *19

If you are curious about the legal implications of this point, go to Frame 19. If not, continue the main body of text as directed.

32 ↑

Resume your reading of the main body of the text at Frame 32.

SKIP TO
CASES ↓ 83

If you are not interested in what is to follow immediately, you may skip ahead and start reading about the sample cases in Frame 83.

REVIEW ↑
RIGHTS 12-15

If you would like to review the concept of "rights," which is mentioned in this frame, return to the original discussion in Frames 12—15. Then resume reading the main body of text with the next frame below this one.

In general, the frame referred to by a starred note will be located at the bottom of that page, separated by a solid line. Frames to which you are directed to turn to check your answers to a question will be located at the tops of the next several pages, also separated by solid lines. Portions that you may skip without loss of continuity will be set off by broken lines across the page.

# Objectives

After completing this self-instructional book, the student should be able to:

1. Given an appropriate clinical case or cases as examples, outline a problem-solving method for dealing with the ethical questions involved. Such a method should include:
   a) identification of the key ethical questions.
   b) formulation of an ethical statement of what ought to be done, in a form specific enough to allow for constructive debate and discussion.
   c) determination of both short-range and long-range consequences of the proposed ethical statement, including consequences on the physiological, psychological, and social levels.
   d) assignment of weights to these consequences according to their relative probabilities.
   e) comparison of these consequences with one's own set of values, to determine the acceptability of the ethical statement.
   f) provision for dealing with a contradiction between one's values and the predicted consequences, either through a revision of the ethical statement or through a reordering of the priorities of one's values.
   g) provision for testing one's personal values for their acceptability, both by reference to commonly accepted morality and by comparison with objective criteria, such as "bioethics."

2. Given a clinical case as an example, identify which aspects of the medical decision to be made are of a technical nature and which are of an ethical nature, and explain how the technical aspects and the ethical aspects are related to each other.

3. Given either a case example or an issue area in medical ethics, be able to discuss the ethical questions raised in terms of:
   a) the nature of the doctor-patient relationship.
   b) informed consent.
   c) criteria for determining quality of life.
   d) determination of the right of participation in the decision-making process; or whatever combination of these is applicable.

4. Given a hypothetical argument on a medical-ethical topic, be able to detect any common errors in ethical argument and explain how the thoughts of the speaker could be better restated. The common errors include:
   a) appealing to empirical data to settle an ethical question, e.g., "Everybody does it, so I ought to also."
   b) arguing backwards from results to the original ethical questions, or, retrospective ethics, e.g., "The operation was a success, so it doesn't matter now that the surgeon didn't get the patient's informed consent."
   c) assuming that a person will have good motives because of his social or professional role, and/or assuming that good motives will lead to good actions, e.g., "As a doctor, I always have the best interest of my patient at heart, so I don't have to ask the patient what he wants done in a particular case."
   d) arguing the ethics of a position by definition, without reference to actual consequences, e.g., "Euthanasia is nothing but a form of suicide, therefore it is wrong."

e) basing one's ethical claims on a "right" without stating where the "right" originates, on what authority it is based, or who has the responsibility to fulfill it, e.g., "As a woman I have a right to bear normal children of my own."

f) arguing that an ethical statement or action is wrong because it may lead to bad consequences, without showing that those consequences are in fact probable (the "domino theory"), e.g., "Abortion on demand is wrong because if you allow it, the next thing you know there'll be total promiscuity and a breakdown of the family."

g) arguing on the basis of a "catch phrase" which is either inherently devoid of meaning or so general and vague as to be inapplicable to specific instances, e.g., "playing God," "primum non nocere."

h) placing great weight on a possible consequence of very low probability, to the exclusion of more probable consequences, e.g., "You should never allow a patient to die without doing everything possible to prolong life, because tomorrow a new miracle cure might be discovered."

# Not Objectives

Because the nature of "medical ethics" is often misunderstood, and is often confused with what is now referred to as "medical etiquette" or rules of intraprofessional conduct, these "not objectives" are mentioned here for clarification.

After completing this book, the student will not be able to:

1)   Recite a set of rules of proper medical conduct, the application of which will assure that one does the ethical thing in any instance.

2)   State an ethical decision-making method which, for any specific case, will yield one and only one "right" answer as to the ethical thing to do.

3)   Cite a "code of ethics" which will give useful guidance in all problematical cases.

4)   Discuss any aspect of medical law, and state how the law would view any action taken in a specific case.

# Ethical Decisions in Medicine

# 1. Introduction: Why Study Medical Ethics?

Mr. L.W., a 54-year-old computer designer, is now in the eighth day of his recuperation from abdominal surgery to repair an ulcer, and is being cared for by his surgeon. While a likable person, Mr. L.W. has a history of neuroses and gives the impression of being a chronic complainer, possibly with a touch of the hypochondriac about him as well. The nurses note that he always requests his pain shot of Demerol, which the surgeon has ordered "every 4 hours p.r.n. (as needed)," and that he regularly complains of recurring pain about ½ hour before his next shot is due.

This morning, the surgeon examines Mr. L.W. and finds that all outward signs point to a routine post-operative recovery. He reminds Mr. L.W. that Demerol, while a very potent pain drug, nevertheless has a high addiction potential if used regularly over too long a period. He notes that "most of my patients" are relatively pain-free by the eighth day after surgery, and suggests that if he were to discontinue the order for Demerol, Mr. L.W. would find that he could really do without it just as well.

Mr. L.W. objects. He insists that regardless of how the other patients respond, he is having real pain, and thinks he could not stand it without medication. He doesn't like the idea of addiction any more than the surgeon does, but he asks that he be kept on Demerol "at least for a few more days."

After a bit more discussion along this line, the surgeon tells Mr. L.W. that he is changing the order to Talwin, a less potent pain drug but one with much less potential for addiction.

Cases like this one occur every day in all hospitals. The decisions such as the one made by the surgeon to change medications are made many times each day with no more than a moment's thought. If this surgeon were asked to elaborate upon the nature of his decision, he would most likely compare the pharmacologic properties of the two drugs, and conclude that "I made the decision according to my clinical judgment." The topic of "ethics" would never arise.

Is the decision really "clinical judgment"? Surely that is a large part of it; the surgeon could not have acted as he did without a purely technical knowledge of the actions of the drugs, augmented by his own experience with large numbers of patients who have used them. But notice that this way of looking at the decision leaves a lot which is assumed but never stated. The surgeon seems to be assuming that Mr. L.W. is not feeling as much pain as he thinks, although he has no way to prove this one way or the other. He has judged Mr. L.W. to be a less reliable reporter in this regard than some of his other patients. Also, implicit in his decision is the judgment that it is better to suffer a certain amount of pain than to become addicted to a narcotic drug.

5    Let's examine that last judgment closer. If the person in fact knows both what it is like to suffer pain and what it is like to be addicted to a drug, as best as he could based on the reported experiences of others, is there any technical knowledge or data which will help him to choose one alternative over the other? In fact, this is a kind of decision to which factual knowledge can contribute, but can never provide the final answer. In the last analysis, a value judgment will have to be made by the individual in order for him to state what is "better."

6    A judgment to which facts may contribute, but which must be decided in the end by weighing values, is a rough definition of an ethical question. There was, in fact, an ethical decision hidden under the surgeon's "clinical judgment." If we had disagreed with the surgeon's decision, chances are that we would have been unable to state our grounds for disagreement, other than to say, "I would have done otherwise." But once the hidden ethical assumptions are brought out in the open, we have a much better opportunity to find the root of our disagreement—or else to reconsider our own ideas and conclude that the surgeon was right after all.

7    And the business of making concealed ethical decisions is not restricted to this particular kind of case. We can generalize all medical decisions to arrive at two conclusions, based on the fact that medicine is an applied art—science of men, applied by men:

    1)   *Every medical decision involves human beings both as the decision-makers and as those who have to live with the consequences.*

    2)   *Every medical decision involves a choice between different outcomes, and human beings are likely to place different values on the different outcomes.*

8    Since both of the listed characteristics are characteristics of ethical questions (a more precise definition of "ethics" must wait until Chapter 2), an obvious conclusion is that *all medical decisions are ethical decisions, or at least that they involve an ethical component in addition to the scientific or clinical aspects of the problem.* If most medical decisions are made without the ethical dimension ever being considered, it is because the ethical issues involved are of a common variety about which there is almost universal agreement. If the ethical question were to be raised as such, most people would solve it easily.

9    Periodically, however, the physician is faced with a dilemma which forces him to recognize the ethical dimension—an unmarried girl requesting an abortion, or a terminally ill patient who requests that the doctor help hasten the end. These cases demand a particularly careful answering of the ethical questions involved. But, if the physician has been in the habit of ignoring the ethical component of his day-to-day decisions, he will find himself at a distinct disadvantage when he faces this large-scale problem. Like anything else, ethical decision-making improves with practice. The physician's entire training since high school has been directed at the techniques needed to make scientific and clinical decisions, but most likely he has never had any formal training in making ethical decisions.

So what then does the physician do? He may choose to follow whatever the current custom of his profession or community happens to be, or he may do what he emotionally "feels" is right at the time, or he may follow the dictates of his religion if they apply. In each of these cases he will take an action. It may be the "right" action according to a subsequent rational analysis. If it is the "wrong" action, chances are that the consequences will be much less dramatic than those of the surgeon whose scalpel slips and severs a nerve, or of the internist who miscalculates the dose of a potent drug. Physicians may lose hospital privileges for technical incompetence, or for violations of "professional etiquette" such as advertising; but they seldom are reprimanded in any formal way for wrong ethical decisions of this nature. 10

↓

So why study medical ethics in general, or this book in particular? We make two assumptions: first, that the physician-to-be would rather be ethical than not; and second, that ethical decisions, like clinical decisions, will be made better if they are made according to a rational methodology rather than haphazardly. 11

The idea of a rational methodology for ethical decision-making may be a new idea. Popular conceptions of "ethics" often picture it either as the following of a set of commandments laid down by the Bible or the A.M.A. or some other authority; or else as a way in which some mysterious feelings deep within our souls magically transmutate themselves into some kind of "force of will" or "will to be" or some such thing. Chapter 2 will go into greater detail about the nature of ethics in order to show an ethical decision-making method which can be usefully applied to problems in medicine. Ch. 2 ↓ 12

# 2. A Method of Ethical Reasoning

Medical ethics is not a branch of medicine, but a branch of ethics. (The question of the definition of "ethics" will be postponed for now.) Before tackling the ethical issues that are peculiar to medical practice, it is best to consider ethics in general, and to ask whether there is some general method of problem-solving which can be applied to any ethical question. This method could then be applied to the ethical issues that arise in medicine.

12

To begin with, one must be able to recognize an ethical, or moral, problem when it arises. We can list two essential ingredients of an ethical problem. The first is the existence of a real choice between possible courses of action. It makes no sense, for example, to make ethical statements about whether or not a surgeon should perform a brain transplant—such action is impossible now, and there are good reasons to believe that it will never be possible, so the choice to do one or not does not really exist.

13

**WHAT ABOUT FUTURE POSSIBILITIES? \*15**

The second major ingredient of an ethical problem is that the person involved must place a significantly different value upon each possible action, or upon the consequences of that action. For example, the question of whether to use silk suture or nylon suture to sew a laceration is, for all practical purposes, not an ethical question; the choice can be made on purely technical grounds. On the other hand, the question of whether to treat a disease by drugs or by surgery has a definite ethical component, since both doctor and patient place a very different value upon taking medication as opposed to undergoing surgery.

14

16

Does this requirement mean that it is not worthwhile to make ethical statements about those types of genetic engineering, such as cloning, which are not now possible? But these technologies might well be developed in future years. In such cases where the implications may have great social import, it makes good sense to get a headstart by thinking of future ethical difficulties right now instead of waiting for the actuality and being caught unprepared.

15

14

5

16      In order to communicate about ethical problems and about our moral judgments, we must use moral statements. (At this point, we are using "ethical" and "moral" as approximately interchangeable terms; a distinction will be made later.) A formula for a moral statement is:

In situation X, person Y ought to do thing Z.

Note three ingredients to a moral statement:
1)  WHAT is to be done (Z)
2)  WHO is to do it (Y)
3)  The CONDITIONS under which the statement is applicable (X)

While moral statements such as "stealing is wrong" do not fit this formula, they can generally be restated in accordance with the formula by filling in the obvious missing elements: "Under no conditions should any person steal."

17      Before discussing how to use ethical statements in problem solving, we will compare ethical statements with various other types of statements. Failure to be absolutely clear about some of these distinctions is a primary cause of errors in ethical reasoning, and of misunderstandings in ethical discussions.

WHY STATEMENTS? * 19

18      A very common type of statement is the EMPIRICAL statement, which asserts that a certain state of affairs does or does not exist. It is likely to cause trouble when it occurs in a form closely resembling that of the ethical statement, such as:

In situation X, person Y often does thing Z.

The key difference is the absence of "ought." The ethical statement, by the use of "ought," both recommends action and suggests that that action is "better" (has a higher value) than the alternatives. The empirical statement is merely descriptive; it makes no value judgments and requires that no action be taken.

20

19      You might wonder why we are starting out with "statements," which are only abstract representations of ideas after all, instead of the ethical judgments themselves. First, we are becoming more aware of the fact that language has a strong influence on the way we think, and that cultural patterns of thinking are reflected in language. (This is why, in order to learn Chinese, a Westerner has to learn not only vocabulary and syntax but also a whole new way of looking at the world.) Second, we find analysis of statements useful for making some important distinctions. Take the difference between our thoughts and our feelings, which can be very important in ethics. In our own minds we are both thinking and feeling together all the time, and it is hard to sort out the two. But by analyzing statements about thoughts and statements about feelings, say, we might gain some new insight into these actual mental processes.

18

Empirical statements have the property of being either <u>true</u> or <u>false</u>. While we sometimes hear these terms used also to apply to ethical statements, it does not seem that a recommendation for action can be <u>true</u> or <u>false</u> in the same sense that a description can. Rather, we would prefer to speak of ethical statements as <u>right</u> or <u>wrong</u>, or, even better, <u>valid</u> and <u>invalid</u>, to remind us that the method we must use to determine an ethical question is fundamentally different from the method of settling an empirical question.

*People trained in the sciences, who are most comfortable with empirical statements, are especially prone to make the mistake of trying to solve ethical problems simply by accumulating data, while ignoring the need to make value judgments. In theory, if we accumulate enough data, we can thereby solve any empirical question. With an ethical dilemma, we can have all the data in the world; we still cannot arrive at an answer until we come to grips with our values and make some value judgments.*

UNCLEAR *23

Other statements besides ethical statements may be said to share the property of being neither true nor false. One is the ESTHETIC statement, such as, "I like to do thing Z" or "Thing Z is beautiful." However, these should not be confused with ethical statements because, like empirical statements, they contain no requirement of action. It is generally understood that "I like to do thing Z" does not necessarily suggest that "I ought to do thing Z."

Another neither-true-nor-false type of statement is the COMMAND, such as, "Do thing Z." Since a command requires action, the difference between it and an ethical statement is not so easy to grasp. The main difference is that a command is meant to apply only to the particular listener at that particular time. The drill sergeant who calls out, "Left face!" may call out, "Right face!" a minute later, and no one would accuse him of contradicting himself.

An ethical statement, on the other hand, implies by its "ought" that in theory it applies to ALL people in similar circumstances. The ethical statement, "The physician ought to provide contraceptives to sexually active minors regardless of whether parental consent is given," implies that ALL physicians should provide contraceptives to ANY sexually active minor who might request them. It is this principle of UNIVERSALIZABILITY that distinguishes ethical statements from commands, and that gives ethical statements their particular force. As we shall see, it also provides a key way of testing the validity of ethical positions.

The reason truth and falsity apply to empirical statements and not to ethical statements is that in order to apply those concepts, we need a principle of verification. We understand how to tell if a statement is true by definition. Likewise, we know how to compare a statement with our observations of the real world in order to tell if an empirical statement is true. However, the way we judge the validity of an ethical statement—which will be shown in the problem-solving method below—is different from the verification process; it involves the weighing of values. There is no "real world" of what "ought to be" available for us to make comparisons—at least, not one that has any degree of universal agreement about it.

20

21

22

24

23

21

24      For a summary of the above, we can construct the following table:

| Type of statement | True/False? | Action? | Universalizable? |
| --- | --- | --- | --- |
| EMPIRICAL | Yes | No | No |
| ESTHETIC | No | No | No |
| COMMAND | No | Yes | No |
| ETHICAL | No | Yes | Yes |

25      Now that the nature of ethical statements is clear, we may briefly consider the types of moral conflicts that can arise. In general terms, these types differ according to the values that we place upon the choices available.

26      The simplest ethical decision is made when one choice is considered to be "good" and the other to be "evil." Because this choice is so easy, it is a common human trait to view ethical issues in terms of "good" and "evil," even when a closer analysis would reveal this to be an oversimplification. In actuality very few ethical problems are genuinely choices of unquestionable good versus unquestionable evil.

27      Another type of ethical conflict arises when one choice is "better" and the other "worse." This type of decision becomes progressively harder to make as the determination of which is "better" and which is "worse" becomes more indistinct. This is especially true where the units of value are very different: is a job that pays $30,000 and entails considerable aggravation "better" or "worse" than one that pays $15,000 and offers peace of mind? Most ethical conflicts fit into this category.

28      A third type of conflict occurs when one must choose between two "goods" which are mutually exclusive. An example in medical ethics is the question of allowing a suffering and terminally ill individual to die; here the two "good" actions of prolonging life and relieving suffering are in conflict. In other cases, the conflict may arise between the doctor's role as a "good" physician and as a "good" citizen of the state, such as when it would seem to serve the public good to violate his promise to keep the patient's information confidential. The problem with these conflicts is that we tend to view the failure to do a good thing as "bad," and so we are forced into doing a "bad" thing no matter which alternative we choose. While these conflicts may not arise often in such clear form, they provide ethics with many of its thorniest dilemmas.

The last type of ethical conflict calls attention to a more general point, the principle of "you can't have your cake and eat it too" in ethics. When there are alternative courses of action open, the decision to do one is also a decision not to do the others. Thus, in ethics, it is easy to "make" a decision in this way without realizing it and which one may come to regret later. Farther on in this book, the question of the allocation of scarce resources will be considered as a separate issue in medical ethics. *For now, however, it is important to note that any ethical decision involves the allocation and expenditure of resources of which there is only a finite amount, such as time. And, of course, the decision to allocate a resource in one place is simultaneously a decision not to allocate it somewhere else.*

29

With all these introductory issues taken care of, we can progress to the major business of outlining and explaining a general method of ethical decision-making. The method is diagrammed in Figure 1 and is explained in the frames to follow.

30

The first step, obviously, is to perceive that a moral problem exists. As was shown in Chapter 1, it is not always easy to sort out the ethical components from the many other types of problems which face us in our daily lives.

31

Next, a list is made of the alternative courses of action that are open to deal with the problem. An error that is commonly made at this step, and which in fact was (deliberately) made above in the discussion of types of moral conflict, is to assume that there must be two and only two alternatives and then proceed to weigh one against the other, possibly ignoring completely the existence of a third course of action which is much more desirable. The human mind prefers "either—or" thinking to the complexities of juggling three or more alternatives, so this error is often made unconsciously. Thus, before proceeding to the next step, it is important to check to make sure the list of alternatives is exhaustive.

32

Having listed alternatives, we next choose one of them as the appropriate course of action. It may seem strange that the choice is made here instead of as the last step of the decision-making process. All that is being done here, however, is a recognition of how human beings actually function. Faced with an ethical choice, in most cases, we immediately WANT to do one thing, based on some gut-level reaction. There is nothing wrong with this, so long as the initial reaction is then analyzed by some rational process, and is rejected if it fails the test. That is the role of the rest of the decision-making process.

33

34     The choice that has been made must next be framed in the form of an ethical statement, with all the ingredients described above: what is to be done, who is to do it, and the conditions under which the statement is to apply. Since the choice has been made, drawing up a detailed statement may seem an unnecessary formality—in fact, in most "ethical discussions," it is never done. The value of this step lies in making explicit the element of universalizability that is inherent in the ethical "ought".

"I have decided to do thing Z" carries no ethical weight; possibly later, under essentially the same circumstances, I might instead decide to do thing W. When cast in the form of an ethical statement, the implication is far broader: "I have decided to do thing Z, and anyone like me, under the same circumstances, ought to do thing Z also." The question then arises: if everyone in fact did do thing Z, what would be the consequences? Would these consequences be desirable or not? In these questions we have the tools for a rational analysis to determine the validity of the ethical decision.

"WHAT IF EVERYONE
DID THAT?" * 36

35     The next step is, in fact, to determine the consequences if the proposed ethical statement were to be accepted. While the first thing that comes to mind are the immediate consequences of my own act, it pays to devote some mental effort to predict the long-range consequences of my own and other's acts as well. The present interest in ecology is teaching us to be particularly sensitive to the aggregate consequences: the consequences of my throwing my beer can beside the road may be nil, but the consequences of everyone doing the same may be disastrous.

Clearly it is impossible to list all the possible consequences, even if we could predict them—just as, in the scientific method, it is impossible to list all the variables that must be controlled for in a particular experiment. Nor can we spend so much time listing possible consequences that we let the time for the action itself slip past. *This means, in the end, that we must always take action on the basis of some degree of uncertainty. The goal is to reduce that uncertainty to manageable proportions, and to insure that we have at least considered all the major consequences which we are able to predict with our current level of understanding of the world.*

37

36     It has been objected that the question of "What if everyone did that?" is not a valid way of judging ethical validity. For example, suppose a medical student is searching for a speciality field, and he learns that there is a shortage of family physicians. He decides he wants to be a family physician. But then he asks, "What if everyone became a family physician? There would be no surgeons, obstetricians, etc. These consequences are bad; therefore, I cannot be a family physician."

This difficulty is gotten rid of simply by stating the more general ethical principle that is to be followed. In the case above, it is something like, "In choosing a speciality, the new doctor ought to choose a field that is presently in need of more practitioners." If everyone did that, there would be no problems.

35

## Figure 1

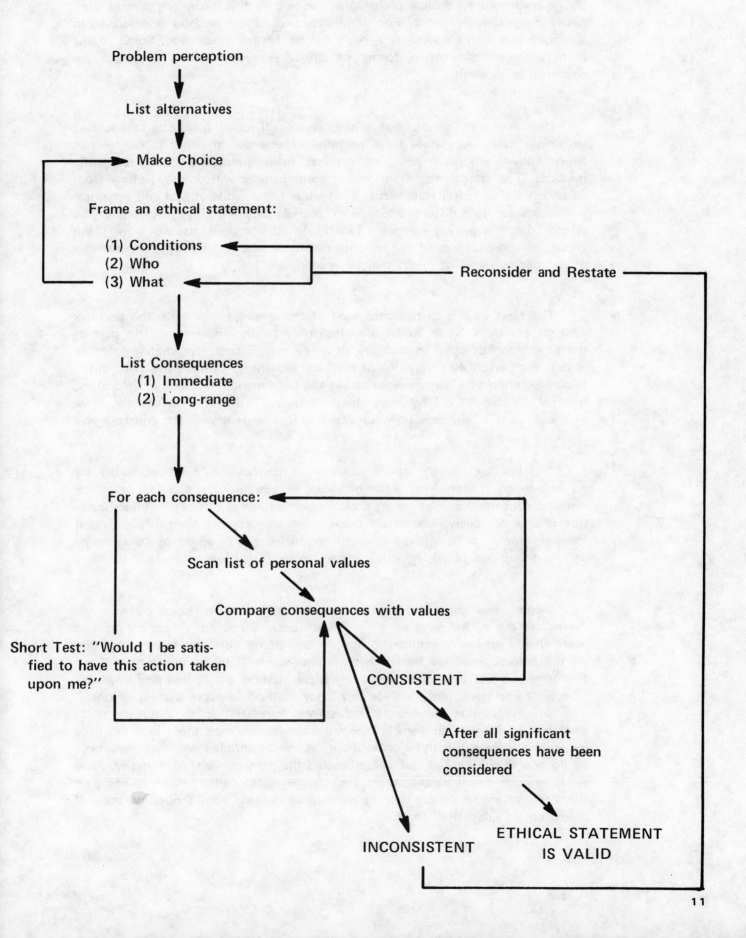

Problem perception

List alternatives

Make Choice

Frame an ethical statement:

(1) Conditions
(2) Who
(3) What

Reconsider and Restate

List Consequences
(1) Immediate
(2) Long-range

For each consequence:

Scan list of personal values

Compare consequences with values

Short Test: "Would I be satisfied to have this action taken
upon me?"

CONSISTENT

After all significant
consequences have been
considered

INCONSISTENT

ETHICAL STATEMENT
IS VALID

37    It should be noted here that this method of testing an ethical act by its consequences (or "consequentialist" ethics) is one type of ethical theory. By no means do all ethical philosophers adhere to this view, and several alternative methodologies exist. For simplicity, one ethical method is described in this book and is then used as a basis for all further discussion. Some of the more common alternative forms of ethical decision-making processes are described in Appendix I.

38    How does one predict what consequences will follow from a certain action? In simple cases, we know from personal experience; in other cases, we can apply known empirical data, or we can make predictions using scientific methods. The statements about which consequences will or may follow from an action are empirical statements. Thus we see that while ethical and empirical statements are two different species of animal, they are closely related in the ethical decision-making process. Clearly, if the statements we now make about the consequences of our act turn out to be false statements, the remainder of our decision-making effort will be wasted.

39    The next step is to compare each of the consequences with the person's own set of values. Since values are often only tacitly understood, this part of the process is less open to scrutiny than the rest. Essentially what is going on is that the person asks himself, for each consequence, "Could I live with this?" If consideration of a consequence causes the person some emotional discomfort, he may ask himself, "Why does this bother me?" and thus eventually arrive at a statement of the specific value which is inconsistent with the consequence.

40    This last set of instructions needs some clarification. First, obviously we do not all go around with a list of values in our pockets ready to be pulled out and consulted as soon as an ethical question jumps out of the underbrush. But just as obviously, we do all value some things more than others, and if someone came to us with a long questionnaire which asked us to compare various things, we could, by our answers, make our values explicit.

41    Second, one might say that we have already made a choice by what we "want" to do in this case, on a "gut-level" basis. Since our values are nothing more than "gut-level" intuitions, are we not doing here the same thing that we did before, when we stated that we just "wanted" to do one thing and not the other? If that were the case, our ethical method would just boil down to, "Do what you want, and then use this fancy method to make it seem rational."
    But that is not the case. If values are "gut-level" in their normal state, they are no longer "gut-level" once we have transformed them into language by stating them explicitly. Furthermore, at the beginning, when we "wanted" to do one thing, we had not yet predicted the consequences of doing so. Now we have both clearly stated values and clearly stated consequences to compare them to; we are no longer dealing with vague desires, even though we are still acting on a "subjective" level.

*In sum, what this ethical method really boils down to is the injunction that we ought to make our values explicit so that we can judge acts by their consequences. We have just seen two steps to this process: 1) stating values and consequences in plain language, and 2) placing values and consequences in close juxtaposition, so that we can make direct comparisons and decide our preferences.* 42

In our ordinary activities, we do not do these things. We allow our values to govern our desires on a subconscious level, without examining the process by which this occurs. In these important respects, then, the ethical method put forth here is a distinct improvement over our "normal" way of acting.

A kind of "short cut" may often be useful in place of an exhaustive consideration of lists of values. If the proposed action affects some other person besides the decision-maker, he may ask, "If I were in that person's situation, and I were like him in morally relevant ways, would I be satisfied in having this done to me?" If the answer is "Yes," it may be assumed that the action is consistent with the decision-maker's own set of values, assuming he has been honest and thoughtful in his answer. 43

The successful application of this technique requires the decision-maker to put himself in the shoes of the other party, and this requires in particular the quality of <u>imagination.</u> In some cases this may be very difficult to apply— for example, in a case in which the other party is mentally retarded.

Once all the consequences have been compared to one's values, and no inconsistencies have been revealed, it may be concluded that the proposed course of action is ethically valid. It should, of course, be borne in mind that possibly all the significant consequences have not been considered, and that new knowledge in the future may cast doubt upon the decision in retrospect. There is no escape from this uncertainty, since all actions have consequences— including the decision not to take action. 44

Much more likely, some inconsistency will be found between one of the consequences and the set of values. When this occurs, the method calls for a reconsideration of the original ethical statement, and a restatement to remove the offending portion. The first thing to try is a modification of the CONDITIONS of the ethical statement. 45

For example, in order to rationalize why a physician should not perform an abortion, one comes up with the ethical statement, "Medical treatment should not be given to a person unless organic illness is present." This suits the purpose since pregnancy is not considered an illness. However, one consequence of this statement is that a physician cannot perform elective plastic surgery. This is inconsistent with one's values, because one has sympathy with people who suffer emotional anguish due to unattractive features. One might therefore modify the original statement to, "Medical treatment should not be given to a person unless organic illness is present, EXCEPT where the danger to life or health is negligible compared to the expected benefits." (What are some consequences of this new statement?)

46    In many cases, changing the conditions will suffice to bring the statement into accord with one's values. However, it may be necessary to change instead the WHAT part of the statement—i.e., the proposed action itself is realized to be inconsistent with one's values. This entails making a different choice, and in turn framing a new ethical statement.

Whatever the case, the modified or the new ethical statement must then itself be examined for consequences, and the process repeated, as shown by the circular arrows in the diagram, until consistency wins out in the end.

47    If one is being really exhaustive, however, the process does not end here. One should investigate the other choices as well; it may be that one or more of them are also ethically valid, as in the "good vs. good" type of conflict mentioned above. One then has a particularly hard decision to make. One must determine which of his set of values are most directly applicable to each of the alternatives. He then must weigh the values to see which he values most highly, and choose accordingly. In the euthanasia example mentioned already, a doctor who would oppose giving a terminally ill cancer patient an overdose of morphine may be saying that he values the principle of preserving life over the principle of alleviating suffering. A physician who decides to give the overdose may be making the opposite valuation.

Note that if one were being thorough in listing the consequences, "Not being able to do the other actions" would have been listed as a consequence of the choice that was made. One could have weighed this against one's set of values, without having to go through the whole process for each separate alternative.

48    So far we have been talking as if each time we applied the decision-making method to an ethical question, we obtained one and only one ethically valid answer. This would be very nice if it were the case, but it is not. In many of the "hard" cases, both because of uncertainties in predicting consequences and because of confusions in how we rank-order our own values, it will be impossible to show that one alternative is clearly superior to the others. Several alternatives will be shown to be equally good, or more likely, equally bad, within the framework of the decision-making method; and we are still stuck with making a choice. We will run across several such cases later on in this book. (Note, in Appendix I, that alternative ethical methods share this problem of sometimes failing to come up with a "right" answer for each case.)

49    When these "hard" cases come up, however, we can learn something from them. If we see that they tend to occur more frequently in certain circumstances, we can try to change those circumstances. For instance, if a physician who sees 60 patients a day in his office is always having to make hard decisions about how to allocate his attention among patients with equally pressing problems, he might decide eventually to try to attract a partner to help with his practice. But in many cases we have no real choice about whether we are to go out on the ethical limb or not; or the consequences of changing the circumstances might be even worse ethical problems than we have now.

14

Now that we have gone through the entire method, we must go back and    50
say a few more things about the so-called "set of values." We have gotten
around one objection by making our values explicit instead of allowing them
to influence behavior on the subconscious level. We still have the objection
that some values, even when rendered explicit, are still objectionable to others.
According to the method as it stands, Attila the Hun could show up, placing
a high value on murder, rape, and pillage, and so long as he made those values
explicit, he could claim that his actions were ethically justified.

Does this mean that we are stuck with whatever set of values we find    51
ourselves with, and there is no way to separate the good values from the
objectionable ones? One preliminary way of testing values is provided in the
ethical method. While we have described it mainly as a way of testing consequences, it can just as easily be used as a way of testing values. Explicate a
value, take some sample cases, and determine how that value would lead you
to act in each case. If a certain value tends to lead you to act in ways which
are generally disapproved of, you would begin to give serious thought to
changing that value, or else giving it significantly lower priority.

If you do no more than accept values which are "generally approved of"    52
and reject those which are not, you are adhering to "common sense morality."
This has been shown to be a useful guide in most simple cases, but a source
of inconsistency and irrationality in complex situations. What one really wants
is some sort of "objective" basis on which to judge values.
    If you accept the doctrines of a revealed religion, your answer is found
there. Your values can be judged according to their consistency with those
doctrines (although there will often be some confusion in applying general
doctrines to specific cases).

We are going to propose that there is a better basis for judging which    53
values are best suited to meet the objective needs of mankind, and we will
describe this basis in a preliminary way in Chapter 18. However, this basis is
not yet so thoroughly worked out as to provide specific guidance on specific
values; and even if it were, many ethicists would not agree with the results.
    For the time being, therefore, we will accept the reality that different
people have different values, and we will leave the ethical method open-ended
to accommodate these differences. We will have to deal with Attila the Hun
later on.

In order to see how this whole process works, it will be illustrated by    54
working through a sample case. Before doing this, however, a few more important
points about ethical reasoning ought to be made.

55      RIGOR. First, discussion of the decision-making process has hopefully dispensed with the common view that ethics is a "soft" discipline, as opposed to the sciences where conclusions are reached by rigorous application of a specific method. While the ethical method certainly differs from the scientific method, it should be clear that the process outlined is an arduous one, which requires every bit as much sustained and disciplined thought as any common scientific problem.

56      PLURALISM. Second, it will have been noted that since individuals have different sets and scales of values, two people, each applying the decision-making method faithfully, may reach two different ethical conclusions. This may bother a reader who has been led to expect that it is the role of ethics to provide unmistakable rules of correct conduct. Actually, such a definition of "ethics" touches only on its very narrowest aspects (if you are still unclear, review the "Objectives" and the "Not Objectives" at the beginning of the book).

A common misconception is that, if we deny the possibility of a system of ethics which clearly tells what is the right thing to do under any circumstances, past, present, and future, then the only alternative we are left with is a totally vague ethics where any one person's opinion is just as good as any other's. In technical terms, this is the conflict between "moral absolutism" and "moral relativism."

57      The "absolutism vs. relativism" way of phrasing the problem, however, falls into the error already mentioned—assuming that there are only two alternatives. *The decision-making process outlined here in fact seeks a comfortable middle ground, which we may call moral pluralism. It allows for differences in personal values and for change in ethical judgments over time, as new knowledge about possible consequences is acquired. At the same time, it prevents a moral free-for-all by insisting that no one can claim ethical validity for his statements until he has subjected them to rigorous and rational analysis. In this way, there may not be one "correct" answer. There will, however, be no more than a few good answers, since the inconsistent or poorly thought out positions will have been eliminated along the way. In any case, it would seem that a statement derived from the decision-making process will prove to be a better guide to action, in important matters, than either one's initial gut reaction or blind adherence to pre-existing rules.*

58      Still, to the ethical philosopher, absolutism and relativism are mutually exclusive categories; so since our pluralistic ethics is not absolutist, it must formally be listed as a type of relativistic ethics. We might also note that an ethical relativist may be saying two different things: either there really is no way finally to resolve a value conflict; or that ideally such a way exists but that in real life it is impractical to insist upon it. Frankena, in his book on ethics (see References), discusses this matter more fully. Here the main thing is to see why a "pluralistic" ethic is not necessarily the same as "do your own thing."

LEVELS. Since, as was noted in Chapter 1, there are potential ethical problems in all aspects of our daily lives (let alone in the practice of medicine), does this mean that we have to stop each time and apply the decision-making method just described in its entirety? Naturally people in practice do not do so. Even "ethical" individuals practice different levels of problem-solving behavior in accordance with the importance of the matter at hand, or in accordance with the novelty of the situation. One useful scheme for categorizing levels of moral activity has been proposed by Henry Aiken.

59

Aiken suggests four levels of moral discourse, each of which is illustrated below by a sample statement on abortion made at that level.

60

| Level | Statement |
|---|---|
| EXPRESSIVE LEVEL | "I hate abortion" |
| LEVEL OF MORAL RULES | "Do not perform abortions" |
| LEVEL OF ETHICAL PRINCIPLES | "The right of the fetus to life is more important than the mother's right to the privacy of her own body" |
| POST—ETHICAL LEVEL | "It is important to respect the rights of others, else human life is not truly 'human'" |

Notice that most daily decisions are made on the first two of Aiken's levels. In simple instances we allow our likes and dislikes to rule; in more complex cases we apply rules which we have come to adopt in the past. Every so often, we are faced with a more complicated problem and have to go through some kind of formal ethical reasoning process. (Note that in this scheme, a person can be moral—acting in accordance with rules of "right" conduct—without being ethical—having gone through a formal reasoning process to decide upon his behavior. In this sense, "moral" and "ethical" are no longer interchangeable terms but refer to different levels of activity.)

61

Any ethical statement raises another potential question——why bother to do what is "right" anyway? Why bother to be ethical? Aiken's post-ethical level deals with attempts to justify the need for ethical reasoning and ethical conduct. Since this book is designed to be on the third level, the post-ethical level is beyond our scope. Our basic assumption is that the physician wants to be ethical and simply wishes to be told how to do it.

62

63      Aiken's levels raise two important points which clarify the objectives of this book. First, it is often the case that conflict on one level requires recourse to the next higher level to resolve the conflict. Thus, we can comfortably operate on the level of moral rules only so long as there is general agreement. If someone questions our decision, or if two of our own rules conflict, we have to either throw up our hands in despair, or else adopt an ethical problem-solving approach to determine what is valid. The goal of this book is not to make the reader use the decision-making process for each moral question, but rather to provide the process as a tool which can be brought into use when required. The ethical person does not use the process continually, but he is prepared to use it at any time whenever one of his decisions requires formal justification.

64      The corresponding point is that, once a new situation has been dealt with on one level, recurrences of essentially similar situations can be handled conveniently on a lower level. The physician faced with his first patient who requests an abortion may have to go through a complex problem-solving process. By the time he reaches his 15th patient, he has adopted a set of "rules" as a shorthand for his previous thinking, and can reach the decision much quicker. However, when the patient presents a novel aspect, e.g., an unmarried woman where all his previous rules had dealt with married women, the physician may have to repeat the decision-making process.

65      CODES. The distinction between "moral" and "ethical" levels of sophistication hopefully explains another point that may have puzzled the reader—why we have begun a discussion of medical ethics without any mention of the various "codes of ethics" that exist in medicine. There have been numerous such codes in the history of the profession, starting with listing of fees and malpractice penalties in the Code of Hammurabi, to the famous Oath of the Hippocratic school, to Thomas Percival's very detailed code (1804) which formed the basis for the first Code of Ethics of the American Medical Association (1847).

66      The limitations of such codes are the limitations of the "moral rule" level as opposed to the "ethical" level—they can apply only to situations stated in the code, not to any new situations that may arise later; and if too detailed, different rules in the code are likely to conflict with each other. In fact, most of the codes mentioned deal with the really hard ethical questions by ignoring them. Instead they deal with the matters that have come to be called "professional etiquette," such as whether a physician should advertise. Note that the entire first half of the famous Hippocratic Oath deals with how a physician should act towards other members of his profession (at that time, a religious cult); the admonitions about service to the patient and about respect for the patient's right to privacy only come later.

LAW. Many of the problems with codes apply also to those who would look to the law as a guide to ethical behavior. In that view, medical ethics can be reduced to one statement, "The physician should obey the laws of the area in which he practices," and all else will follow. One problem is that even the most patriotic physician will envision a few instances in which he would find it ethical to violate a particular law. A possible example occurred in the 1960's in Connecticut, where an archaic law from the Colonial era, never repealed, prevented physicians from giving any kind of contraceptive information. Civil disobedience by some physicians led to a landmark Supreme Court ruling which overturned the law.

67

A more basic point, however, is that the law, as it pertains to most medical matters, is designed to be permissive rather than comprehensive. Unlike a set of traffic ordinances, the law generally prohibits the extremes of behavior, and leaves the subtleties to individual or professional judgment. Thus, in the majority of sticky choices that a physician may have to make, he is not liable to indictment under the criminal law in either case, and he could conceivably be sued under the civil law in both cases; so the law as such is little help to him in making up his mind.

68

At various points in this book, we will mention various points of law when they have particular interest for a specific ethical issue.

We have now reached the conclusion of our discussion about "ethics" without ever having defined "ethics." As a self-test, which of the definitions below is the best summary of the points which have been attributed to "ethics" so far?  Check your answer. . .

69

1)  Ethics is the study of right conduct.

↓ 74

2)  Ethics is the study of rational processes for determining the best course of action in the face of conflicting choices.

↓ 71

3)  Ethics is a set of guidelines which, if followed, will always lead to correct behavior.

↓ 75

4)  Ethics is the study of how people act in the face of difficult choices.

↓ 79

We will now illustrate the problem-solving method by working through a sample case. If you feel that you understand the method thoroughly without any illustration, go on to Chapter 3.

70

Ch. 3 ↓ 99

↓ 72

71

70

By choosing Definition no. 2, you have summarized the major points of the preceding discussion. Now go on to the sample case which illustrates the application of the problem-solving process.

---

## CASE 1

72

You are a pediatrician in private practice. A mother and father bring in their 4-year-old daughter, who has been complaining for three days of slight fever, runny nose, and irritability. Some of the irritability has rubbed off on the parents and they demand rather abruptly that you prescribe an antibiotic for the child.

According to your diagnosis, the child, with high probability, has a viral infection. At any rate, the infection seems to be selflimiting and you feel that no medication is required. You know that antibiotics can do no good in viral conditions, and that the indiscriminate use of antibiotics is considered poor medical practice. Your first inclination is to explain that to the parents and prescribe no medication, while encouraging them to call back if the child gets worse. However, you see that the parents have a hostile attitude, and you are aware that it is standard practice among many pediatricians to prescribe antibiotics just to save themselves the explanation and to "make the parents happy." You are certainly not looking forward to taking the time to give the parents a full explanation, and even so they might call another doctor or go to an emergency room.

What should you do?

---

73

76

The ethical problem has been identified for you. The next step is to list the alternative courses of action open. What are they, and how many are there? Answer this for yourself before proceeding to the next frame.

---

74

69

By choosing Definition no. 1, you have selected what may be right by dictionary standards but which says very little about ethics. What is "right" conduct? How is it to be determined? Is the same conduct always "right"? Go back to the list and try again.

75

↑ 69

By choosing Definition no. 3, you have shown that you are confused about the distinction that was made between "moral" and "ethical," or about the objectives of this book, or both. Review the sections on levels of moral activity, on "codes," and the original objectives; then return to the list of definitions and make another choice.

---

76

Technically, there are almost an infinite number of choices, since one of the questions is what to tell the parents, and there are innumerable ways of phrasing the exact words. For example, it may be ethically a different matter to tell them, "I will not give her any medication," as opposed to, "I will not give her any medication, because she has a viral cold and antibiotics are no good for that." As to alternatives which are both generally stated and realistic, we can identify at least these:

1) Prescribe a mild antibiotic; no explanation.

2) Try to explain why an antibiotic would not be indicated, without committing yourself to any action. If, after a few minutes, it seems that the parents do not understand or are still dissatisfied, give up and prescribe a mild antibiotic.

3) Explain to the parents the pros and cons of prescribing an antibiotic, ask them what they want, and follow their wish.

4) Same as (3), but in addition to giving the pros and cons, add that you strongly recommend against prescribing. However, you will do it if they desire.

5) State, "I am not going to give your daughter an antibiotic because..." and then explain, taking as long as required to answer all the parents' questions.

6) State, "I am not going to give your daughter an antibiotic because in my professional judgment it can't do any good and may do some harm." Answer a few questions, but if they are dissatisfied after you have spent a few minutes with them, end the conversation by saying that if they don't like it they can see another doctor.

↓

77

Which of the positions listed would you choose? Or would it be a different one? Write out for yourself a formal statement of your ethical decision for future reference. Now you have to list the consequences of your action. Try to spend some time thinking of the long-range consequences as well as the immediate ones, before going on to the next frame.

↓

78

We can't list all the significant consequences of all the choices listed, especially since choices which are combinations of actions will have consequences for each part. For the sake of simplicity, a list of some of the more obvious consequences of prescribing an antibiotic and of not prescribing are listed in Table 1. If the consequences have different probabilities of occurring, these are indicated in the table as "high," "low," etc.

↓ 80

# Table 1

## Partial List of Consequences for Case 1

### Prescribing

1. The parents will be satisfied with your action.

2. Parents will expect you to give drug each time in the future when they bring child, will be dissatisfied if you don't. (high)

3. Parents will be dissatisfied later if they find out that antibiotics are not indicated for viral disease. (low)

4. If your diagnosis was wrong, the patient may be cured. (low)

5. Patient may develop an allergic reaction to drug, possibly a serious or fatal one. (low)

6. The child may become sensitized to drug and suffer allergic reaction upon a subsequent exposure to it. (low-medium)

7. Use of the drug may aid in the natural selection of new strains of bacteria that are resistant to the antibiotic. (low)

8. You will be personally dissatisfied by having abandoned your principles.

9. The parents will have to pay for the drug.

10. You will reinforce the parents' erroneous notions about proper use of drugs.

11. The patient may develop a side effect from the drug. (low-medium)

### Not Prescribing

A. The parents will be dissatisfied with your action. (high)

B. You will have the personal satisfaction of following your principles.

C. Parents may take child to an emergency room to get drug, depriving child of the better follow-up care a private physician can give. (?)

D. There will be no chance of the child developing an allergic reaction to the drug.

E. By avoiding indiscriminate use of antibiotics, you are helping to avoid the emergence of new, more resistant strains of bacteria. (high)

F. The parents will be saved the price of the drug.

G. If parents decide to seek another doctor, you will lose their fees in the future.

H. If parents complain about you in the community, your reputation may suffer. (?)

I. You will have made a contribution to the education of the parents on the appropriate use of drugs. (high-medium)

J. If your diagnosis was wrong, the patient may get worse. (low)

By choosing Definition no. 4, you have indicated that you may not be 79 clear on the distinction between empirical and ethical statements. Statements about how people actually act are empirical statements, and are the subject matter of the behavioral and social sciences, not of ethics. Ethics is instead the study of how people <u>ought</u> to act. Go back to the list of definitions and make another choice.

↓ 69

---

The next step is to compare the list of consequences with the individual's 80 set of values. Of course, you can do this for yourself privately. However, since the purpose of this book is to make explicit things which we usually do without thinking about them, try this exercise instead. Suppose you adhere to the following set of values, that is, you value those things in the list below very highly. Which of the consequences listed in Table 1 are consistent with these values? Which are inconsistent? Are there any value conflicts that must be resolved by assigning relative weights to different values?

List of Values:  Therapeutic conservatism (i.e., giving only treatment that is necessary and no more)
Education of patients toward correct health habits
Having other people like you

↓

Consulting Table 1, we see that for the value of therapeutic conservatism, 81 4, D, E, and F appear to be consistent with it while 2, 5, 6, 7, 9, 11, C, and J are inconsistent. For patient education, I is consistent while 2 and 10 are inconsistent. For having others like you, 1 and 4 are consistent while 2, 3, 5, 11, A, H, and J are all inconsistent. There are no specific value conflicts, i.e., consequences that are consistent with one value and inconsistent with another. Note, however, that if the high-probability consequences are given greater weight, the value of having other people like you would tend to guide you toward prescribing the drug, while the value of therapeutic conservatism would lead to not prescribing. In the total decision-making picture, the primary conflict might be between these two values.

(Is having other people like you a good value to have? Is it particularly likely to conflict with other values?)

↓

Please note that there is one way <u>NOT</u> to reach a decision: that is, by 82 counting up the number of "consistents" and "inconsistents" and deciding by "majority vote." This is both because some consequences are more important than others, and because of the different probabilities. Is a favorable consequence of low probability more or less important than an unfavorable consequence of high probability?

This problem is a fatal error in all "arithmetic" approaches to ethics so far proposed, such as the situation–ethics rule of taking the number of people to be helped by an action minus the number of people hurt. A mathematical approach to the manipulation of values may yet be devised, but it will have to be more sophisticated than this.

↓

83    By now you should be able to see whether the choice you made is consistent or inconsistent with your values. Recall, however, that so far we have only been talking about the consequences of this one case. Your formal ethical statement, which you wrote out, must apply also to all similar cases. You cannot accept this statement as a valid guide to behavior unless you think of some of the other cases that it would apply to, and satisfy yourself that the consequences in those cases would also be acceptable.

For instance, suppose you had decided not to prescribe the drug, and had phrased your statement, "A physician should never prescribe a drug that is medically contraindicated merely because the patient would be made happier by it." You might then envision a case in which a mentally ill patient is requesting a harmless therapy, and threatens suicide or some other bodily harm unless it is given. It might well be in accordance with your values to give the patient a placebo for a while to buy time for the treatment of the underlying mental illness. You might then change the statement to, "A physician should never prescribe a drug that is mentally contraindicated merely because the patient would be made happier, unless the patient may suffer grave consequences as a result of a mental condition." Can you further refine this statement by thinking of new cases that it would apply to?

84    In complex issues, you might end up with an ethical statement that has so many conditions tacked on that it would take up several pages. In such cases, you might well conclude that a general ethical principle will not apply, and that each case presents so many unique features that it must be decided on its own merits. The ethical statement may then be shortened to simply list the basic criteria which you will apply to each unique case in order to guide your decision.

85    Without giving any "right answer," we have outlined an approach by which the ethical decision-making process can be used for a rational analysis of Case 1. Before concluding this chapter, we will go into one other point which might have been raised by the application of the ethical method to this case.

86    RATIONAL DECISION THEORY. As you went through Case 1, you may have been dissatisfied with the rough way in which the consequences were compared according to their consistency with values and also according to their high or low probability. It may have occurred to you that there ought to be a mathematical way of comparing these factors in order to obtain a more quantitative answer. There is such a method, the basis of which is called Bayesian decision theory, which can be very useful in some instances. A full description of this theory and its modifications is given by Jeffrey (see References), but we shall outline it here by giving one example.

Let's suppose that we are trying to decide whether it is better to treat a 87
certain patient by surgery or with medication. For simplicity let's also assume
that we can list just three consequences that may follow each action, and that
these consequences are mutually exclusive; we can call these the "good,"
"bad," and "very bad" consequences for each. In the case of surgery, say that
the patient might have a complete cure, or he may suffer side effects from the
surgical procedure, or he may die from the surgery. In the case of medication,
the best he can hope for is a partial cure; and he also might have side effects,
or might die from the drugs. Let's assume also that the side effects of the
drug (unless they are fatal) are treatable with other means, but that the side
effects of surgery are untreatable and permanent.

Now we construct a table, listing at the front of each row the various 88
actions we might take, and at the head of each column, the possible contin-
gencies that might arise outside of our control. Such a table for the case cited
is shown in Figure 2A.

Now we have to determine the probability of each of these possible conse- 89
quences. We can assume that we have the data to do this. Using the convention
of 1.0=complete certainty and 0=impossibility, we can state that with drugs,
there is a .70 chance of a good outcome, a .28 chance of non-fatal side effects,
and a .02 chance of side effects causing death. Say that the surgery is of a
relatively dangerous sort: there is only a .50 chance of a good outcome, with
.40 of the cases having a bad result and .10 directly resulting in fatality.
We can substitute these values to obtain the table of probabilities shown
in Figure 2B.

We also need a term to represent the value, or desirability, placed on each 90
of the outcomes. Presumably we would have to obtain this from the patient
by asking some carefully designed questions. Let's say that we get the following
results, also on a 0—to—1 scale: complete cure is highly desirable, at 1.0;
a partial cure is worth .7; treatable side effects are .5; untreatable side effects
are .2; and death is at the bottom of the list with 0. (We could adopt any other
scale, calling death 0 and complete cure 100, for instance; so long as the
relative spacing between items and their rank ordering are the same, the final
results will be the same.)
These desirability values are entered in the table in Figure 2C.

As we saw in Case 1, we want to weight the consequences differently 91
depending on their relative probabilities. In mathematical terms, we do this
by multiplying the probability value in each square of the table by the corresponding desirability value; the product is called the weighted desirability. This
is shown in Figure 2D.
Since the events shown by the column headings are outside of our control,
any of them may occur. Therefore, to decide what to do, we have to add the
weighted desirabilities for all the columns in each row. As Figure 2D shows,
this gives us a sum of .63 for drug therapy and a sum of .58 for surgical therapy.
We conclude, then, that drug therapy is superior to surgical therapy. Another
way of saying this is that drugs come before surgery in this patient's preference
ranking.

Figure 2A. Summary of Case

|  | Good | Bad | Very Bad |
|---|---|---|---|
| Drug therapy | Partial cure | Treatable side effects | Death |
| Surgical therapy | Complete cure | Untreatable side effects | Death |

Figure 2B. Probability Table

|  | Good | Bad | Very Bad |
|---|---|---|---|
| Drug | .70 | .28 | .02 |
| Surgery | .50 | .40 | .10 |

Figure 2C. Desirability Table

|  | Good | Bad | Very Bad |
|---|---|---|---|
| Drug | .7 | .5 | 0 |
| Surgery | 1.0 | .2 | 0 |

Figure 2D. Table of Weighted Desirabilities

|  | Good | Bad | Very Bad | Sum |
|---|---|---|---|---|
| Drug | (.70) (.7) = .49 | (.28) (.5) = .14 | (.02) (0) = 0 | .63 |
| Surgery | (.50) (1) = .50 | (.40) (.2) = .08 | (.10) (0) = 0 | .58 |

92    Now we know what we want to do in this hypothetical case. To show the other possible applications of the Bayesian system, let's take it one step further. Suppose you are a surgeon who wants to improve the surgical technique for this disease, so that it will be superior to the existing drug therapy. Assume that for some reason the .10 mortality rate is relatively fixed, but that you can possibly alter the surgical technique so that you lower the rate of side effects and increase the rate of complete cure by a corresponding amount. Question: How much do you have to increase the probability of cure to make the surgery preferable to drug therapy?

93    We solve this problem by noting that the sum of the probabilities right now for complete cure and for side effects together is .90. Then, if we raise the probability for cure to some new rate x, the probability for side effects will be .90−x. We also know that to make the preference ranking of surgery and drugs exactly even, we want the sum of all the weighted desirabilities in the "surgery" row to be .63. Keeping the same desirability values, the new row in the weighted desirability table would be:

$$(x) (1) + (.90-x) (.2) + (.10) (0) = .63$$

Solving,    $$x + .18 - .2x = .63$$
$$.8x = .45$$
$$x = .56$$

These calculations tell us that the enterprising surgeon must aim at making     94
the chance of complete cure greater than .56 before his surgical therapy will
be preferable to drug therapy.

We have indicated that Bayesian decision theory has a number of advantages.     95
Why do we not adopt it as the central ethical method?

First, remember all the simplifying assumptions that we had to make in
order to get our sample case to fit into a simple matrix of six squares. In a real
case, we might have five or six possible actions and each could have ten or
twelve contingent consequences; we would have to go to a computer to solve
the problem. (With increasing uses of computers in medicine this may in fact
occur; indeed decision-theory programs might be added on to computer-
diagnosis programs. How would you view such a development?)

But a more basic problem is deriving the desirability values. Once these     96
are given, the calculations are easy. But do we always know what desirability
values we place on things? We might know that we would prefer some degree
of disability to death, but can we say just how much more we prefer it?
If we can't, then our assignment of desirability values is nothing more than
pulling numbers out of the air. There are several strategies to get around this,
but none of them dispenses with the element of subjectivity.

Because of this problem with desirability values, we are often no better     97
off using the supposedly quantitative Bayesian system than we would be using
the qualitative method described above. In that case, we would prefer to use
the qualitative method, to avoid giving our decision an appearance of "objectivity" which it does not deserve.

We can conclude that we ought to keep the Bayesian rational decision
theory in mind as a useful strategy to apply when values of probabilities and
desirabilities are readily obtainable, but that this system cannot replace a more
general, qualitative ethical decision-making method.

This completes our discussion of the ethical decision-making method.     98
This method will be used in the discussion of medical-ethical cases which follow.
Because of the requirements of space, we will not be able to go into each case
in as much depth as we did Case 1; instead we will pick out those facets of each
case that bear most directly on the particular issue we are discussing at the
time. However, the complete ethical process could be applied to each of the
cases; and you will gain practice in decision-making by trying to apply it
yourself rather than simply being content with the discussion given for each
case. As you do so, turn back to this chapter whenever you need to refresh
your memory about the way the method works.                          Ch. 3   99

# 3. Key Issues in Medical Ethics

No doubt you are now eager to come to grips with some of the critical ethical issues facing medicine today—abortion on demand, distribution of scarce resources, brain surgery to control behavior, and a host of others.

99 ↓

Unfortunately, there is no guarantee that the critical issues of today will still be the critical issues in the years to come when you are actually practicing medicine. Most books on medical ethics start out by listing such specific issues and considering each in turn. Since this book is more interested in giving the tools to deal with new and unfamiliar problems, rather than giving out the "answers" to current problems, we will take a slightly different approach.

100 ↓

A study of the many issues in medical ethics suggests that there are a few key issues which keep cropping up in most or all of these discussions. Thus, while what one learns from a careful analysis of abortion may not be applicable when one turns to the issue of behavior control, there are some more basic ethical issues that apply to both abortion and behavior control. It seems logical to start with these key medical-ethical issues before going on to the specifics.

101 ↓

This book considers the key medical-ethical issues to be four:

102

1) The nature of the doctor-patient relationship
2) Informed consent
3) Determining the quality of life
4) Determining the right of participation in decision-making

A chapter will be devoted to each of these in turn.

Ch. 4 ↓ 103

# 4. The Doctor-Patient Relationship

A good place to start with medical ethics is to examine the human context out of which the ethical questions arise—the doctor-patient relationship. Any relationship between two parties carries with it a set of mutual expectations. The special nature of the expectations in the doctor-patient relationship give rise to a number of problems, as well as a few solutions.

103

To start with the obvious, we might state that the doctor-patient relationship is a relationship of one human being toward another human being. While it does not seem to tell us much, it is an important beginning, and serves to alert us to some of the more extreme misconceptions about the medical context. For example, the statement, "The physician ought to have no emotional involvement with his patients," becomes highly suspicious when the human nature of the doctor-patient relationship is considered.

104

Obviously, however, the doctor-patient relationship entails a number of features that other human relationships do not share. A man carving on the body of another person in a dark alley is a despicable criminal, while someone doing the same thing under the lights of an operating room in sterile garb is a respected savior. The exact nature of these unique features, however, is not always clear, and different authorities hold up different factors as being the most crucial to the doctor-patient relationship. A quick beginner's guide to this territory has been provided by Robert Veatch, who has cited several idealized models of the doctor-patient relationship.

105

In Veatch's "Engineering Model," the physician acts as a scientist who believes that he must deal only with facts, and must divorce himself from all questions of value in order to remain "pure." His role is to present all the facts to the patient, let the patient make up his mind, and then carry out those wishes. Morally, he is no more than the plumber called in to clean out the drain. A Roman Catholic physician, who in his private life believes abortion to be an act of murder, will, in this model, perform abortions upon the request of his patients in his role as "applied scientist."

106

In the "Priestly Model," on the other hand, the physician plays a role that is frankly paternalistic. The patient (who, we might say, has somehow "sinned" by getting sick) comes for treatment, counsel, and comfort. The decision-making is placed in the physician's hands, and the patient who does not follow the doctor's orders is adding an even greater "sin" on top of his illness. According to Veatch, a chief sign of this model is the "Speaking-as-a" syndrome: "Speaking as your doctor, I feel that it is definitely time for you to undergo surgical sterilization." The decision here is a moral, not a medical one; but the priest-doctor is presumed to have competence in both areas by virtue of his M.D. degree.

107

108    Each of these two models has features which most doctors and patients would consider undesirable. Each also has some desirable aspects. In many cases, it is well for the doctor to view himself as the agent responsible for carrying out the patient's desires. In many cases, it is well for the doctor to feel that he has a responsibility to provide emotional support and comfort to the patient. As a result, most real doctor-patient relationships are a mixture of aspects of both models, depending on the immediate needs of both doctor and patient.

109    However, is it possible instead to devise a third model—an idealized model that can provide better guidelines for behavior while avoiding the bad features of both the other models? We think that the best candidate for this is Veatch's "Contractual Model."

110    *In the "Contractual Model," the contract between doctor and patient is a non-legalistic statement of general obligations and benefits for both parties. This calls for a sharing of decision-making responsibility. The physician acknowledges that the patient ought to have control over his own life whenever significant decisions are to be made. Once the important, value-laden aspects are dealt with, however, the patient recognizes that the physician has the requisite skill to make the technical decisions needed to implement the general goal that the patient has agreed to. The patient expects that the physician will take no major action without allowing the patient to make the decision, but does not expect to be consulted on all the technical details. The physician also retains the right not to enter into the contract, or to end the contract, if the implementation of the patient's wishes would force him to perform an act that he, the physician, finds abhorrent by his own moral values.*

112  FINANCIAL CONTRACT    *111

111    Some writers refer to the doctor-patient "contract" when they wish to discuss the method by which the physician is paid, and of course in practice this is an important part of the mutual expectations between physician and patient. However, we will be using "contract" in this book in such a way as to exclude the purely financial part of the picture. The question of the extent to which certain social schemes of physician payment hinder the establishment of an ethical doctor-patient relationship will be taken up in Chapter 16.

You can see why we referred to this model as "idealized"; obviously very few doctor-patient relationships fit this description. Very often the doctor makes no inquiries into the patient's wishes until a crisis occurs; and then there may be no time for inquiry, or the patient may be unable to communicate.

However, we can contend that if doctors and patients at least made an attempt to aim at this ideal model, the resulting doctor-patient relationship would be one that would provide a better atmosphere in which to act ethically, with a greater likelihood of long-term satisfaction for the patient.

We will accept the "Contractual Model" as the best single statement of the ideal doctor-patient relationship, and illustrate its applications in the cases which follow. Before doing this, however, we must provide some justification for doing so. The model itself has eliminated the possibility, which most physicians would find hopelessly impractical, that the patient ought to have a say in all medical decisions. The question, then, is whether he is to have input into any medical decisions; and if so, how those he ought to be involved in can be distinguished from those in which the doctor has the final say.

Most people would agree that the patient has some rights to participation in the major decisions affecting his own life and body. At least, if it were to be widely known that doctors everywhere had adopted a totally paternalistic model, very few patients would go to doctors. Also, to return for a minute to the legal realm, the courts have consistently recognized a legal right of the patient to make decisions affecting his control over his body. The trend in recent court decisions has been indeed to broaden the area to which this legal right applies, as we shall see in the discussion of informed consent. Therefore, a physician who makes it a habit to exclude patients from decision-making, whatever his moral justification or lack of it, may eventually find himself in legal trouble.

The question still open, then, is how to distinguish the morally significant decisions from the purely technical ones. The model itself does not provide much guide; we can only attempt to point out some general principles by means of case illustrations.

*What we are saying in the "Contractual Model" is that the patient has the right of participation in medical decisions that are morally significant to his life.* We must immediately qualify this to apply to the conscious, rational patient who has passed the "age of understanding" (usually taken to be about 14 years of age).

In Chapter 7, when we discuss "Rights of Ethical Participation," we shall take the right of the patient for granted. We shall consider instead when others in addition to the patient have the right of participation, and who can assume this role for a patient who is irrational, unconscious, or a minor.

112

113

114

115

## CASE 2

116     You are a partner in a urology practice. Your associate, Dr. X, tells you of a patient who came in yesterday asking for a vasectomy. Mr. M.Q., apparently an intelligent and well-read man of age 32, has two children, aged 7 and 4, which he considers to be the ideal family size. His wife has a condition contra-indicating the use of oral contraceptives, and has expelled several IUD's. They are presently using the condom for birth control and both find it unsatisfactory. M.Q. states that he and his wife are agreed that it would be best for him to undergo vasectomy.

     M.Q. further states to Dr. X that he realizes that the operation must be considered irreversible. He has read in the papers of a case in which a sterilized man lost his wife and children in an auto accident, remarried, and then regretted not being able to father more children of his own. M.Q. says that he has pondered such possibilities, but upon weighing all the factors he has decided to undergo sterilization and accept any possible consequences.

     Dr. X says he does not want to perform the operation. Before joining you in partnership, he had a case where the tragedy alluded to by M.Q. did indeed occur. The other man, who had cheerfully consented at the time of surgery, afterwards bitterly attacked Dr. X for performing the sterilization. Dr. X feels that M.Q.'s present statement is worthless, since no one can predict how one would actually feel in the face of such a tragedy until it occurred. For all these reasons, Dr. X has made it a personal rule never to do vasectomies on patients of Mr. M.Q.'s age, who still have as many potential child-conceiving years ahead of them. However, he wants your views before making a final decision.

     Would you perform the vasectomy?     Yes ↓ 117
                                           No ↓ 118

---

117     By agreeing to perform the vasectomy, you have shown accord with the "Contractual Model." By just about any standards, whether or not to be sterilized is a morally significant choice for the patient and thus earns his right of participation in the decision. As a physician, you have the duty to make sure M.Q. knows all the important facts about vasectomies and their consequences, since, as we saw in Chapter 2, ethical judgments made on the basis of inaccurate data are worthless as practical guides to behavior. Since vasectomies have been the subject of much attention in the popular press, and since M.Q. has illustrated a grasp of the most relevant points, you seem justified in engaging him in a minimum of questioning and explanation before agreeing to do the operation.

118     If you refuse to do the vasectomy, you are apparently putting decisive weight on the arguments raised by Dr. X. Let's examine them. First, what is the actual probability of the hypothetical auto accident actually occurring? How does this compare to the number of men who were quite satisfied with the results? If the probability is sufficiently low, is it correct to give that consequence so much weight in the final decision?

     While all negative consequences must be considered, it is in general an ethical "error" to allow a bad consequence of very low probability decide the question by itself. An example of this error from another medical issue is to refuse to allow a terminally ill patient to die by withholding extraordinary means of therapy, "because who knows, tomorrow they might discover a new drug that would have cured him." In this case it is a good consequence instead of a bad one, but still of very low probability.

But more important than this is the difference of opinion between Dr. X and M.Q. on the matter. Dr. X's statement that no one can really predict how he would act in a hypothetical situation he has not experienced is factually true. But it does not follow logically from that that Dr. X ought not perform the vasectomy—unless one makes the assumption that Dr. X knows better than Mr. M.Q. how Mr. M.Q. would act in that hypothetical situation. This is the element of paternalism that we found fault with in the "Priestly Model", and which we specifically excluded from the "Contractual Model."

This is not to say that in some cases Dr. X might not know the patient's true mind better than the patient. But then it is incumbent on Dr. X to demonstrate by the patient's words or behavior that the patient knows his mind poorly. On the other hand, M.Q. presented as a rather uniquely rational and thoughtful individual, so these proofs would be hard to come by in his case.

119

As this case illustrates, it is easier to remove paternalism from one's ideal model of medical practice than it is to avoid unconsciously slipping into it in one's actual activity. This is because the "Priestly Model" has traditionally been very powerful in medicine and has shaped patients' expectations of their doctor's behavior. Also, the paternalistic role fits in well with the average physician's own emotional needs.

120

While many patients allow their doctors to act paternalistically by default, because the patient is unaware of any alternative, some patients genuinely want this relationship, due to their own inability to, or fear of, making important decisions. If, early on in the relationship, the patient says something like, "You're the doctor, so just do what you think is best and don't bother me with the gory details," he has made his own moral decision as called for by the "Contractual Model," and the physician may then be justified in making subsequent major decisions on his own.

## CASE 3

The population of a very small country in Asia is doubling every 21 years. This growth is negating economic gains and hindering meaningful economic development.

121

The country's Family Planning Council, after a massive study, concludes that continued rapid growth jeopardizes the very existence of the country and the health and welfare of its citizens.

They have recommended drastic action: that every citizen who voluntarily agrees to accept sterilization be given coupons redeemable for 100 kadis ($20 U.S.) worth of food. Any individual who voluntarily requests sterilization after no more than two children will get another 100-kadi coupon. And to increase recruiting, a similar coupon would be provided for persons bringing to a government clinic anyone who subsequently accepts sterilization.

121 cont.    In defense of its proposal, the Council argues: "No one will be penalized for having children; no one will be forced to refrain from having children; no one will suffer. In accord with the U.N. Declaration of Human Rights, every citizen should have available to him those means of controlling family size which are consistent with his own values and religious beliefs."

The traditional religious beliefs of the country apparently offer some resistance to limitation of family size on the grounds that such matters should be in the hands of God. However, studies have suggested, in past population programs in that country, that in practice, the religious objection was limited to a very small minority of the population.

You are a high official of the World Health Organization, charged with recommending whether WHO will provide assistance to this program. Since WHO money is vital to equipping the sterilization clinics, you have considerable leverage over the provisions of the plan. Do you recommend WHO participation? If not, what changes, if any, in the proposal would you require in order for it to get your approval?

(Adapted from: Case Studies in Bioethics, Case No. 139. Hastings Center Report, February, 1973.)

---

22    Case 3 was included to remind you that paternalism can exist on the social level as well as in individual relationships, and this will become increasingly important as social policy in medical areas becomes more widespread. While there are a number of pros and cons on either side, one question we could ask here is: Does the Council know what is good for the people of Kadi-land better than the people? (How does the fact that they are poor, uneducated Asian peasants influence your decision?) If the program is really good for the people, why is it necessary to "bribe" them to participate? Especially, why is it necessary to pay some of them to recruit others?

This case is well worth discussion in a small group—especially since, within your professional lifetime, you may be called in to judge a similar proposal for some community in the U.S.

TRUTH TELLING

123    Let's now examine some of the consequences of the "Contractual Model." *If the patient has a right to participate in decisions which are morally significant for him, and if a correct ethical decision depends on the accuracy of the relevant data, it follows that as a general rule, the patient must at all times be told the truth about his medical condition.* This brings up the issue of what to tell the patient, especially one who is dying or who has a potentially fatal illness. This is a problem on both the ethical and emotional level—even after making an ethical judgment about what we should divulge, we may not have the nerve to actually face the patient and say it. While this applies to every communication with the patient, consideration of the more dramatic cases highlights the crucial issues.

CASE 4

As a new intern in a large city hospital, you take the initial history and physical of Mrs. P, a 54-year-old, post-menopausal Jamaican-born woman who comes in complaining of severe pain and a mass in the right lower quadrant of the abdomen. After the interview and after establishing some initial rapport with the patient, you elicit from Mrs. P. the fear that she has cancer. You reassure her that she will get a complete workup with laboratory tests. She replies sadly, "I know if it was cancer you doctors wouldn't tell me." You end the conversation by saying that you and the other doctors will know much more after the initial lab tests are done.

A tentative diagnosis of degenerating fibroid was made and the patient underwent surgery. Later, the pathology report showed that in fact Mrs. P. had Stage IV cervical cancer. While the surgeons had removed all the tumor they could see, the spread was such that distant metastases were very likely, and all they could do would be to try radiation and chemotherapy. The five year survival rate of Stage IV cervical cancer is 0–20%.

Your first response is to want to go to Mrs. P. and explain to her that she has cancer and that she has a limited time to live, although everything possible will be tried to prolong it. You want to try to help share her grief and offer continued moral support. Since you are new, however, you want to ask your chief resident how to proceed.

The chief resident says that you should "never use the word 'cancer' to a patient or they lose all hope; it's best to use a lot of medical jargon to soften it." You reply that somehow or other you feel that Mrs. P. has to be told her survival chances. After an increasingly angry interchange, the resident exclaims, "Look, how would you like it if you told her she had incurable cancer, and she walked over to the window and jumped out? Just let me handle this on rounds."

Later the resident tells you shortly that he has informed Mrs. P. that she had a malignant process and the surgeons had removed it.

Are you satisfied with this? If not, what do you do now?

(Adapted from: Case 101, Columbia University Program in Medical Ethics, Courtesy Dr. Robert Veatch)

Case 4 illustrates that the problem of what to tell the patient is one where general rules are least likely to be of benefit. The resident's rule, never tell a patient they have cancer, clearly saves him a lot of hard thinking, but it displays a singular disregard for the individual emotional states and emotional needs of patients.

Incidentally, the idea of a patient "jumping out of a window" after being told bad news seems to have widespread exposure, and is one of the more commonly cited defenses for not telling the whole truth. In one study of a large number of suicide reports, a group from the Hastings Center was unable to find a single case of a person committing suicide as a result of being told that they had a fatal illness. (Another instance of decision-making by a single, low-probability consequence?) In our experience, we have been able to verify one such suicide case.

126      On the other hand, the rule "Always tell the patient the whole truth" can be just as inhumane if applied uncritically. Many patients are very adept at denying an obviously terminal illness, and may be using their denial as a defense against a total psychological breakdown. Is it consistent with the "Contractual Model" to state that the patient does not have the right to deny his reality?

127      Case 4 has another point worth pondering. Consider the statement of Mrs. P: "If it was cancer you doctors wouldn't tell me." Mrs. P. did not make up this idea out of thin air; she has been exposed to instances in the past, her own or those of friends, in which the doctor withheld information which was later found out. This shows that we cannot decide whether to tell the truth or not on an ad hoc basis, without considering the future consequences both for our relationship with that patient and for the trust placed by all patients in the doctor-patient relationship in general. Any decision made with the eye toward getting us out of a temporarily sticky situation may come back to haunt us in several forms later on.

     Some of the unanticipated consequences of medical deception are nicely illustrated in Case 5.

---

CASE 5

128      "The prize fighter J.J. Corbett had died of cancer, and The New York Times ran the story with this headline: 'Ex-Champion Succumbs Here to Cancer. He Believed He Had Heart Disease.' Such was the conscientious lie with which Gentleman Jim's doctors had let him live out his last days. However, other doctors soon began to violently protest the open publication of the deception in a news story, one physician complaining to the editor that several of his own patients with heart diseases were wild with fear that they too had cancer of the liver."

(Joseph Fletcher, Morals and Medicine)

---

129      *The "Contractual Model" would seem to suggest the following ethical rule: "The physician should tell the patient the truth about his condition, in language he can understand, unless the physician has reason to believe that a degree of harm, more serious than merely a temporary emotional depression, would follow as a result."*

     This means that the burden of justification of not telling the whole truth rests on the physician; and that, in order to avoid slavish adherence to truth-telling as a rule, he must be alert to any signs or "messages" from the patient that would indicate that the patient would be better off not having the entire truth thrust upon him at once. In particular, the physician dare not take, "Tell it to me straight, Doc, I can take it" at face value.

     Case 6 is described by Dr. Bernard C. Meyer in Torrey, Ethical Issues in Medicine.

## CASE 6

A hospitalized man has had a biopsy taken of an enlarged cervical lymph node and you are awaiting the results of the pathology report. The patient appears to be rather agitated by these proceedings. He finally states that if the biopsy showed cancer he wouldn't want to live; and if the report came back negative, he would be convinced that you were lying to him in order to spare him the shock.

The biopsy report indicates a malignant lymphoma. Furthermore, a more thorough physical exam has turned up a mass in the patient's abdomen, and all indications point to its being of lymphatic origin and also malignant. Lymphomas of this type, in general, respond fairly well to chemotherapy; but it is difficult to predict the outcome of any individual case before a course of therapy is attempted.

What do you tell your patient?

---

If you tell the patient he has cancer, you are either adopting the general rule of always telling the truth; or else you are assuming that his statements do not reflect his true mental status. Possibly he might really want to know and would be happier knowing. Possibly if he really did not want to know, he would simply deny the truth when it is told to him ("they must have gotten my specimen mixed up with someone else's in the lab") and no harm would have been done, except possibly for some anger at you.

If you elect not to tell, either you have adopted the general rule of not telling patients they have cancer; or else you are taking at face value the fact that revealing the true diagnosis would send the patient into a significant depression. Or possibly you wish to avoid an emotion-laden confrontation.

In the actual case, the physician did neither of the above. Instead, he adopted a procedure which ought to be used much more in medicine. Sensing his own inadequacy to evaluate the patient's possible emotional reaction, he called in a psychiatrist to advise him as to how to proceed.

Meyer reports that after evaluating the situation, the psychiatrist advised the physician to tell the patient: that the biopsy of the cervical node showed cancer; that he also had a growth in the abdomen which was very likely cancer; that the type of cancer involved tends to respond well to chemotherapy; that if chemotherapy, in turn, were to cause him any discomfort, he could receive medication for its relief; and that the doctors were very hopeful of a successful outcome. The physician, a surgical resident, was "both appalled and distressed" when he learned what he was to do, but he steeled himself and spoke the required formula with conviction.

39

134    While happy endings are not reliable indicators that the original ethical decision was correct, this case has one anyway. Says Meyer: "The patient, who, it will be recalled, had declared he wouldn't want to live if the doctors found cancer, was obviously gratified. Immediately he telephoned members of his family to tell them the news... That night he slept well for the first time since entering the hospital... Just before leaving he confessed that he had known all along about the existence of the abdominal mass but that he had concealed his knowledge to see what the doctors would tell him. Upon arriving home he wrote a warm letter of thanks and admiration to the resident surgeon."*

135    Several points about this case deserve comment. First, it provides an excellent example of how empirical findings can be "fed in" to the ethical decision-making process without making the error of assuming that the ethical question is an empirical one. The resident realized the ethical question at stake, but also saw that information about the patient's emotional state, with predictions about his reactions, were essential empirical data upon which the ethical question was based. Accordingly, he called in a specialist who was best suited to supply the missing empirical data.

136    The second point is that "telling a patient" something takes place over a span of time, and is not a one-shot affair. Thus, the shading of the phrases used, whether the truth is delivered all at once or in small doses, and the kind of follow-up are all important parts of the ethical decision, as well as "tell" or "don't tell." A decision to reveal a grave prognosis, which may be "ethical" in itself, may become "unethical" if the physician tells the patient bluntly and then withdraws, without offering any emotional support to help the patient resolve his feelings. In fact, the assurance that the physician plans to see it through along with the patient, and that he will always make himself available to offer any comfort possible, may be more important than the bad news itself. In many of the "sour cases" that are offered as justification for withholding the truth, it may well be the absence of this transmission of compassion, rather than the telling of the truth, that produced the unfortunate result.

### CONFIDENTIALITY

137    What are some of the other consequences of the "Contractual Model"? We might consider also one of the terms of the implied contract—that the information gained by the physician in the course of the relationship will be kept confidential. While many patients may not be aware of any "right" to be told the truth, or to avoid a paternalistic physician, the "right to privacy" is very well known because of its existence as one of the most ancient traditions in medicine. As the Hippocratic Oath held, what the physician hears "which ought not to be noised abroad" will be kept in confidence. Of course, the Oath offers no clarification as to what ought not to be noised abroad. The corresponding statement in the A.M.A. code is qualified: "unless the law requires it or if necessary to protect the welfare of individuals or the community." It is in deciding when these "loopholes" apply that many of the ethical dilemmas related to confidentiality arise.

*From B.C. Meyer, "Truth and the Physician."   In: <u>Ethical Issues in Medicine</u>, ed. E.F. Torrey, Boston, Little, Brown, 1968.

## CASE 7

This was Mr. G's second admission to the Brooklyn Psychiatric Clinic for acute paranoid schizophrenic break. After three days of round-the-clock cramming for his doctoral exams in political science at Columbia, he had been found claiming that the Nazis had been infiltrating the Columbia political science department, and had assaulted three innocent passers-by on the street whom he accused of being part of the Nazi conspiracy. He was subdued and taken to the clinic. You, a staff psychiatrist, examine him and conclude that this break has been related to the pressure of exams, and that the prognosis for recovery after a short stay is very good.

As you are filling out the record, Mr. G demands to see what you are writing, and you obligingly give him a blank copy of the admission form. This computerized form has blanks for the patient's name, address, social security number, "problem appraisal," and diagnosis to be entered in the form of the code number from the American Psychiatric Association code manual.

"You mean you are going to feed my entire life into a computer?" asks Mr. G. "Where does this carbon copy go?"

"To the Department of Mental Hygiene in Albany. It's required by law as part of a multi-state information system."

"I have been planning a career in the foreign service after finishing my degree. That's the whole reason I've been going to school for the past four years. Do you realize what happens to my foreign service career once this gets into the government computer?"

"These records will surely be treated with strict confidence; they are only for statistical purposes." But you have been reading about recent government wiretapping and snooping in the papers, and your voice lacks conviction.

"Well, I say you can't send my name in," says Mr. G. "It violates my rights of confidentiality. I do have rights, don't I?"

"I'm violating the law if I don't send it in," you say.

Mr. G. declines to offer sympathy.

What do you do with the computer form?

Send in the form         ↓ 140
Don't send in the form      ↓ 142
Send in form without name ↓ 145

(Adapted from: Case 117, Columbia University Program in Medical Ethics, courtesy Dr. Robert Veatch.)

---

Case 7 is an excellent case to practice listing and weighing the consequences of the two opposite courses of action. (Don't forget an additional alternative: postponing sending in the form in the hopes that the patient will be more "rational" later and will agree.) However, on the emotional side, there are several factors that might tip the scales in favor of actually going the confidentiality route, even with insufficient ethical justification. First, the actual chances of going to jail are small. Second, harm done by breaking confidence is to be done to Mr. G., whom you know personally, while the harm of not sending in the form is harm to the impersonal "system" with whom you have no sympathy. Third, "civil disobedience" is after all in the grand tradition of Thoreau, Gandhi, et al. Fourth, after all, he may never have any further psychiatric problems anyway, so the imagined harm may be unreal.

What about a case where the harm is real and clear, and where both parties are known to you and deserve your sympathy?

↓ 141

140     Sending in the form means that Mr. G's diagnosis is fit to "be noised abroad," regardless of any adverse consequences upon his career. (It seems reasonable to assume that his guess as to the possibility of the State Department getting hands on the "confidential" file is accurate, especially where national security could be concerned.) You could justify this decision on several grounds. First, you are, as a doctor, doing a great service to humanity, and if you were locked up in jail you would be depriving your future patients of this service. Second, this man ought, in fact, to be denied a foreign service career because he might have another break at an inopportune time and thus jeopardize foreign policy; therefore, you are doing your duty as a citizen.

    Restate the two above justifications as formal ethical principles. Do you think, in such form, they are generally valid? (For example: Suppose Mr. G. ends up in a desk job in Washington. Would a schizophrenic break in a person of that position be a large enough threat to national interests to justify ruining his career?)

139

---

CASE 8

141     As genetic counselor for the community Tay-Sachs disease genetic screening program, you have good news for Mr. and Mrs. E., a young couple of Ashkenazic Jewish extraction who plan to start a family soon. They are aware that the recessive gene for Tay-Sachs disease, a degenerative disease of nerves which usually kills children before the third year of life, occurs in 1 in 30 people in that ethnic group, and so wished to be tested. They also know that if the parents are known to carry the gene, amniocentesis can be carried out on the unborn infant to detect Tay-Sachs disease, and that child could be aborted. Once a child is born with the disease there is no treatment.

    You are happy to tell Mr. and Mrs. E. that there is no risk of them having a baby with Tay-Sachs disease. You also tactfully tell them that you have, however, discovered that Mr. E. carries a recessive gene for the disease. This, you explain, will in no way affect his health; and since Mrs. E. carries no such gene, none of their children can inherit the two recessive genes necessary for the disease to develop. Mr. E. seems to understand but looks worried.

    You know that Mr. E. has two younger brothers, also approaching childbearing age. You suggest that they also be tested for the gene, since one of them might chance to marry a carrier, in which case each of their children would have a 1 in 4 chance of developing the disease. You also recommend that his parents be tested to determine which side of the family the gene comes from.

    Mr. E. finally speaks up. He knows that he is in no jeopardy, but he is struck by the knowledge that each of his cells is marked by this terrible disease. Somehow he feels that he is "not quite a man" if half his children will also have that "sickness in their cells," even if they have no clinical disease. Maybe he was being foolish, Mr. E. continued, but he could not bring himself to tell his brothers that he was carrying this gene. Further efforts on your part to persuade him to change his mind only make him more adamant; he forbids you to do anything that would reveal his condition to his family, regardless of the possible consequences to his brothers' families.

    What do you do now?

(Adapted from: Case 121, Columbia University Program in Medical Ethics, courtesy Robert M. Veatch)

143

Not sending in the form means, in principle, that you have decided to be prepared to go to jail, and are prepared to deprive the psychiatric profession of one practitioner when there is already a shortage of psychiatrists, and to deprive your family of your financial support and charming company. It also means you have no compunction about Mr. G., with his history of two schizophrenic breaks, one involving physical assult, entering the foreign service and possibly achieving a post of high responsibility. Do you feel that the advantages of preserving confidentiality outweigh these considerations? Also, what probabilities do you assign to the consequences just listed, that you may be sent to jail and the rest? How do those influence your answer?

142

139

---

At the point in your application of the decision-making method where you listed the alternatives open to you, how many alternatives did you list? Whatever they were, they should have taken into account your answers to two questions:

143

1)  Is it necessary to take action now or can it be postponed for a period of time up to several weeks?

2)  Is the attitude expressed by Mr. E. likely to be his final word on the subject, or is it open to modification?

The first question is an important thing to note for any ethical decision. Just as it is in error to try to convene a committee to draw up a report on whether to resuscitate a patient who has just stopped breathing, it is in error to rush headlong into immediate action on an ethical issue that will permit of more lengthy reflection and possibly consultation with others. It is as important in medical ethics as it is in clinical medicine to learn to distinguish the emergencies from the situations that will allow more thought and the gathering of more data.

The second question shows why, in this case, waiting a few weeks might be of benefit, assuming, of course, that the brothers of Mr. E. have not yet actually started their "family planning." Mr. E's response to genetic counseling is not unusual. In fact, in one study, a few fathers went so far as to deny paternity of their offspring rather than admit that they carried a dangerous recessive gene. It is also possible that Mr. E. will remain set in this view for the foreseeable future. However, it is at least probable that after he recovers from the initial emotional impact, Mr. E. will be approachable in the issue of his responsibility to his brothers, and will give his voluntary consent to divulge the information. If he does not, then the ethical issue recurs in a more black-and-white form: tell or don't tell?

144

A comparison is interesting between Cases 7 and 8. The decision of Mr. G. the Nazi-hunter, while creating problems for the doctor, was nevertheless completely rational from Mr. G's point of view. Why should the doctor's legal scruples bother him when his entire career is at stake? On the other hand, very likely Mr. E. himself would admit that his own behavior is irrational, if he could separate himself for a minute from his emotional involvement. Thus the prognosis for a later change of decision seems better in Mr. E's case than in Mr. G's.

146

145     Sending the form in without name and social security number is a compromise that satisfies neither side. Actually it is the same as not sending in the form. For statistical purposes, the study needs to know if this is a new admission of a new patient or the return of a patient who has been treated in the past. Forms without names might as well be no forms at all. Also, the law requires that the form be sent in fully filled out, so this is as much a violation of the law as not sending in the form. Sending in a form without a name might have validity only as a symbolic act of civil disobedience. In that case, you would have to be taking the position that the law is bad in all cases, not just in Mr. G's.

139 ↑

---

146     Before leaving Case 8, here are some further points to ponder:

1)   If, after the course of action proposed, Mr. E. still refuses consent to divulge, would you tell the brothers or not?

2)   Does the "loophole" in the ethical codes, "when necessary to protect the welfare of individuals or the community," apply here?

3)   Suppose Mr. E's brothers were already patients of yours in the counseling program, instead of mere acquaintances as originally stated. Would your duties and/or approach to the problem change?

4)   What would be the long-term consequences for the counseling program, if any, were you to write to the brothers without Mr. E's consent?

147     One question that might have occurred to you is: would Mr. E. have any legal course of action open against you if you divulged the information?

    While the legal system has long held the lawyer-patient relationship to be inviolate, because the system itself could not operate without such a provision, it has had less self-interest in giving legal protection to the doctor-patient relationship—especially since such protection could deprive the court of significant evidence. The result in the U.S. has been a significant variability among the states as to whether a statute exists granting such a privilege, and as to how the courts apply it to specific cases. The result offers good opportunities for legal and ethical responsibilities to go separate ways, as Case 9 illustrates.

---

## CASE 9

148     You have been treating Mr. Z. for two years in your office for severe back and leg pain which you have diagnosed as sciatica. You learn by chance that recently Mr. Z. slipped and fell while getting out of a cab; and, claiming that he never had a backache for a day in his life before the accident, is suing the cabdriver for injuries.

    You are aware that one word from you in court could blow Mr. Z's case, as well as losing you a patient (whom you now consider no great loss). Your attorney, whom you consult, however, points out that in your state, your knowledge of Mr. Z's condition is "privileged communication" unless Mr. Z. himself releases you from legal responsibility. If Mr. Z. were suing you for malpractice, you would be released in order to defend yourself; but you are not released by Mr. Z. suing someone else. The attorney agrees that as things now stand the judgment will surely go against the hapless cabdriver—"but that's the breaks."

Do you take your attorney's advice to keep still, or do you attempt to communicate with the cabdriver's lawyer regardless of the legal consequences to you?

(Adapted from: H.A. Davidson, in Torrey [see references]).

One apparently reasonable compromise between self-respect and the law would be for the physician in Case 9 to refrain from involving himself in the legal proceedings. However, at Mr. Z's next visit, the physician might inform him that he has heard about the court case; that he regretted not being able to testify; and that Mr. Z. should go shopping for another doctor. Would this, in your view, be a justifiable compromise, or merely a hypocritical gesture by way of salving the physician's conscience?

What may happen where there is no statute granting privilege to doctor-patient communications?

## CASE 10

In Hague vs. Williams, the court, in the absence of a privileged communications law, supported a physician who told an insurance company that a baby's death had been due to a congenital defect. Since the insurance policy contained a clause excluding congenital defects, the parents sued the pediatrician for revealing this information without their consent and against their interests. The court held that in some cases the public interest supersedes the right of privileged communication: "In this case, the public's interest in an honest result assumed dominance over the individual's right of non-disclosure." Presumably it was felt that the physician had acted not out of malice, but out of a genuine impulse to see justice done.

Do you agree with the court's reasoning, from the ethical point of view?

(Adapted from: H.A. Davidson, in Torrey [see references]).

A physician (quoted by Davidson) noted about Case 10: "This case lays down a much lower standard than that which is required by the ethics of the medical profession. The case illustrates that once a disclosure is made, the courts will go far in searching for a principle of 'social importance' to rationalize the disclosure. I do not agree with the results of this case. The doctor should not have made a voluntary, out-of-court disclosure of this nature. The law should have granted redress." *(Note that this authority never stated exactly which principle of ethics was violated.)

In comparing your reactions to Cases 9 and 10, was your decision swayed at all by the fact that in one case, the person who stood to lose was an innocent cabdriver with whom you could sympathize, while in the other case the loser was to be the large, impersonal, and doubtlessly wealthy insurance company? Are such considerations ethically relevant?

In the discussion so far, we have taken for granted two things: *First, that the right of the patient to privileged communication is recognized as highly desirable; and second, that the right is not absolute. We have thus sharpened the ethical problem to that of determining "how much" public welfare concern is necessary before the right is superseded. This is a question about which individuals' differences in personal values are likely to be very significant.*

*From H.A. Davidson, "Professional Secrecy." In: Ethical Issues in Medicine, ed. E.F. Torrey, Boston, Little, Brown, 1968.

153 At the very least, the physician invoking "public welfare" to justify disclosure has to accept the burden of proof of defining what the disastrous result of non-disclosure would have been. In another of Davidson's examples, a doctor was upheld by the court when he informed the U.S. Air Force without the consent of the patient that one of their civilian employees, an accountant, was an alcoholic. It may be argued that if the patient were a pilot, there might have been no question about the justifiability of the disclosure; but since he was an accountant, it is hard to see exactly what the danger was that demanded this extreme step. Merely that he worked for the Air Force was not enough.

(Some corporations get around this by making the "voluntary" release of such medical information by the employee a condition for his continued employment. This gets the doctor off the hook but raises other ethical questions.)

---

## CASE 11

154 Your patient is a New York City bus driver with a known heart condition; it is your medical opinion that he could have a fatal heart attack while driving and you advise him to quit his job. He refuses since driving is his only means of livelihood.

Should you inform the bus company?

(Adapted from: H.A. Davidson, in Torrey [see references].)

---

155 In the actual case, the doctor did not inform the employer. Subsequently, 30 people were killed when the bus driver had a heart attack and plunged his bus into the East River.

Of course, it is possible that the driver might have gone his way without trouble for another 10 years. If that had been the case, would it have made the doctor's decision ethically correct? Is the fatal outcome ethically wrong?

Note that, according to the decision-making process, the ethical validity of an action is judged according to the consequences of the formal ethical statement. However, the statement is ethically valid or not at the time that the decision is made; and does not become valid or invalid later because of the results of that action.

157 UNCLEAR *156

---

156 It may sound like doubletalk to say that a thing is ethically valid or not because of the consequences, while the consequences do not make a thing ethically valid. However, in the first instance, the reference is to the consequences of the formal ethical statement, while in the latter it is the consequences of the particular act. In "situation ethics" the consequence of the individual act is what counts, but in Chapter 2 we specifically rejected this view.

Recall that the formal ethical statement is universalizable; that is, it should apply to any similar case. Suppose my neighbor's dog barks too loud one night, and I determine that I wish to cut off one of my neighbor's ears. If we consider only the consequences of this act, I find that it is quite consistent with my personal set of values, since I do not like my neighbor too much.

160

## RIGHTS

Before leaving the doctor-patient relationship issue, this is as good a time as any to mention the nature of these "rights" about which we have been blithely conversing. The word "rights" can be used in a number of senses, some of which have much less ethical justification than others.

The main feature of a "right" is that the conferring of it on one person automatically confers an obligation on another, sometimes hypothetical, person. To say that A has the right to life, or the right of free speech, is to say in the same breath that the person who might be planning to kill A, or to prevent A from speaking his convictions in public, has an obligation not to do those things.

157

The most obvious kind of "right" is that which is stated in a constitutional right, and which has official legal recognition. In that case, there is no question where the authority comes from to bestow the right and the concurrent obligation. Fortunately or unfortunately, the number of rights specifically granted by the Constitution is less than what many people assume. We have already mentioned that there is no constitutional right to privacy in a doctor-patient relationship; where such a right exists, it is by a statute of the legislature, which is subject to repeal.

158

What about the "rights" that are not specifically granted by law, but which people claim to have anyhow? One important thing to consider in this regard is the nature of the (often unspoken) obligation which accompanies the right. In most of the rights that are universally recognized, such as the right to life and to free speech, the obligation is being imposed NOT TO do something to the person possessing the right—a relatively easy obligation to anyone not bent on establishing tyranny. Many of the invented "rights," on the other hand, such as "I have a right to attend the college of my choice," carry an obligation for someone else TO DO something—while, of course, leaving entirely unresolved how that person or persons are to find the resources to do it. The "right to health care," which even the A.M.A. has recently come to recognize, falls into this latter category.

159

161

---

However, just by saying that that is what I want to do, I cannot claim to be acting ethically. To do so, I must subscribe to the formal ethical principle, "Anyone whose dog barks too loud at night should have one ear cut off." Now since I have a dog who might very well sound off one evening, and since it is not consistent with my set of values to go around doing Vincent Van Gogh imitations, I must reject this ethical statement. By doing so, I am constrained from carrying out the proposed mayhem upon my neighbor.

It is important to see by this that comparing the consequences of an action to one's own set of values could lead to all sorts of evils being justified—IF we forget the nature of formal ethical statements and look at one case only.

We must also remember that at the time we make the ethical decision, all our predictions as to consequences are only probability estimates which may prove wrong. We do not have the luxury of waiting to see whether the bus driver has a heart attack at the wheel, and then going back and making our decision afterward.

160

157

161    Another way of looking at the "rights" issue is a pragmatic one: what purpose is served by calling something a "right" rather than a desire? Certainly, on the plus side, there is a rhetorical benefit of using a newly formulated right as the slogan for a policy of social change. "Right to health care" has been used in this way. Another example is the "Patient's Bill of Rights" established by the American Hospital Association (see Appendix II). The A.H.A. does not, in fact, offer a means of redressing a denial of any of its listed rights other than to express its hope that individual hospitals will feel bound by them. However, many of the rights listed are already recognized in law. The formulation of a "Bill of Rights" is a rhetorical means to call to the attention of patients that they do not, in fact, have to put up with certain behavior which they may have thought was their inevitable lot.

162    There is also a disadvantage to labeling "rights" which becomes clear when we consider the important role of rational argument in clarifying one's ethical principles and decisions. Suppose in an argument, your opponent states, "I have a right to X." While carrying a moral connotation, in the form of the unstated obligation, the appearance of the sentence is that of an empirical statement, and seems to beg for a judgment of true or false. You therefore reply, "No, you don't." The argument is immediately completely polarized, and no agreement is possible without open warfare.

Suppose your opponent had stated, "I think it would be good if you were to do X." You may then ask, "Why?" and get into the substantive issues involved. This alternative way of phrasing the issue makes it much more likely that the argument will be constructive, and that the disputants will come to find a common ground.

163    Of course, it is much easier to say, "I have a right" than it is to think about one's real reasons for wanting something, which may in fact be rather inadequate from an ethical standpoint. That is why we hear today of so many "rights" from all sides.

*But for purposes of ethical reasoning, it is wise to stay away from all "rights" other than those actually granted by legal means. If a person tries to end an ethical argument prematurely by claiming a "right," it is appropriate to ask, "By whose authority?"* On the other hand, a non-"right" statement can be shown ethically valid just by showing that the consequences of establishing it as a universalizable ethical principle are good ones and outweigh the disadvantages.

164    However, there will be occasions in which discussion of ethical issues in terms of "rights" is appropriate or may be preferred. In those instances, you can use the comments above to help analyze the ethical arguments. For example, it is always wise to spell out the obligation that is implied by the right. Is this an obligation to do or not to do something? Does the person who is claiming the right in fact recognize the obligation, and is he prepared to accept it?

It might also be recalled that most rights can be waived under certain 165 circumstances. Just what are those circumstances for the right in question? Do some special features of the doctor-patient relationship apply?

An important social issue related to rights and the associated obligations is whether these are spread over the entire society or whether they are applied in practice only to certain minorities.

In the following pages we will mention many "rights" and will have occasion to investigate them by asking such questions as these.

One final comment on the doctor-patient relationship is necessary. You 166 may have been disturbed that in all the sample cases cited in this chapter, the social context was that of one doctor in private practice seeing one patient. A number of developments are now occurring in the field of health care delivery that make it likely that, inside of 20 years, such a social relationship will be in a minority status within the health care field. Which of the ethical principles that are valid for the one-on-one relationship will still be applicable in, say, a health care delivery team concept is an open question, which will have to be worked out as these future developments take a clearer shape. For example, experimental use of computer storage and recall of patients' medical records have already raised significant questions about the future of the "right to privacy."

For an example of a problem that could arise within a health care team setting, see Case 27 in Chapter 7. Ch. 5  167

# 5. Informed Consent

The "Contractual Model" of the doctor-patient relationship, as we discussed in Chapter 4, carries as a major feature the obligation of the physician to allow the patient to make the decisions that are morally significant to his life and health. The consideration of how this is done leads to the issue of informed consent.

167

To start with an obvious point, the two-word phrase "informed consent" indicates the two ingredients of this issue, each of which may give rise to ethical questions. First, we might want to ask whether the patient's consent was obtained, and whether this consent was truly voluntary. Second, when consent has been established, we might ask whether the patient was adequately informed beforehand.

168

The comment about being "adequately" informed points out an important consideration—that there is no such thing as "informed" consent in a strict sense. We might say that if each patient were to take a complete course of study in medical school, he would be "informed" enough to give truly informed consent. But even this neglects the fact that most medical decisions are made with a considerable degree of uncertainty on the part of the doctor himself. How does one inform the patient about what one does not know? All of these suggest that "informed consent" is an ideal to which medical ethics seeks close approximation rather than rigid adherence.

169

Some people have used the impossibility of getting informed consent in a strict sense as a justification for not trying to inform patients about possible consequences of a proposed treatment. Do you think this is valid? (A common ethical "error" is to invent impossible criteria, and then reject a proposed course of action because it fails to meet them.)

The fact that "informed consent" is an ideal to be approached clarifies our ethical task in deciding whether a particular consent is informed consent. In no case in medicine is absolutely no information given to the patient. The ethical task, then, is to decide whether enough information was given to allow the patient to make up his mind in a rational manner. If we assume that the patient will want to apply the ethical decision-making process for himself, this means that we will have to give him all the major consequences that are morally relevant.

170

171    However, in much of the daily practice of medicine, "getting the patient's informed consent" is treated as the equivalent of getting the patient to sign his name to one of a number of standard forms, under the assumption that this is sufficient to prevent any legal repercussions. This leads us to ask whether the legal sphere has anything to say about informed consent, and whether this is an adequate standard for medical ethics in this area.

172    To start with, we might observe that getting the signature on the form is not in itself a guarantee that legal liability will not follow. If the patient can show in court that he did not read the form, or that he was under the influence of some potentially mind-altering medication at that time, or that he was under some form of duress to sign, the form has no legal weight. In a questionable case, the physician or the hospital might well find it hard to convince a jury that none of those factors did occur. It is much easier for the patient to allege that such things happened than it is to prove conclusively that they didn't.

173    More basic than that, however, is the fact that motives are going to play a large part in the way the individual doctor actually performs with regard to informed consent. The doctor who believes in informed consent because he wants to stay out of court is going to approach his task of informing the patient differently from his colleague, who believes in informed consent because he adheres to the "Contractual Model" and feels that the patient has a moral right to make these decisions for himself. The latter motive is much more likely to bring about ethically valid behavior, because it reminds the doctor of the ethical component of his task.

174    Further, recall the comment at the beginning of the last chapter, that the doctor-patient relationship is basically a relationship between two human beings. Strictly from that standpoint, it would seem to be preferable to treat the patient as someone whose consent is valued because of respect for him as a person, rather than to treat him as a potential litigant in court whom one suspects of wanting to take advantage of any slip the doctor might make.

175    What do the courts in fact have to say about informed consent? A typical case would be one in which the doctor tells a patient that he requires surgery, that the surgery has some complications possible, but that these are remote so he need not worry about them. Subsequently one of the complications does in fact occur. The patient sues the physician for negligence in performing the operation and for failing to obtain informed consent for the operation.

       This shows why informed consent cases are hard to deal with from the standpoint of extracting the issues of ethical importance. The jury has to decide the issues of negligence and informed consent separately. If expert testimony establishes that there was no way that the complication could have been prevented, the jury may find that the physician was not negligent and still assess damages against him for failure in obtaining fully informed consent.

Also, lack of informed consent does not by itself entitle a patient to collect damages. He must prove to the jury, not only that his consent was not "informed," but also that had he been fully informed he would not have gone ahead with the treatment. That is, he must prove both that informed consent was lacking and that he suffered material harm as a direct result.

Therefore, if the jury finds in favor of the doctor, it is not always possible to tell if they felt that the consent was informed; or if they found the consent lacking but determined that the patient would have gone ahead with the treatment in either case.

For all these reasons, specific court rulings are of limited value in helping to clarify ethical principles in informed consent. However, the matter of general judicial policy in informed consent is presently undergoing a change, which is of interest to the medical ethicist. What is happening is that an established precedent is being overturned and is being replaced, apparently, by legal principles which are much more in line with the "Contractual Model" of medical practice. Thus, except for the business of assessing financial damages, the new court decisions promise to be much more in keeping with the decision-making process that an ethical physician would use to determine informed consent.

As summarized by Rubsamen, the old judicial standard was, and in most areas still is, the common practice within the medical community with regard to informed consent. That is, the doctor is free of legal liability so long as he can show that he gave the patient the same information that is commonly given by practitioners in his community, no matter how inadequate that amount of information might be. If the patient is to prove his case, he must come up with an opposing expert witness to testify that the standard of practice is different from what the accused doctor says it is. Now, doctors are usually reluctant to testify against other doctors; and even if a doctor will stick his neck out and testify against a colleague who had prescribed an obsolete and dangerous drug, this same doctor might be unwilling to testify against a colleague on such a vague and judgmental matter as informed consent. The result is that under the old judicial standard, the cards are stacked heavily in favor of the doctor.

By this standard, the court was essentially saying that whatever the medical profession chose to do regarding informed consent was good enough for the court. The court was in effect making the ethical error of "generalizing expertise." Failing to distinguish a largely ethical question from the more common technical ones, the court assumed that just because the doctors were experts in clinical medicine, the same sort of expert testimony that was used to judge medical competence or incompetence in a malpractice suit could be applied to the matter of what the patient ought to be told. And if the courts were mistaken in this view, the physicians were unlikely to go out of their way to complain about it.

176

177

178

179

180     Recently, however, the new mood of the country seems to have infected at least a few courts, who have adopted a new standard. Applying the legal convention of a hypothetical "reasonable man," these new decisions have held that the doctor is obligated to tell the patient all the information that a "reasonable man" would need in order to make up his mind in a rational manner. Furthermore, how much information this includes is subject to testimony from lay individuals, as to whether disclosure of a particular possible consequence of therapy is material or not to making a decision. (Expert medical testimony is still needed to establish that that is a consequence of the therapy, however.) This standard is strikingly in accord with the ethical decision-making process we have described here. According to several legal authorities, these new decisions represent the current trend in the U.S. and will, over time, be accepted in other jurisdictions also.

181     So if—as is not always the case—the legal and ethical considerations are both pulling in the same direction, where could opposition to the practice of fully informing the patient and obtaining his consent arise? Of course, the tradition of paternalism is active in this regard. Again, the problem is mainly one of unconscious paternalism rather than an overt decision to be paternalistic. For example, a surgeon may agree in principle that patients have the right to make informed choices on "important" questions. He then tells a patient, "You have to have your gall bladder out," and neglects to list the possible complications of surgery as well as failing to mention alternative medical treatment. In the surgeon's mind, since he does several such operations each week, this is a "routine" matter; the patient's consent is a foregone conclusion; why burden his mind with trifles? He forgets that things look very different from the patient's point of view, where no surgery is "routine."

182     An example of a frankly paternalistic attitude is found in this testimony from a 1961 Missouri case, Moore v. Webb. An attorney is questioning Dr. Webb, a dental surgeon, about his approach to getting informed consent:

183     Q:  Couldn't [the patients] have [a partial plate] if they wanted that?
        A:  That all depends. I don't think so. I think you should strive to do for the patient what is the best thing over the long period of time for the patient. We tried to abide by that.
        Q:  Isn't that up to the patient?
        A:  No, I don't think it should be. If they go to a doctor they should discuss it. He should decide....
        Q:  Isn't this up to the patient? If I want to pay $800 for a partial, I hope the dear Lord lets me keep my teeth. If I want to keep these teeth, can't I do it?
        A:  You don't know whether they are causing you trouble.
        Q:  That is up to me, isn't it?
        A:  Not if you come to see me it wouldn't be.

Other factors standing in the way of informed consent include the time problem, since even an additional five minutes spent answering the questions of a not-overly-bright patient may tax a busy practitioner's schedule. A common way around this problem is to delegate the task of "obtaining informed consent" to anyone from the office nurse to the receptionist. This solution may be highly satisfactory or the opposite depending upon the training and the degree of responsibility given to the party performing the task.

Not only does it take more time to inform the "not-overly-bright" patient, but conversation with this patient is also likely to be less congenial for the doctor, who is likely to spend more time talking with patients closest to his own social and educational level. This helps explain the finding in several studies of doctor-patient communication, that often the amount of information given the patient is inversely proportional to the patient's need for information.

In addition, another factor is operating in the physician who chooses not to inform a patient of the risks and alternatives. While betraying something of a paternalistic attitude, this practice has unique aspects, which demand separate examination. There is the idea that it is bad to describe all the risks because, in many if not in most cases, the patient would then be scared off and would refuse to consent to treatment that is definitely in his best interests.

While this argument assumes that the doctor knows what is in the patient's best interests, by raising the question of fear in the patient's mind, it is able to cast doubt on the patient's ability to make rational decisions. Given an irrational patient, paternalism on the part of the doctor is more easily justified.

This idea is held as an article of faith by many practitioners, as illustrated by this portion of the testimony of Dr. Brown, who was being sued for failure to inform the patient of the risks of dermabrasion. (The appeals court in this case, Hunter v. Brown, Washington, 1971, set one of the precedents for the new standard of informed consent.) Dr. Brown stated:

"Now, if we go into the risks involved, I would be talking the rest of the day about risks...Risks are minimal, and they are never mentioned to a patient... A patient would walk out of everybody's office if you would say there is a danger of anything. This is never done...It is not good practice to frighten a patient by telling them a dozen different things that might happen as a result of dermabrasion."

(By using terms such as "it is never done" and "it is not good practice," is the physician trying to mask the distinction between ethical questions and clinical judgment, in order to protect his status as as "expert" on the matter?)

No one would quarrel with the proposition that some patients might be dissuaded from needed treatment out of fear if told the risks. But the proposition that many patients would be so dissuaded need not be treated as an article of faith—it is an empirical statement which can be investigated scientifically. An attempt to do this was made by Alfidi, who set out to prove that most patients would refuse the "routine" procedure of angiography if the risks were fully explained. He accordingly drew up a "horror sheet" consent form which listed in great detail all the possible complications, such as loss of an organ and possibly death, while noting that the rate of serious complications is about 1 in 500 procedures. Patients were requested to read this through and sign.

**188**      The results surprised the investigator. Of 232 patients, 228 consented, or about the number of refusals that might be expected in any case for a diagnostic procedure. Furthermore, on a subsequent questionnaire, about 85% of the patients indicated that they had appreciated being given the detailed information, even though in many cases it increased their anxiety.

However, in a later study, Alfidi adopted the alternative approach (which we will discuss below) of asking each patient whether or not he wanted to know the risks; in a variety of x-ray procedures, nearly two-thirds stated they did not want that information. Again, even among those requesting the risk data, only a very few refused consent. Thus it appears that even when patients are forced to sit through a recitation of risk factors "against their will," as it were, there is little evidence to suggest that refusal to consent will automatically follow——unless the particular patient's past behavior provides evidence to the contrary.

**189**      Thus we are in the same boat as with deciding what to tell the patient in other circumstances. Adopting a general rule to tell the patient as much as he needs to know to make an informed choice does not relieve us of the responsibility to pick out those occasional patients who do not desire such knowledge and who would be better off without it, in their own view. "Don't describe the risks unless the patient asks," seems too passive an approach, since it can be amply be demonstrated that many who would want the information would not ask out of fear of taking up the doctor's valuable time or for other reasons. Still, it is important to leave the patient an out, so that he knows what you are willing to tell him and yet can still refuse to hear it.

**190**      *What seems a very workable formula has been suggested by the physician-lawyer Rubsamen. He recommends that the doctor say to the patient something like, "There are significant risks involved, and even though they are remote in your particular case they can be serious. Do you want me to outline them for you?" If the patient says no, it would ·seem that the physician has met his ethical obligations by going no further. Rubsamen adds that if the doctor then notes this conversation in his records, he would seem to have fulfilled his legal duties as well.*

ETHICAL TO LET
PATIENT BE PASSIVE? * 194

**191**      Before going on to consider cases, it should be noted that two important related issues will not be treated in this chapter. One is the right to refuse treatment. This is assumed by the right of informed consent, or else there would be no reason for informed consent. This issue will be taken up in the next chapter under "Quality of Life."

The other issue arises when informed consent is being obtained, not for a procedure that is established and for which only the usual degree of clinical uncertainty applies, but for an experimental procedure in which an additional degree of uncertainty has been deliberately added to the situation. The entire issue of human experimentation will be taken up in Chapter 11.

## CASE 12

A 14-year-old girl is referred to you, a general surgeon, with a complaint of severe abdominal pain of one week's duration. Based on a thorough workup, you narrow your differential diagnosis to several conditions, all of which require surgery, and you decide that the best course is exploratory laparotomy as soon as possible.

Of the several diagnostic possibilities you are considering, the most likely one can be corrected only by a procedure that carries with it a 50% or greater risk of subsequent sterility, as a result of compromising the ovaries and uterus. The results of mortality and serious complications are otherwise those of any surgical entry into the abdominal cavity.

The girl's father is deceased and her legal guardian is her mother.

What will be your procedure for obtaining informed consent for the surgery you propose?

Will you direct this procedure at:

The girl only?

The mother only?

The girl and mother, in separate interviews?

The girl and mother, both in the same interview?

---

**193**

Your primary question as to how to proceed is: who is the patient? This is not as silly as it may sound. The girl will have her belly cut open and will have to live with whatever consequences arise. However, since it is the mother, as a fellow adult, that the physician is most comfortable communicating with, and since it is the mother who pays the bills or who will withhold payment if not satisfied, there is a natural inclination to treat the mother as the real patient and to relegate the girl to secondary status when it comes to explaining risks.

Once you have determined that the girl—who has reached the so-called "age of comprehension"—is the primary target of your efforts, the question of exactly what to say, and whether to tell the mother (who must sign the legal consent form) at the same time, will be determined by your reading of the circumstances. In general, it might be best to tell both at once, and then to check with each individually later on to see if they have any questions they were not willing to broach in front of the other.

---

**194**

Is it right if the patient wants to cop out as a moral agent with control over his own destiny, and you do nothing to dissuade him from this attitude? To say that you have an obligation to make him "be a man and face his responsibility squarely" smacks too much of the "Priestly Model." You can, however, at future interviews when the pressure is off, try to explore his reasons for taking that attitude. It might be that some patients adopt that role because that they have been led to believe that that is the socially expected behavior of patients; and once you show them that you do not expect such behavior and in fact prefer the opposite, they might come to take a greater role in decision-making. Other patients may still be scared stiff at the idea of making a significant decision; and if their passivity makes you too uncomfortable, you would not be unjustified in advising them to seek another, more paternalistic, doctor.

REVIEW

"PRIESTLY MODEL" | 107

195        You obtain consent from the mother only and do the surgery.

With the girl convalescing well and ready for discharge the following day, you consult with the girl's mother in your office to discuss your follow-up management plan. You explain that while the girl has not been informed of her chances of sterility—you did, as it turned out, have to do that procedure—you feel that her well-being can best be safeguarded by telling her as soon as possible. Thus she will have been able to assimilate this fact gradually by the time she reaches the age of wanting a family.

You are surprised to learn that the mother regards your plan as cruel and that she feels that it would expose her daughter to constant emotional anguish; that it would destroy any of the "joy of youth" she might experience in her adolescence. The mother feels that she would be clearly deficient in her maternal role were she to allow you to tell the daughter.

Upon further prodding by you, the mother agrees that it might be unjust to allow the girl to enter into marriage later in ignorance of her condition. She says that she would just attempt in subtle ways to discourage her daughter from marrying. If, however, the girl did become engaged, the mother states that she would tell the girl after the wedding had taken place.

Since you note that the mother is stating her views calmly, with an appearance of having thought through the situation, you try, as gently as possible, to dissuade her from her proposed action. As you proceed, however, she becomes hostile and expresses her fear that you will upset her plans by telling the girl without her consent. She forbids you to say anything and threatens legal reprisals if you ignore her injunction.

193        What do you do now?

---

CASE 13

196        You, a urologist, are being sued by a patient upon whom you performed a trans-urethral resection to correct a urinary problem of several years' standing due to enlarged prostate. It is usual in doing that type of procedure upon a patient of this age (67) to sever the spermatic cords, which results in sterility. At the time of the surgery, you conducted a cystoscopic exam of the bladder under local anesthetic. You then went to the head of the bed and told the patient what you had found, and that the resection would be required. He replied that you should do what was necessary.

The patient is now very upset over being sterile and contends that he did not know and was not told that this was included in the procedure. Had he known, he says, he would not have given consent.

Did you act ethically in this case or not?

---

197        In a case of this nature in Minnesota in 1958 (Bang v. Charles T. Miller Hospital) the court placed great weight upon the fact that there was nothing of an emergency nature about the operation, and that the various alternatives, including the possibility of sterility, could be known in advance. The court saw no reason not to have informed the patient that the most usual procedure would result in sterility; that there was another procedure possible; but that this other was less satisfactory in terms of long-range prognosis and possible post-operative infection. The patient could then have made up his own mind. You lost.

Note that, for an expert, it is easy to forget that the average layman does not know that sterility results from trans-urethral resection. It is also easy to assume that sterility can be of no consequence to a 67-year-old man. Both assumptions follow from failure to extend the imagination necessary to put yourself in the patient's place.

## CASE 14

A woman comes to your surgical practice with a lump in her right breast which, to manual palpation, strongly suggests malignancy. You explain that you would like to take a surgical biopsy and that if it is positive you feel that only removal of the entire breast will give a hope of cure. The middle-aged woman states that she wants you to do the biopsy, but that she will not have her breast removed and will only give permission for removal of the lump. You decide that this is another of those women who are so emotionally messed up about their breasts that they would die of cancer rather than lose one, and you determine to cater to her present whims without giving up your option to do what is in her long-term best interests once she is under anesthesia.

On the day of surgery, you note in the chart a consent form for the operation of mastectomy, duly signed by the patient. As you see her just before surgery, she again repeats her desire that you are to remove only the lump and not the breast.

Do you have consent to perform right mastectomy when the biopsy comes back positive?

In this case, you have a lot of evidence that the patient does not want to lose her breast. The only evidence that you have consent is a piece of paper which says "mastectomy" which she signed. Assuming she read it before signing, it is at least worth knowing whether the patient knows what "mastectomy" means; in one court case in which such a sequence of events occurred, the court held that the fact that no one told the woman what a mastectomy was or allowed her to ask constituted failure to obtain informed consent.

Another point raised by one side in that case was that, even if the signing of the document constituted informed consent, the woman still had the right to withdraw her consent at any time prior to surgery. Therefore, her statements immediately before surgery should have constituted a valid withdrawal of consent. In any case, from an ethical point of view, the patient's earnestly expressed wishes ought to be given more weight than a standard form.

The next case also deals with withdrawing informed consent.

## CASE 15

201    You are a psychiatrist. Mrs. R.L., a 56-year-old widow, voluntarily hospitalizes herself to be treated by you for psychotic depression. You explain to her that such a condition as she has often responds best to a series of electroshock treatments, and after explaining the procedure, you obtain her verbal and written consent. Mrs. R.L., however, finds the first treatment a very frightening experience. When the attendants come to get her for her second shock, she refuses to go.

You can have the attendants forcibly take Mrs. R.L. to the treatment room and administer the shock. Do you zap her or not?

1) Zap—because she is, after all, psychotic, so you can't place much weight on her expressed wishes.

▼ 203

2) Don't zap, yet. But get a court order to have her committed as mentally incompetent, then proceed with treatment.

▼ 207

3) Don't zap. Talk to her, get at the basis of her fears, remind her that such an experience is not abnormal with shock, and explain again the benefits you hope for. Try to get her to agree voluntarily again.

▼ 211

4) Don't zap. Mrs. R.L. has withdrawn her consent for the therapy. She has a right to do this, so you might as well send her home.

▼ 214

(Adapted from Hastings Center Report, June 1972)

---

202    Regarding the option of having Mrs. R.L. legally committed, it has been the case that just about anyone with an M.D. after his name can go into court and emerge within 24 hours with an order to commit practically anyone as mentally incompetent, for practically any reason. That this may be changing is reflected in the new Michigan mental health code enacted in 1974, under which, in order to commit a person involuntarily, it must be shown either that he is a clear danger to the life of others or himself; or that he is incapable of performing the basic life functions necessary for his own survival. Further, these must be shown by acts the individual has actually performed, not by a physician's guess as to what he might later do. By these criteria, what would

204 ↓    Mrs. R.L.'s legal rights be?

If Mrs. R.L. is psychotic and therefore she cannot give true informed consent, what right did you have to start treatment at all? She is no crazier now than when she came in; since she had one treatment, she should actually be a little better.

Or you may have reasoned that since she has refused beneficial therapy, she is now crazy and can be ignored when she refuses. The practical consequences of this view are two. First, you are in effect denying the right of any psychiatric patient to refuse treatment. Second, you are saying that the psychiatrist always selects the best possible therapy and is never mistaken.

Is mental illness, of any sort, an automatic indication that a patient cannot make a rational judgment for informed consent? Go back and choose another alternative.

203

201

---

## CASE 16

204

You are an American physician in the jungles of Nigeria, and you are there to try out a new vaccine for measles, a disease which is causing significant childhood mortality in the region. The vaccine that you will be using causes encephalitis on rare occasion. It also has the potential of sensitizing the child to proteins in the vaccine besides the measles material itself, so that the child might have an allergic reaction to a subsequent vaccination of a different type. The relation of such sensitization to various auto-immune diseases is not known at present.

The mothers are all uneducated and speak their tribal language, which you do not. How do you go about getting informed consent, or do you bother to do it? (This case is intended for thought and/or discussion.)

(Adapted from: Francis D. Moore, cited in Katz)*

---

Having reviewed some specific cases, we might go back and look over some of the arguments against informing the patient of risks, or those arguments designed to distinguish the patients who should be told from those who shouldn't. First, we know that a person given too much information may worry, and that worry can adversely affect a patient's illness or his post-operative recovery. How much worry is grounds for withholding information? In deciding this, it is important to remember that worry may also serve a useful psychological function, by allowing the patient to prepare better for his ordeal. (Does a patient have a "right" to worry? Is not a doctor's desire to spare the patient worry and to take all the worry upon himself frankly paternalistic?)

205

A related but distinct argument is that disclosing negative possibilities deprives the patient of the effect that a doctor can bestow just by saying confidently, "Don't worry, nothing will happen, you're going to be just fine." Whether this effect is called the "placebo effect," suggestion, or whatever, there is empirical evidence that it works, and that in some cases it works better than standard therapy alone. If we are not ethically justified in withholding a drug from a patient who could benefit from it, how can we withhold this self-fulfilling suggestion which may be more powerful than a drug, and with fewer harmful side effects?

206

208

*J. Katz, Experimentation with Human Beings. (Russell Sage Foundation, 1972; cited by permission of the Russell Sage Foundation.)

207

What is the practical and ethical difference between this alternative and No. 1, even though there is a great legal difference? You are still administering shock to Mrs. R.L. against her will. Therefore, you must be willing to accept all the ethical implications of choice No. 1 if you go this route. Either go back and read the frame for choice No. 1, or make another choice.

201

208

While we might hope that the patient who is most dependent on this self-fulfilling effect of optimism would be the one to signal to us that he does not desire full disclosure of risks when we ask, this may not always be the case. Where the risks are rare or minor, we can give full disclosure while laying great stress on the low probability and on the many patients who have no trouble. Where the risks are of high likelihood or are serious, and the patient has not explicitly asked not to be informed in reply to your question, we might be forced to ask whether the patient's right to make his own decision does not outweigh his right to the placebo effect. And don't forget that after consent has been obtained, we can still be as optimistic and encouraging as possible in our further visits with the patient.

209

Earlier we cited empirical evidence that patients seem to want information by way of supporting the idea of full disclosure. Can empirical data about what patients do with that information be used as an argument that disclosure is a waste of time? In one set of interviews with relatives of patients with kidney disease, who had agreed to serve as donors for kidney transplants, it was found that in most cases the donor's mind had been made up as an on-the-spot judgment as soon as the possibility was mentioned. By the time, later, when the physicians got around to explaining all the risks in order to get official informed consent, the patients' minds were permanently set. When confronted with the offhand way they had made this crucial decision as compared to the way they made other major decisions in their lives, the donors tended to say that this was a special situation which could not be compared to ordinary decision-making. In this group, if any of the information given by the doctors was ever heard at all, it seems to have played no role in any rational decision-making process.

210

We might reply to that in two ways. If we want to call it a "right" to make an informed decision, then a right is not negated just because a number of people decline to exercise it at a given time. If, on the other hand, we want to avoid the hangup with "rights," we can ask what are the consequences of assuming in advance that the information given will not be put to good use. If even a minority of persons would in fact have used the information to make rational decisions, can we weigh the loss of this opportunity to them against any time or effort that might have been saved by not disclosing the information?

212

You seem to have chosen the ethically most acceptable course of action. However, to a certain extent, you are postponing your decision. What if Mrs. R.L. still continues to refuse?

211

↑
202

---

If the question is one of saving time by not talking to patients whose minds are already made up, it would seem that this could be accomplished almost as well by the application of Rubsamen's formula of saying that there are risks and then asking the patient if he would like to have them described.

212

↓

This concludes our discussion of informed consent. We might summarize a few of the major points in this chapter:

213

*1)    A genuine desire to provide the patient with the information he needs to make a decision is more likely to lead to ethically valid behavior than the mere desire to stay out of court.*

*2)    An assertion that fully informed consent will scare a patient off cannot be taken on faith, but requires empirical justification.*

*3)    A right to be informed implies a right not to be informed; a good formula for informed consent will leave the patient an out.*

*4)    Informed consent for a therapeutic procedure requires revealing both the risks of the procedure, and any alternative forms of treatment that are possible.*

*5)    Informed consent can be withdrawn at any time.*

*6)    "Mental illness" does not by itself preclude the possibility of obtaining informed consent.*

*7)    Divulging full information does not necessarily conflict with use of the "placebo effect" in the form of subsequent emotional support and reassurance. It need not be brutal.*

Ch. 6 ↓215

---

By choosing this course you seem to be saying, in effect, that Mrs. R.L. by refusing her treatment has rejected you, so now you will get even and reject her.

214

Mrs. R.L. has refused to undergo this treatment, but she did come in voluntarily to be treated. Possibly if you explain matters further to her she will change her mind. If not, there are some alternative forms of treatment for depression that might, while not as satisfactory as electroshock, still be better than nothing.

Is it ethically valid, where genuine treatment options exist, for a doctor to insist that the patient agree to the doctor's choice or else go elsewhere for care?

↑
202

# 6. Determination of the Quality of Life

You have noticed that so far this book, while attempting to emphasize processes instead of listing rules of behavior, has nevertheless suggested general guidelines and has taken sides on specific issues. This will not stop here, but you are cautioned that in this chapter anything offered as a conclusion must be taken with a larger grain of salt, and with more critical appraisal, than anywhere else. The area of quality of life, which embraces the issues of allowing to die, "mercy killing" or euthanasia, abortion, and refusal of treatment, is one of the most controversial ones in medical ethics; and the decisions that the medical profession makes in this area in the next few years will have a profound impact on the very meaning of the words "doctor" and "medicine." In fact, at the start, we have to justify using a phrase such as "quality of life" in the first place.

215

Presumably a major reason for talking about the quality of life is to be able to reach the conclusion that some sorts of life are better than others, and that some sorts of life are in fact so bad that death would be preferable. And supposedly the only reason we would have for wishing to reason this way is because we want to take action to implement our conclusion. Why would physicians, who are in the business of preserving life, want to justify bringing about the death of a patient? The motives fall into two general categories. One is the injunction, dating back at least to Greek times, to relieve suffering. The other is the more modern concern about conserving scarce resources (Chapter 12), which has been given impetus by the realization that continued overpopulation may produce the extinction of our civilization.

216

Everyone in medicine will be presented with a situation in which, because of one or both of these motives, he finds that what he regards as his ethical duty is inconsistent with keeping the patient alive. Stripping away all the language and getting to the heart of the matter (even though it may sound brutal), he wants the patient to die. If he is a sensitive and ethically minded person, he may then have one of two reactions, depending on his value background and the nature of his previous experience. If he finds that his desire is not evil in itself, but he is still mindful that he has a particular responsibility to act consistently with clear ethical guidelines, he will then be led to some type of "quality of life" approach, which we shall spend most of this chapter describing.

217

On the other hand, he might be so horrified by his desire that the patient should die that he rejects it immediately, and in fact looks for ways to prevent such an evil desire from even occurring to him in the future—fearing that in a moment of weakness his emotions may get the better of his reason. This person will find ethical justification in the principle of "absolute sanctity of life," which in turn gets its major support mostly from religious ethical systems.

218

219     Since, so far, we have not given much attention to religion as a source of ethical principles, it is worth quoting at length from a particularly precise statement of "sanctity of life" as viewed by an orthodox theologian—in this case, Dr. Moshe Tendler, professor of Talmudic law at Yeshiva University, in a 1972 Symposium on Ethical Issues in Human Experimentation:

"As you know, the ethical foundation of our society of Western civilization is a biblical one...There are certain indispensable foundations for an ethical system and one of them is the sanctity of human life. This concept has a corollary; that is that human life is of infinite value. This in turn means that a piece of infinity is also infinity and a person who has but a few moments to live is no less of value than a person who has 70 years to live.

220     "And likewise, a person who is handicapped and cannot serve the needs of society is no less a man and no less entitled to this same price tag—a price tag inscribed with an infinite price. A handicapped individual is a perfect specimen when viewed in an ethical context. This value is an absolute value. It is not relative to life expectancy, to state of health, or to usefulness to society....

"When does man become man is the real definition of the problem of the morality of abortion. When is man no longer man is similarly the real definition of the problem of euthanasia, and all of it depends on your concepts of the rights of man....

"Another principle germane to the discussion is that the protection due your fellow man is directly proportional to his helplessness. The more helpless he is, the more he must be protected. This is the key to the ethical principle of man imitating God, illustrated in biblical literature by the men who care for the orphans and widows, and for the helpless and defenseless....

221     "It is not necessary in a system of ethics to which I adhere—a biblical system of ethics—to have informed consent if you know for sure, with the best of your scientific and ethical ability to evaluate, that the action is for the benefit of the patient. Just as a man cannot commit suicide under our ethical system, he cannot refrain from benefiting from medical advances and by doing so forfeit his life passively. If indeed a procedure is looked upon as a proper medical procedure, it will be proper to institute it even without informed consent. It is only when there is a question of probability—odds on the chance of helping, or on the chance of hurting—that we expect adults to be able to make a consental decision...."

What are the implications of this statement for the nature of the doctor-patient relationship?

In light of what we have discussed up to now, one of the features of        222
Dr. Tendler's statement that should be very striking is the extreme degree of
paternalism that he injects into the doctor—patient relationship. In particular,
the focus of decision-making responsibility is almost completely removed from
the patient. In most medical matters it is the physician, "imitating God" by
helping the helpless, who has the say in the matter. But in life and death
matters, lest "imitating God" turn into playing God, the responsibility is
removed from both doctor and patient and reserved for God alone. While it
is possible to take a sanctity-of-life stand without embracing such an extreme
degree of paternalism, when it comes to life-and-death matters any such stand
is likely to be more paternalistic than the "Contractual Model" we have been
using.

At any rate, how a sanctity-of-life physician should proceed in a particular        223
case is clear. He has to determine that the object in front of him is a man and
that he is alive. It then follows that he is prohibited from any action which,
according to his medical knowledge, would shorten or jeopardize that life.
Is he also enjoined with the responsibility to do everything within his medical
power to preserve that life? Pope Pius XII's 1957 encyclical says that he may
not necessarily be required to use "extraordinary means"; other views differ.

Before finding fault with the sanctity-of-life view, it is only fair to note        224
that it is seldom held in pure form. Most of its adherents would accept the
killing of plants and animals, and the killing of another man in self-defense, or
the execution of a criminal. Therefore, it is most commonly held in the form
of "sanctity of innocent human life."

Our basic objection to the sanctity-of-life principle should be predictable        225
from the emphasis we have placed all along on rational decision-making processes. In practice, sanctity-of-life becomes a decision-avoiding tool; decisions
are made in advance for all cases without any consideration of individual
circumstances. It may not be completely fair to accuse sanctity-of-life adherents
of wanting to get out of doing their moral homework, but that is one way of
looking at the end result. The objection against this view is the same as the
objection against any absolutist stand, which claims to be stating a moral
principle that is valid for any person, place, and time.

In this light, the concept of "sanctity of life" has been analyzed in some        226
detail by Clouser. His conclusions support the notion that the concept, where
it is so defined as not to be totally vacuous, generally leads to implications
that the proponents of the view would usually not accept.

227    The sanctity-of-life principle can, however, be restated in a consequentialist form more in keeping with the principles we have been using—that is, that one ought never kill an innocent human being because following such a course would have undesirable consequences. As emotionally stated by certain vocal proponents of sanctity-of-life views, the undesirable consequences are as follows: first you allow abortion, then you open the door to mercy killing, then you start shooting inmates of mental hospitals, and eventually, in short order, we will have resurrected Nazi Germany.

228    We can label this strategy a "domino theory" or "foot in the door theory" of ethics, which argues that while the action proposed may not be all that bad in itself, it will <u>inevitably</u> or at least with high probability lead to evils of a far greater magnitude. This last statement is, of course, an empirical one, and can be argued as to whether it is true or false. In this case, we would argue that, even though many systems in the past which did not adhere to sanctity-of-life principles did end up producing vast evils, there is no reason to assume before the fact that a system which we might propose in the future will be unable to avoid like consequences. (This DOES suggest, however, that when we propose such a system, we had better be damned careful to specify exactly what we mean by all our statements and to build in as many safeguards as possible.)

229    In particular, the assumption that allowing physicians to allow certain patients to die or to kill them would lead to widespread abuse seems to be implying that most physicians right now have a genuine desire to do away with many of their patients and are presently being restrained only by sanctity-of-life considerations. This idea is at least highly arguable. A more realistic objection is that, certainly, right now physicians do not want to kill patients, but if in the future they should get into the habit of doing so, they would become very lax about applying ethical considerations to each individual case. From the example of the Nazis again, we may assume that somehow the executioners in the gas chambers were able to do their jobs day in and day out while still keeping their sanity. As far as doctors go, this kind of habitual disregard is probably already present in areas where abortion is allowed, as regards the ethical rights, if any, of the fetus. However, when we get to patients after birth, it seems highly unlikely that the situation in which it would be admissable to kill a person or allow him to die would arise so frequently as to give rise to habits. Doctors still want to save most of their patients.

230    In the final analysis, however, we can give the lie to the "domino theory" view only by actually coming up with an ethical system which condones the death of certain patients in certain circumstances while still protecting the rights of individuals and upholding humanistic values. What do quality-of-life approaches have to offer in this regard, and how well do they measure up?

The first clue that the quality-of-life people may not be all that sure of
themselves is the fact that they tend to start out by manipulating definitions of
words. One trend is to decide upon some very minimal criteria for a level of
quality of life that should be preserved; and choosing a word such as "person"
to describe someone who possesses at least these criteria. Then, anyone who is
a human being but not a "person," while not someone to be taken lightly
from an ethical viewpoint, may nevertheless be allowed to die or may be
killed without the ethical stigma that would attach to the case of a "person."

Another view suggests that we agree that all human beings are "persons;"
however, that we change our ethical principles to state that some persons in
some circumstances ought to be allowed to die. The reasoning behind what
may seem like nitpicking is the observation that previous societies bent on
committing injustices have commonly defined the victims outside of humanity
as a preparatory step, either by calling them "non-Aryans" or "gooks" or
whatever. Therefore, this view goes, we are more likely to avoid injustices if
we adopt an ethical strategy that specifically reminds us of the humanhood
of all people, even those whom we are about to deprive of life.

The test of both views, of course, lies in the specific ethical guidelines
created. The "person" definers have to come up with a list of criteria that
can be applied without value biases, that include the categories that we might
wish to be included (such as fetuses in unwanted pregnancies, people with
severe mental defects, people with terminal illnesses undergoing great suffering,
etc.), and that exclude all those whom we want to consider worthy of preserving
through medical efforts. This is a tall order. A most common mistake in such
lists of criteria is allowing hidden value biases to creep in without realizing
that many segments of society might not agree. For example, a frequently
mentioned criterion is that a "person" must be capable of rational thought,
and this is often given great weight. One wonders if rational thought would
be placed so highly if such lists were made up by the "man on the street"
instead of college professors.

One of the most extensive and detailed of the proposed "person" lists is
the original list of 15 criteria by Joseph Fletcher, which is given for illustration
in Appendix III. Fletcher subsequently concluded that one of the 15 criteria,
cerebral function, was in fact basic to all the others and thus could stand alone
as the primary personhood criterion. An individual without any functional
brain cortex, even if he is spontaneously breathing, is thus not a person.

235    It is important to note, however, that such "person" definitions do not in themselves solve the problem. Recall that an ethical statement cannot be deduced from an empirical one. There is no logical connection between "X is not a person" and "I ought to condone the death of X." It is generally agreed that dogs are not persons, but we do not go around wantonly killing dogs as a result. A counter argument could be based on Dr. Tendler's appeal to helplessness: because human beings who are not "persons" lack certain important traits or capabilities, they are less able to fend for themselves and thus deserve our special protection.

236    Or take another argument as follows: A child who was born with a severe mental retardation as well as other physical defects is, by your particular definition, not a "person." However, his parents have become very attached to him and, even though his prognosis for any great life expectancy is nil, they want him kept alive as long as possible. Now (one could argue) if this child were a "person," his own interests would overshadow that of his parents, and we would be obligated to put him to death painlessly in order to relieve his suffering and because his quality of life is so low. However, since the child is not a "person," we have to consider the wishes of other "persons," his parents, above his own interests. Therefore, we ought to keep the child alive for his parents' sake. It should be clear from this that "person" definitions, while maybe a good aid to begin thinking about such issues, leave open as many questions as they solve.

237    *Whatever definitions one employs, it still stands that any quality-of-life person who allows a patient to die or who kills a patient (including a fetus) has taken an irrevocable action and is obligated to be able to defend it ethically at some length. In particular, it would appear, he is obligated to show that he is acting under some coherent and internally consistent ethical framework and has not simply made up his rationalizations to excuse his actions in this one particular case.* This requirement for consistency is why we have lumped such matters as abortion and allowing terminally ill patients to die under the title of quality of life, instead of considering them as separate issues. *Any value judgments made about events at the beginning of life should also be applicable to judgments made about the end of life, and vice versa, if we are to have a quality-of-life framework consistent enough to overrule the sanctity-of-life objections.*

238    This consistency requirement is where most present ethical attempts fall down, and it is probably the case that no present theory adequately meets it. The general tendency is to be much more concerned and scrupulous about cases involving a newborn, who has his whole life ahead of him, than in cases involving an elderly person who has passed his productive years. Such distinctions are less likely to be ethically valid than to be a reflection of the death phobias and the general prejudices against aging and the old which characterize our society. For example, we might feel that being unwanted by its mother-to-be is sufficient grounds for aborting a fetus, which is either a human being or a potential one. Can we then conclude that being unwanted by the family is sufficient cause to put to death a half-senile 85-year-old lady in a nursing home (especially if the family is named in her will)? Whatever criteria we choose for quality of life are going to have to be applicable equally to both ends of the spectrum.

Despite these problems, however, there is one other distinct advantage 239 to a quality-of-life approach. What does sanctity of life tell us about whether or not we can operate on a man's brain to eliminate antisocial behavior? Or whether it is all right to grow human embryos in a test tube? Or how much the state ought to know about the genetic traits of its individual members? On the other hand, if we were able to come up with a coherent and consistent set of quality-of-life criteria, they would help us answer all these questions, in addition to matters of allowing to die. How this occurs will be shown in later chapters on specific issues in medical ethics.

↓ 243

HAVE WE FOLLOWED
ETHICAL METHOD? * 240

It may have seemed to you that this discussion of quality-of-life criteria 240 contradicts the ethical method of Chapter 2, where we stated that an act must be judged by its consequences. Presumably we wanted to say this to avoid the possibility of ethics deduced from a priori rules. Yet now we are setting up just such an a priori rule in the form of a set of criteria, instead of doing our ethical homework and determining the good and bad consequences of allowing the patient to die vs. prolonging life.

While one can get this impression, this is not actually what is occurring. Remember that we are supposed to determine consequences of rules, not of individual actions, because our ethical judgments are supposed to be universalizable. We feared that if we looked at just one case instead of at the universal rule, we might be overly influenced by our emotional involvement and by selfish interests. In an emotion-charged issue such as death, this fear is especially realistic.

↓

There are a number of rules available to us, which we have already rejected 241 on the basis of their consequences. First, we saw that use of the sanctity-of-life view results in a rigidity of action without regard for individual circumstances, in some instances causing the production of significant suffering. Next, we saw that to make ad hoc decisions on each case, without general guidelines, was very likely to produce a great inconsistency of behavior, leaving the patient unsure of what to expect, and leaving the public unsure of the trust that it has placed in the medical profession. We rejected these consequences as inconsistent with the values espoused by our doctor-patient "contract."

↓

By exclusion, we have been led to a rule which takes individual circum- 242 stances into account, but which relies on general guidelines; and we proposed some set of quality-of-life criteria as these guidelines. Life, as we all know, has its good consequences and its bad consequences. For most of us the former far outweigh the latter. But (unless we have a priori accepted the sanctity-of-life view) we can imagine circumstances in which the reverse would be true. A good set of quality-of-life criteria would serve to indicate to us when that point is reached when the bad consequences start to outweigh the good ones.

↓ 245

In the absence of an ideally coherent and consistent framework, what kinds of distinctions are made in practice by physicians confronting these issues? Doctors naturally shy away from Philosophical niceties such as "quality of life criteria" and make judgments instead based on what it is that they are required to do. Therefore, abortion questions become separated from death questions. On the latter, various people distinguish a number of stages of involvement, ranging from strict sanctity-of-life to complete acceptance of euthanasia:

### Anti—euthanasia

1) Treat vigorously
2) Treat with ordinary means but withhold extraordinary measures

### Passive Euthanasia

3) Decline to initiate treatment
4) Stop ongoing treatment, having obtained consent of patient beforehand
5) Stop treatment without consent of patient

### Active Euthanasia

6) Give patient means to kill himself
7) Directly bring about death, with patient's consent beforehand
8) Directly bring about death without patient's consent

It is curious to see how far down the list physicians will go, and what ethical justification they offer for stopping where they do. To the sanctity-of-life believer, all the "euthanasia" items are out of bounds, although some of the most liberal might allow (3). (Incidentally, euthanasia is from the Greek meaning "good death" and originally meant easing the patient's death suffering. The modern interpretation of "mercy killing" is not strictly correct.) Some doctors will go to (3), for example, saying it is okay not to attempt resuscitation of a newborn with obvious gross deformities, but state that once treatment has begun the doctor is obligated to stick it out. Possibly the greatest gap is between passive and active euthanasia, or between (5) and (7) with (6) up for grabs in the middle. Doctors who are proud of their "bravery" in pulling the plug on the respirator of a patient with no brain function left will turn tail and flee when it is suggested that a terminal patient be given an overdose of morphine. (In one study, 59% of doctors would consider the former acceptable, but only 27% the latter.)

---

Once we have a set of criteria proposed (such as Fletcher's in Appendix III), we must immediately test it by determining its consequences—that is, by listing all the specific instances we can think of, and then seeing whether the criteria apply the labels of "personhood" or "nonpersonhood" to each. If we find the criteria labeling as "nonpersons" people who should, by our values, be worthy of protection and preservation, then we see that we must modify the criteria. Furthermore, since we would not wish others to impose their personal values on us over so central a matter as life and death, it follows that we must not only judge the criteria by our own values, but must also judge them by the values that seem to be most widely held in society.

If you are still unclear about the role played by rules in a consequentialist system of ethics, see the discussion on act-utilitarianism and rule-utilitarianism in Appendix I.

One current and very difficult ethical debate is whether there is any moral     246
difference between passive euthanasia and active euthanasia, since the result
in either case is a dead patient. Those physicians who have already accepted
the principle of active euthanasia in their own minds want quite naturally to
say that there is no difference, so that the much larger group of passive-euthanasia
adherents will be forced to agree with them. The latter, however, contend
that there is a clear difference between allowing death to occur and acting to
produce it. But most of these men, in a manner similar to that of John Fletcher,
take this difference for granted and are mostly unable to specify precisely where
it lies. This leads to the suspicion that the difference may be an emotional and
not a moral distinction.

This leads to the possibility that ethical philosophers, whose business it is     247
to analyze distinctions and confusions and who operate at a distance from the
emotionally laden clinical realm, might have a valuable contribution to make
here. A short digression is worthwhile to see how they approach this issue.

MAY SKIP TO 258

One philosopher who denies a killing-letting die moral distinction is     248
Jonathan Bennett, who wants to distinguish between actions (such as killing)
and the consequences of actions (such as the death of a patient by refraining
from treatment), but wants to deny any moral weight to this distinction in cases
such as we are interested in. He argues that in killing, one has many moves one
can make, of which a few entail the death of the victim, and one chooses to
move in one of those ways. But in letting die, of the many moves one could
make, only a few can bring about the continued existence of the patient, and
one chooses not to act in one of those few ways.

Thus for Bennett, the difference between killing and letting die boils     249
down to the proportion of the ways one could move to the ways of bringing
about an end, and he states that no moral weight can be given to what is at
best a relative difference.

Not unexpectedly, critics have found Bennett's analysis in terms of numbers
of moves insufficient to get at the real problem.

250    A re-definition by Dinello seems much more to the point: A has let B die if conditions are such that B is going to die; A knows how to do some things that will change those conditions and is in a position to do so, but chooses not to do so. As we will see below, Dinello states that re-defined this way, there is a clear moral distinction between killing and letting die, but that this distinction does not have <u>absolute</u> moral weight; that is, it is to be taken into account along with other factors.

251    Rachels joins Bennett in denying the moral distinction, but does so without getting bogged down in the "moves." Rachels starts by noting that usually we think of "killing" as something done in back alleys for bad motives, while "letting die" is done in hospitals by white-coated lovers of humanity. The problem is to construct a hypothetical test case in which motive, settings, and all other emotionally laden variables are held equal, and the <u>only</u> difference is between killing and letting die.

252    Suppose, Rachels says, Smith wants to kill his 6-year-old nephew to get an inheritance, and decides to drown him in the bathtub, and in fact enters the bathroom with that purpose. But by coincidence, at that moment the nephew slips, hits his head, and falls unconscious with his face in the water. Smith could save him by picking his head up out of the water, but instead Smith just stands by while the child drowns.

253    Now, if Smith tried to excuse himself by saying that after all he did not kill the child but only let him die, we would hardly be inclined to change our moral assessment of his action as a result of that distinction. Therefore, Rachels argues, if in practice in a particular case we do make such a distinction, it must be on grounds other than the killing-letting die difference. And in cases where <u>only</u> the killing-letting die difference applies, it may well be more humane to to choose the quicker course—see Case 44 as an example.

254    Dinello, in order to rescue the killing-letting die moral distinction, proposes a counter-example against Bennett which, if correct, would hold against Rachels too. Dinello hypothesizes a case in which Tom and Dick are in a hospital suffering from terminal heart failure and terminal kidney failure, respectively. Tom will die in two hours if he does not get a heart transplant; Dick will die in four hours if he does not get a kidney transplant. No other donors are available. (To make the case even more slanted in Dinello's favor we may add that Tom and Dick are identical twins, so that their tissues are sure to match; and that any kidney machines in the area are inoperative.)

Dinello states that if Bennett and Rachels are correct, we would find no moral difference between allowing Tom to die and then removing a kidney for Dick, and killing Dick to get a heart for Tom——the motives are the same, and either way one of them must die regardless. But surely killing Dick to get a heart for transplant would be wrong.

Our first reaction to Dinello might be that indeed, by following the logic of Rachels, there would be no moral difference between letting Tom die and killing Dick. If this judgment runs counter to our moral intuition, so what? The entire case situation runs counter to our intuition. If Rachels' argument seems to hold for the case of the terminally ill patient where we want to alleviate suffering, that is all we need for our purposes.

But in fact we can attack Dinello more directly than that. Look back at his definition of "letting die" above, which includes the stipulation that one must be in a position to change the conditions. Elsewhere Dinello seems to accept social roles as part of that "position," and in medicine that ought to include medical ethics. Now we can surely construct an ethical argument, by the method in Chapter 2 or most others, that it is wrong to hasten a person's death solely for the purpose of obtaining an organ for transplant. But since doing this to Dick is the only way to save Tom's life, and since an ethical doctor would not be "in a position to" do this, then it is not the case that the doctor has "let Tom die," by Dinello's own definition. Dinello's counter-example fails.

- - - - - - - - - - - - - - - - - - - - - - - - - - - - - - - - - - - -

In conclusion regarding stages (5) and (7), we have seen that anyone who wants to lump passive and active euthanasia under the same moral category does have philosophical justification to back him up. However, this justification might not be of the conclusive type to sway someone who has strong religious or other leanings in the opposite direction. Thus the ethical debate on this issue is sure to continue.

Another argument, going back to the question of creating unfortunate habits among medical practitioners, would accept (4) and (5) while rejecting (3). The emphasis here is upon the sometimes emergency nature of the way a patient comes in and the lack of time to decide. This argument holds that if the doctor had to stop and think before starting mouth-to-mouth resuscitation, for example, many completely deserving patients would die as a result of delay. Better, in this view, to make it a routine to start emergency treatment. Then, if it is later decided that the patient would have been better off dead, treatment can be stopped.

255

256

257

258

259

260    Rather than approach it this way, it seems better to make a distinction based on the amount of time available to make a choice. In many cases it is known beforehand that a certain patient is likely to have cardiac or respiratory arrest, and it can be decided whether or not to resuscitate if this occurs. Of course, a valid rule is: when in doubt, give treatment.

261    It should not be forgotten in this discussion that (7) and (8) are clearly violations of U.S. criminal law, while (6) might also be depending on circumstances. But even this does not give as much support to the killing-letting die difference as many physicians seem to think. Murder statutes are generally worded so that all that is required is that one has, through direct action, brought about the death of an individual. Thus "pulling the plug," the classic case of passive euthanasia, would also count as murder, if done in the absence of the "brain death" laws we will discuss later.

262    But in any case the legal question does not render the ethical question moot. First, euthanasia of both types does occur in practice without anyone reporting them, although active euthanasia is probably rare. Second, bills have been introduced into several state legislatures which would legalize (7), and a pro-euthanasia lobby seems to be growing under the "death with dignity" banner (as we shall see in Chapter 13). Third, some civil suits have been brought in the courts alleging "wrongful life," in cases where it was argued that the patient's best interests would have been served by hastening death. If courts accept this argument, a conservative physician might find himself sued for not having performed euthanasia.

263    As we try out these principles on specific cases, another warning is useful. Recall the two different kinds of motives for condoning a patient's death—relieving suffering vs. conservation of resources, or the interests of the individual vs. those of society. While the two motives can coexist, it is still useful to identify which is operating in any specific case. It is common in argument for a person condoning death for one reason to use the arguments of the other reason in order to win the sympathy of the audience. For example, our real motive for abortion may be that the mother can't afford another child, but we may end up exaggerating the hypothetical suffering faced by an unwanted child in order to avoid the stigma of appearing to support society's rights over those of the individual. Laying the motive or motives on the table helps to get to the heart of the issue.

CASE 17

The patient is a 73-year-old man who was diagnosed as having cancer of the colon 2 years ago and underwent colostomy. After recurrence of the malignancy, x-ray therapy was instituted, apparently unsuccessfully. By this stage in the natural history of the disease, metastases of the cancer to other sites are almost inevitable, and in fact the latest liver function studies are suggestive of possible early liver metastases. Your medical opinion now is that, with no more than purely supportive therapy, the patient's life expectancy is no more than two months. Now the patient has developed a productive cough, and the chest x-ray indicates bronchopneumonia.

While usually drowsy and sometimes obtunded, the patient is still able to communicate. He has said a number of times over the past week that he has nothing to live for, that he is weary of all the hospital procedures, and that he would prefer that the doctors "just leave me alone."

As physician in charge, do you institute antibiotic therapy for the pneumonia?

If you decided to acquiesce in the patient's desire, two factors may have made it easier to do so than it would have been to allow a patient to die under other circumstances. First, this would generally be regarded by physicians as a don't-start-treatment case as opposed to a stop-treatment case (although a logical argument might say that the treatment began when you accepted the patient, not when this new problem turned up). As we mentioned, this distinction seems in practice to carry great emotional weight for the physician. Second, we could describe this as "voluntary passive euthanasia," since we are allowing the patient to make his own assessment of the quality of his life, and are not imposing any values of our own upon him.

In the actual case upon which Case 17 was based, cited in Fletcher's essay in the book by Torrey, the physician was able to keep the patient alive for an extra 10 months, by treating with antibiotics as well as a large number of other procedures, until the man finally succumbed to liver failure. His justification for this was that he was opposed to "letting the patient go" under any circumstances. He based this rule of behavior on the fact that it was always possible that at the last possible minute a new treatment might be discovered, or that one of the infrequently recorded "miraculous remissions" might occur.

How do you appraise the validity of this justification?

In the course of this unit we have been occasionally pointing out ethical "errors" which seem to occur most frequently in discussions on these topics. This chapter will provide especially good material along this line, since no other medical issue is as likely to prompt physicians to adopt flimsy rationalizations to cover up the truly emotional basis for their decisions. The "something may turn up" argument is in this category. Either it is being used as a smoke screen for a pure sanctity-of-life view, or else it must also be applicable to other medical situations as well. And, certainly, in no other cases do competent doctors base their hopes on something statistically so unlikely as the sudden appearance of a new miracle drug. Competent doctors base all their other medical decisions on the likely, not the unlikely, probabilities, and on the treatment they have at hand at the present time.

268    Rejoinder: "How would you feel if you had, in the late 1940's, just mercifully allowed an advanced tuberculosis patient to die, and the next morning you picked up a paper and read about the discovery of streptomycin and its availability for use?" Answer: presumably you would feel badly. You would also feel badly, or should, if you allowed the patient to linger on and no new drug had appeared in time. The statistical chances of the latter are far greater than those of the former; so why, unless you were already committed to a rule of preserving life for totally unrelated reasons, would you give the former so much more weight? (Also remember that new drugs, today, seldom burst upon the scene. Their experimental development is usually known years in advance of their being made available.)

269    Another reason that could be given for preserving the life of the 73-year-old cancer victim is that withholding therapy at his request would be the same as the patient's committing suicide, which is both ethically and legally wrong. The objection to suicide, as the previously quoted remarks of Dr. Tendler would suggest, frequently indicates a general sanctity-of-life view. Saying a thing is "wrong because it's the same as suicide" is making a moral judgment by definition of words; whereas, in the ethical method we have adopted, it is the consequences of the ethical principle and not definitions that form the basis for judgment.

270    The fact that suicide is legally wrong is of some greater interest as well as practical consequence. In John F. Kennedy Hospital v. Heston, New Jersey 1971, a 22-year-old woman of Jehovah's Witness faith ruptured a spleen in an auto accident and refused the blood transfusion that would have allowed her to survive the surgery that was indicated. (Jehovah's Witnesses interpret one passage in the Bible to mean that blood transfusion constitutes a contamination of the soul and would prevent a person from entering Heaven.) The hospital went to court to get a legal guardian appointed with direction to consent for the surgery. The court appointed the guardian and gave as its reason that suicide was a violation of common law as well as present New Jersey criminal statutes. A person who attempted suicide and survived could be found guilty of a criminal act, though such charges are seldom brought; and the court ruled that the woman's refusal of transfusion constituted attempted suicide. Note, however, that had the hospital acceded to the patient's wishes without going to court, the chances of later being charged with a criminal act would have been exceedingly remote. (The woman had the operation and survived.)

271    Another anti-suicide argument can be easily disposed of: the idea that anyone who wishes to end his life must be mentally unbalanced and is therefore incompetent to consent or not to consent to medical intervention. Granted, many people who wish to end their lives suffer from mental illnesses such as depressive states (which, however, can be diagnosed psychiatrically with some degree of confidence). However, in order to accept this argument, one must accept the conclusion that follows logically—that there is no instance in which a rational and sane person could wish to put an end to his life. Most of us could imagine such an instance, and thus an "any" or "all" statement with regard to suicide is rendered invalid.

## CASE 18

You are the physician in a hospital in Georgetown, Washington, D.C., called in to treat a 25-year-old female auto accident victim. The woman tells you she is a Jehovah's Witness and strongly refuses to consent to the blood transfusion that you feel is absolutely necessary to save her life. The woman is married and has a 7-month-old daughter.

Would you go to court to seek permission to administer the transfusion?

272

---

In your attempt to come up with a response to this case, did you decide to ask the husband for his opinion, and possibly his assistance in changing his wife's mind? Why or why not?

273

In the actual case (Application of the President and Directors of Georgetown College, U.S. 2nd, 1964) the court ordered the hospital to proceed with the transfusion on the grounds that child desertion was against local law, and thus the state had an interest in preventing the woman from (indirectly) committing the crime by allowing herself to die.

This is one of those cases in which it becomes important to ask whether legal conclusions coincide with or differ from ethical considerations. The legal justification for this sort of action is described by the New Jersey court in the Heston case alluded to: "....the Constitution does not deny the state an interest in the subject. It is commonplace for police and other citizens, often at great risk to themselves, to use force or stratagem to defeat efforts at suicide, and it could hardly be said that thus to save someone from himself violated a right of his under the Constitution subjecting the rescuer to civil or penal consequences.

274

"....Religious beliefs are absolute, but conduct in pursuance of religious beliefs is not wholly immune from governmental restraint."

Another way of looking at this same court decision, however, is to recall the comment of one authority in Chapter 4. Apparently the idea that courts will go out of their way to find reasons to justify a medical act applies to cases where the act is proposed, as well as those in which it has already taken place. Viewed this way, the courts' reasoning often takes on an aura of post-facto rationalization which ought to be kept distinct from true ethical reasoning.

275

It ought to be pointed out, incidentally, that there is ample court precedent for refusing to grant the hospital permission to give a Jehovah's Witness patient a blood transfusion against his will, so long as the patient is a competent adult and no minor dependants are involved. (In several cases the patient had stated that he was opposed to transfusion on religious grounds, but if the court ordered one he would submit. What is the true "will" of the patient in a case like that? At least one court apparently read this as a tacit request for the transfusion and granted the injunction.)

## CASE 19

276    You are treating an 80-year-old widow suffering from diabetes and advanced arteriosclerosis. She has been in a home for the aged for the past two years and has just recently been admitted to the hospital with diabetic gangrenous infection of one foot. You can solve the present problem by doing an above-the-ankle amputation. You know, however, that this cannot be a life-saving procedure; that there is no chance of the lady ever walking again; and that, as often happens in diabetics, the same infection may recur above the amputation site later. You might, by doing the operation, give the woman another one or two years of life.

The patient, from an overall view of mental function, is probably mentally incompetent. However, she can communicate desires and is aware of her body. She tells you that she wants to keep her body intact and is totally opposed to amputation. She does not specifically state that she wants to die—which might easily follow within a month or so if the gangrene is not treated—and you cannot be perfectly certain that she perceives that this is a consequence of refusing to have the surgery.

You speak with your patient's three sons. Two of them tell you that they feel that everything should be done to prolong their mother's life, and are willing to go to court, if necessary, to be appointed her legal guardians for the specific purpose of consenting to the operation. The third son, himself a physician, says that he is opposed to the surgery because he fears that the anesthesia might prove a greater risk to a compromised circulatory and respiratory system than the infection would.

You are also aware that if you do the surgery and the patient wakes up to find her foot gone, she might either accept it, or go into a depressed state which in itself might hasten her demise considerably. However, you are not willing to predict her emotional state in that hypothetical event.

Do you do the amputation or not? (If you decide to do it, is the consent of two sons sufficient, or do you have to go to court?)

---

277    We had another case previously where a psychiatrist called in as consultant provided valuable input for the physician's ethical decision. Did you think of a psychiatric consult to evaluate this patient's status?

This case presents a number of uncertainties, which probably means that it is closer to the usual reality than a number of the cases discussed so far. For one thing, how competent does a person have to be to refuse consent in a life-and-death situation? One argument might be that since this decision is so important, one must demand a very complete degree of mental power, and reject any decision where mental competence can even be called into question. Another would be that since whether one wants to live or die is so basic a decision, a person should be able to express his true wishes on that score even if his mind is unable to grapple with more sophisticated problems. In sum, it seems that this woman is making a quality-of-life judgment that has to be given considerable weight in the final analysis. Exactly how much weight may be debatable.

REVIEW
PSYCHIATRIC CONSULT 131-134

This case did come to court as Petition of Nemser, New York, 1966. The court's decision was peculiar. First, the court refused to appoint guardians, but it denied that by doing so it was acting to end the life of the patient. Apparently, the court felt that this could have been construed as an emergency situation (since failure to amputate now might have made an above-the-knee operation necessary instead of the above-the-ankle one); and that the hospital should have gone ahead simply on the consent of the two sons, without being so super-cautious of possible legal consequences. In effect, the court chided the medical profession for dumping the decision on the legal doorstep instead of dealing with it.

The court, it seems, was expressing a fear similar to the one already mentioned as an argument against not initiating treatment. In an emergency, a physician who has gotten into the habit of pausing to consider all the legal consequences (as well as the ethical ones) may by his delay cost the lives of some patients who deserved to live. However, this is a case—as we shall discuss more in Chapter 7—of getting hung up on "who decides" and forgetting about "what to decide." The court decision seems to fail completely to speak to the basic issue of whether the woman should be allowed to die.

---

CASE 20

"All you're doing is turning him into a vegetable," exclaims the wife. "I forbid it. Let the poor man die in peace."

Your patient is a 79-year-old man with an implanted pacemaker whose battery has run down. If he does not have the relatively minor surgery needed to replace the battery, he will most likely die inside of three months. As far as you can tell, the wife's description of his mental state is accurate. The man has no comprehension of his condition and cannot make any decisions.

The chief resident tells you that failure to replace the battery would be unethical. "The man does not have to die yet," he says. "If you make it your business to end his life before his time has come, you are playing God. Who gave you that right?"

The hospital attorney says that if it should come to that, there might be some chance of getting a court order for the operation, in case the wife as legal next of kin will not consent.

Do you do the operation or not?

---

How do you assess the quality of life of the patient in this case? It is interesting to see where this patient would fit under Fletcher's criteria for "personhood" (Appendix III). As we mentioned, most people's quality-of-life criteria demand some degree of conscious self-awareness as a minimum condition for a truly human existence. Therefore, most quality-of-life arguments would support the non-replacement of the battery.

Was this case harder than the three previous ones in this chapter? In it we crossed the line into the world of involuntary passive euthanasia—where the patient can no longer give even a questionable expression of his own wishes. In such cases we have a major overlap with the topic of the next chapter—who is best qualified to speak for the patient's best interests.

This case did come to court (Bettman, New York, 1972). In a possibly controversial decision, the court overruled the wife's objections and ordered the surgery performed.

281      What is your reaction to the statement of the chief resident which condemns "playing God"?

The accusation, "If you do so-and-so then you're playing God," is heard with amazing frequency in discussions of medical ethics, considering that it is almost totally devoid of meaning. Such a statement only makes sense if we assume a picture of a God who takes an active interest in, and intervenes in, the daily lives of individual human beings. It then follows that either medicine is totally ineffective in accomplishing its goals, or else that physicians are "playing God" every time they interfere in the "natural" course of an illness— in fact, every time they practice medicine. If you do not object to "playing God" by giving antibiotics for a sore throat, you have no business objecting to "playing God" when the question of allowing to die comes up.

The question "Who gave you the right?" is indeed an interesting one, but it applies across the board to all medical interventions, not just passive euthanasia.

If it were agreed upon to forbid the use of the expression "playing God" in all arguments on medical ethics, the quality of such discussions could be enhanced significantly.

---

## CASE 21

282      A 10-year-old boy, severely injured in an auto accident, is rushed to Sparrow Hospital in Lansing. Shortly after he has been put on a mechanical respirator, and has received a unit of blood to combat shock, it is observed that his pupils are fixed and dilated and that he shows no spontaneous movement or reflexes. While you are able to maintain his respiration by mechanical means and his blood pressure is stable, electroencephalograms taken 24 and 48 hours after admission show no electrical activity of the brain.

As attending physician, you discuss the situation with the family. They agree that it would be better to turn off the respirator than to keep the patient alive as a body without a brain. At this point, the hospital transplantation team interpose and express a desire to harvest the kidneys for renal transplant. Before they do this, they will have to do blood studies to type the tissue in order to choose the most appropriate recipient. The parents consent to have the child kept on the respirator another 36 hours so that the tests can be done while keeping the kidneys fresh.

At the conclusion of the 36—hour period, you seek the family's final consent to turn off the respirator and remove the kidneys immediately there-after. However, the father says that in thinking the matter over more thoroughly now, he has developed serious reservations about this, and relatives have also planted doubts in their minds. He now feels that the proposed action would be the same as murdering his child, and he feels quite mixed up about the whole matter. His general inclination at this point is to refuse to sanction turning off the respirator. His wife, uncertainly, agrees.

What do you do now?

Your first emotional response to this case may be, "Dammit, the parents gave their consent, and we went through this whole expensive tissue-typing based on that. They can't back out now." It must be clear that this is an emotional reaction. At the outset, you accepted without question the fact that the parents were competent to speak on behalf of their unconscious son. If they can speak for him, they can change their minds for him. People may make a decision and stick to it forever after in the pages of ethics textbooks, but that is seldom the case in real life. 283

↓

The boy in this case, by most quality-of-life definitions, is no longer a "person." But here an even more basic issue may be at stake: is he alive? It may make a great deal of difference whether you are removing the kidneys from a dead body, or allowing a patient to die so that you can subsequently remove them. 284

Note that if you allow him to die to remove his kidneys, your motive is that of societal benefit, so you cannot claim to be acting in the boy's benefit. You can, however, argue that it is a matter of indifference to the boy since he cannot have any awareness in either case. If the boy is already dead, there is no individual left whose interests can be considered. Societal benefit is then the only legitimate consideration, and the only sort of objection to removing the kidneys might be a religious or sentimental desire on the part of the parents to preserve the body intact.

↓

In most states of the U.S., the boy as described is legally alive, since he is breathing and his heart is beating; these are the traditional legal criteria to establish that artificial legal concept called the "time of death." But in a few states (four at this writing), laws have been passed with new criteria for death. The new alternatives proposed are based on the work of a Harvard Medical School ad hoc committee to investigate "brain death." This group recommended, based on empirical studies of irreversible coma, that a person should be considered dead if he exhibits:  1) total unresponsiveness to external stimuli,  2) no spontaneous movement or attempts to breathe, and  3) no elicitable reflexes. A flat EEG tracing is of "great confirmatory value" but is not required if no EEG machine is available. These criteria, to confirm death, must be repeated 24 hours later with no change. They are considered inoperable in cases of hypothermia (body temperature below 90° F) or overdose of depressant drugs such as barbiturates—in both those instances patients have had all these signs for 24 hours and still have recovered later. 285

↓ 287

HOW IS CONCEPT
ARTIFICIAL? *286

Why do we say that "time of death" is legal fiction? From a medical or biological point of view, it is clear that different components of our bodies die at different times. Most of a person's cells are still alive after heart and lungs cease functioning. One could even say we start to die the moment we are born. A medical view based on empirical evidence is forced to view death as a continuum. In law, however, it is still important to fix a precise time of death in order to handle matters such as inheritance and insurance benefits. If death were treated as a continuous process in law as in medicine, such matters would become completely muddled. 286

↓ 287

287     Brain death, according to the Harvard criteria, is a very demanding definition; many individuals in coma who realistically have almost no chance for
recovery of any useful function will nevertheless fail to meet the criteria.
Presumably if we were to wish to implement Fletcher's revised criteria and call
death coincident with cessation of cerebral function, we would demand a flat
EEG but not be concerned about spontaneous respiration or the other signs.
The insistence on very strict criteria is typical of the caution with which those
seeking to redefine death have proceeded.

288     By the Harvard criteria, the boy is dead. In such a case, the parents could
be told that their son is dead, and permission could be requested to preserve
the body for 36 hours to remove the kidneys. This might well have alleviated
the parents' concern that they would be a party to the "murder" of their son.
It would also make it unnecessary to go through the formality of unplugging
the respirator before removing the kidneys, since that would make no difference
if the boy were already dead.

     Notice how most of the ethical dilemma here—even for a strict sanctity-
of-life advocate—is neatly solved by changing the criteria for death. In fact,
the solution is so neat that it alarms some people for just that reason. The same
danger applies here as with the criteria for "personhood"—can we not extend
the definition of death, say, to include mentally retarded individuals as well as
those with complete loss of brain function? (The care with which the Harvard
group based their criteria on proven indicators of irreversible coma makes
such an abuse very unlikely.) It is also of concern to many that the brain
death criteria arose in the first place as a means of getting hold of more donor
organs for transplant, and not out of any concern for the rights or best interests
of the "dead" individual.

IS THIS NEW DEFINITION
OF DEATH? * 290

289     The death-as-process view has been well argued by Morison. We should
add that Kass has objected that while dying is indeed a process, that should be
distinguished from the event of death; the fact that we find it hard to measure
when an event occurs does not mean that it doesn't. For Kass, throwing out
the idea of death as a discrete event has many unwanted consequences. He also
accuses Morison of failing to keep straight on two different questions: when
an individual's life is no longer worth living, as opposed to when he is in fact
291     dead.

290     A number of supporters of the brain-death concept have cautioned about
the importance of avoiding any confusion between "definition of death" and
"criteria for determining whether death has occurred." They feel that this is
important if the public is to accept the new criteria that the medical profession
is proposing. That is, it must be made clear that brain death is not a new kind
of death, or that other new kinds of death may be added on later. Rather,
dead is dead. It just so happens that new means of prolonging life, such as
respirators, make the old signs of death unreliable, so medicine has had to
discover new signs for that minority of cases where the traditional heart and
lung criteria can no longer be useful. The actual event of death is the same
regardless of what means are used to detect it.

For this reason, some authors have found fault with the Kansas statute, which tends to suggest that brain death and heart-lung death are somehow different things. The Michigan statute follows a model law proposed by Capron and Kass, which makes it clear that there is only one kind of death, but that in different circumstances different criteria may be needed to detect it.

290 cont.

289

291

Before leaving Case 21, consider the following argument:

It has been admitted that the major motive operating in this case is the desire to obtain kidneys suitable for transplant purposes. This is true whether you are allowing the patient to die or whether you are applying "brain death" criteria, since in the latter instance the desire for donor organs was the motive for formulating the criteria in the first place. While obtaining donor organs to save others' lives is a laudable goal, to allow it to take charge of our decision-making in this case would be the same as saying that the end justifies the means. In ethics, we can never allow this to be the case, so we have to try to keep the boy alive as long as possible.

What is your reaction to this argument?

292

At first glance it is hard to favor a position which seems to hold that "the ends justify the means," since in our experience this sort of moral position has always been associated with such undesirables as social violence, fascism, etc. This, however, is an emotional reaction. What is the logical validity of this view?

On analysis, we find that what is meant by "ends" must be some of the consequences of the particular action-specifically, those consequences which make up the intended outcome. Unless you wish to adopt a deontological view of ethics (see Appendix I), we have shown that it is only by the consequences of an action that one can justify it. Thus, so far as it goes, "the ends justify the means" is an accurate description of the decision-making method of Chapter 2.

293

But what is it that a person really means when he invokes the ends-can't-justify-means line? Say that a political group wants to commit an illegal act to further some socially good cause. An onlooker admits that their goal is beneficial, but objects to the means employed, which must necessarily contribute to the breakdown of social order. Therefore the illegal act is wrong, since "the ends can't justify the means."

294

All that the above says is that our "end" is but one of the consequences of the action, while the action must be justified on the sum total of all the consequences. Even where our intended outcome is good, the bad "side effects" may far outweigh it. Thus it seems that "the ends can't justify the means" is simply a more clumsy way of making a point we have emphasized all along: one must consider all the consequences, not just the desired ones or the short-range ones.

## CASE 22

295      You are in charge of the obstetrical wing of a New York hospital when a 24-year-old woman comes in in labor. You learn that on the previous day an abortion had been induced at a clinic in another part of the city by the saline method (withdrawing amniotic fluid from around the fetus and replacing it with equal volume of saline). At that time the duration of the pregnancy had been estimated at 22 weeks. From what little you are able now to learn from the mother, she does not want the baby and desires to carry through with the abortion.

     A while later the woman delivers a fetus, which you estimate by visual inspection to weigh about 1700 grams. As you are about to turn away, a nurse suddenly notices that a heartbeat is present in the fetus.

     Normal policy in your hospital calls for attempted resuscitation of any child with a birth weight as low as 1000 grams. There is no policy for attempted abortion resulting in live birth, since this has never happened before in this hospital.

     Do you attempt to resuscitate the fetus or not? In either case, what do you tell the mother?

     (Adapted from: Case 104, Columbia University Program in Medical Ethics, courtesy Robert M. Veatch)

---

296      This fetus, while still in the uterus, was defined as a "nonperson" both by the mother, in her desire not to have it, and by the New York law which permits abortion up to the 24th week of pregnancy. The fetus has now, in effect, put in an application for "personhood," and you have the power to reject or to attempt to accept that application.

     Take the last question first. If you elect, no matter what happens, simply to tell the mother that the abortion has been completed (regardless of the ethics of that), you still have to decide what to do now. If you tell the mother the truth, she is likely to be equally dissatisfied if you tell her that she had a live baby but that you allowed it to die; or that she has a live baby which you saved for her, and she now has to take it home and care for it; or that she had a live baby which you attempted to resuscitate, but after a few days it died anyway, and she now owes a $4000 hospital bill for your efforts. None of these later consequences makes any of the immediate decisions more attractive, so you have to decide the immediate question on its own merits.

297      From a quality-of-life standpoint, one might frame three arguments. Which do you find most acceptable?

     1)   The decision as to the child's "personhood" was already made by the mother when she decided to have an abortion. You have no business interfering at this late time. Let the baby die as planned.     ↓ 298

     2)   The original decision of "nonperson" status was made while the fetus was still in utero and by presumption unable to sustain an independent existence. Thus the mother could bestow "nonperson" status upon it. Now the situation has changed, and you see that the fetus-child is in fact potentially capable, with your assistance, of a life on its own. Thus earlier decisions do not apply     ↓ 299 and the fetus has become an individual human being over whose body the mother no longer has any right to pronounce.

     3)   It would be presumptuous for you to make such a complex decision on your own. Assuming that the mother is in good enough shape to give an opinion, you should ask her whether to resuscitate the infant or not.     ↓ 302

You have made the choice that was actually made by the physician in the real-life case—and a choice that has been rejected by a number of other physicians in similar situations. While the act of not resuscitating the fetus might be justifiable, the argument used in no. 1 suggests that once one ethical decision is made, you are bound to carry it out come hell, high water, or new information. This view is a cop-out. We saw in Chapter 2 the various points in which empirical data influence the ethical decision-making process. That carries with it an obligation to reconsider the original ethical decision whenever new data appear that could influence the decision in those ways. If the particular action is already final and irrevocable, the obligation is to reconsider for the benefit of cases you might run into in the future. In this case, however, the decision has not reached the final stage. Since you have new data and you still have a chance to save the fetus, you have an obligation to reconsider, even if you have less than a minute to do it.

298

↓ 299

Choice no. 2 correctly perceives that the situation has changed since the original decision was made, and that a rethinking might be in order. It also perceives that if the fetus is now a "person" by virtue of attempting to breathe and have a heartbeat, your decision to save its life or not can no longer be subject to the mother's wishes in a negative way—the fetus' "right to life" now clearly takes precedence over any rights of the mother. However, presumably the original decision to abort was made, or ought to have been made, on the basis of some sort of quality-of-life criteria. This original argument may have taken one of two general forms:

1) The fetus in utero is a "nonperson" but we cannot kill it unless we are able to justify it in view of that fetus' own interests as a potential person. In this case we decide that the quality of life to be experienced by this person-to-be, due to the family financial situation, emotional problems, or whatever, is such that non-existence might well be preferable. Therefore the fetus should be aborted.

2) The fetus in utero is a "nonperson" while the mother is a "person," so the wishes of the mother take precedence over any presumed interests of the fetus. In this case the mother does not want to have a baby, so the fetus should be aborted.

Notice that if you argued as in no. 1, the fetus' heartbeat does not negate the poor quality-of-life that you have predicted it will have to face, so a decision to resuscitate it would be questionable. In argument no. 2, the new data represented by the heartbeat has materially changed the respective "rights" of fetus and mother, so you would be justified in resuscitate the fetus as a new infant.

299

↓

300

↓

301

↓ 303

You have tried to duck the decision but you are not going to get away with it. Recall the general principle reached earlier in this chapter—in an emergency situation, when in doubt, treat. A newborn with a heartbeat but no respiration represents a medical emergency. If the idea of resuscitation even crosses your mind, it must mean that you have at least a doubtful opinion that the newborn object might be a "person" worthy of having its life saved. As long as that degree of doubt exists, you are not justified in delaying treatment even long enough to call the mother's attention to the situation and get a statement from her. This is not even taking into account the shape the mother must be in after just completing labor and being, most likely, under the influence of various medications which dull her senses—under such conditions, how well will any opinion she might give reflect her true desires? Go back to the original list and choose another alternative.

302

↑ 297

303      If you did not choose no. 2 above, go to the frame referred to and read the two arguments to justify abortion of the fetus. It should be clear from these that "abortion" is not a single medical issue about which neat judgments can be made (other than either a blanket ban, or an "Engineering Model" injunction to do whatever the patient asks for and don't raise any objections). When appeal is made to the quality of life of the prospective person, it is clear that even if the reasoning is faulty, some attempt at least is being made to consider that person-to-be's best interests. In such a case, which is most clear when the fetus has been diagnosed as having a genetic defect, abortion might be classed as prenatal euthanasia.

      In the other argument, appeal is made only to societal needs—either the need to restrict population growth, or the more specific emotional or financial needs of the mother. The ignoring of the best interests of the person-to-be is justified by the "nonperson" status of the fetus. This is clearly a different ball game, and the two distinct motives for abortion ought to be kept clearly separate in one's mind.

REVIEW
"ENGINEERING MODEL" 106

CASE 23

304      Mr. and Mrs. H.D. are the parents of four healthy, normal children and one 2-year-old child who was discovered at birth to have the appearance characteristic of Down's syndrome or Trisomy 21; further chromosomal tests confirmed this diagnosis. The child was noted early to have a loud systolic heart murmur and now has progressive symptoms of heart failure. As the H.D.'s family physician, you refer the patient to a cardiologist, who reports that the child has a large ventricular septal defect and possibly other heart defects. Correction would require inserting a catheter into the heart through a vein in order to determine the precise extent of the anomaly, then cardiac surgery. This cardiologist is of the opinion that since the family already has four healthy children, and since this mentally retarded child can never be a functional or significant member of society, it would be a waste of funds and manpower to do either the catheterization or the surgery. In this case the child would most likely be progressively unable to tolerate exercise, be confined to bed, and die from a secondary infection within one year or so.

      With the parents still uncertain, you refer to another cardiologist who confirms the first one's diagnosis and prognosis. However, he says that he would go ahead and correct the defect if possible. In fact, referring to the age-old medical dictum of  primum non nocere  ("first, do no harm") he states categorically that it would be unethical for you to do harm by allowing the child to die.

      You again confer with the H.D.'s. It is clear that they are thoroughly confused at this point and your injunctions that the decision is theirs to make have been to no avail. They are looking to you for the decision, and any preference you suggest one way or the other, no matter how many reservations you tack on to it, is probably going to sway them.

      Incidentally, while the family is not destitute, they cannot afford such complicated surgery and the cost would have to be financed publicly through Michigan Crippled Children's funding.

      Do you favor cardiac catheterization or not?

This case can be approached as a straightforward quality-of-life decision. Analogous to the abortion case, two justifications are possible if you elect to allow the child to die. Either the quality of life of a child with Down's syndrome is so poor that it would be kinder to let the child die; or the child's "nonperson" status allows one to let it die in order to conserve societal funds and medical resources. The major difference between this and the abortion case is the different quality-of-life criteria needed to define a Down's syndrome child as a "nonperson" as opposed to those required for a fetus. (Do Fletcher's criteria in Appendix III exclude this child from "personhood"?)

A few of the phrases encountered in Case 23 are worth looking into in more detail. First, we read that the H.D.'s are the parents of "four normal, healthy children" besides the infant with Down's syndrome. This phrase has a tendency to come up in case descriptions of genetic problems. Why? If all that is needed is data about how many other children the H.D.'s must care for, in order to determine how much time and energy they have to take care of a mentally retarded and sickly youngster, it would be sufficient to say "four children." There is at least an implication here that since the H.D.'s have other children who are well, they would be less likely to miss the "defective" one if you were to allow him to die. Not only is this not true empirically, but it reduces all the children to the status of pets—they are considered in terms of how good they make the parents feel, not as individuals with needs of their own.

Next we come to the first cardiologist who states that a mentally retarded child "can never be a functional or significant member of society." Can one make a categorical statement about the entire field of mental retardation? Even within the one disease category of Down's syndrome (or "mongolism") one can find individuals who are of low-educable I.Q., who can perform simple tasks and can do routine work, and who are capable of giving and receiving love within their family units. We also find severely retarded individuals with multiple physical defects as well. We have no data here about where the D. child fits on this spectrum as far as mental competence goes, so it is premature to make judgments about his worth as an individual.

(If you are not familiar with Down's syndrome, and with the range of mental retardation in general, you might wish to read a little in standard genetics or pediatrics texts.)

Finally we encounter cardiologist no. 2 who tells us what is moral and immoral based on the age-old dictum of "primum non nocere." This seems to be invoked as a supposed last word in ethical discussions about as often as the adage about "playing God," and so we must subject it also to a similarly close inspection. First, assume that "harm" simply means "hurt." Who is to say that we would be hurting this child more by letting him die than by keeping him alive? Moreover, much of medicine involves doing a small amount of hurting in anticipation of a greater good to follow. Are we to interpret "primum non nocere" as prohibiting any sort of surgery, or prescribing a drug with a known side effect, or puncturing a vein to draw blood?

REVIEW
"PLAYING GOD" ¦ 281

305

306

307

308

309 But a philosopher might object that strictly speaking, "harm" and "hurt" are not equivalent, and that "harm" means "wrongful hurt" or "hurt deliberately done without any accompanying benefit." By this definition, "primum non nocere" is the same as "don't hurt anyone unless the good consequences outweigh the bad consequences," which is really no more than a recommendation to use a consequentialist ethical method, such as we proposed in Chapter 2. But the ethical method is just the beginning, and gives no answers until we fill in the relevant data and values. Thus, "primum non nocere" can never be accepted by itself as the "last word" in an ethical argument; and, like "playing God," we might decide that an agreement to ban it from ethical discussions would be an improvement and a clarification.

---

### CASE 24

310 As her family physician, you accompany Mrs. M.K. to the Regional Perinatal Center when, at the 28th week of her pregnancy, you discover during an office physical that she is in heart failure and that she has a rhythm disturbance (ventricular tachycardia). It is found that drug therapy is unable to convert her to normal rhythm; and because of the danger of the tachycardia progressing to fatal ventricular fibrillation, the specialist wants to convert the heart with DC current. You ask about the effect of the electric current on the baby's heart rate; no one seems to be sure although healthy infants have been delivered after the mothers had DC cardioversion earlier in pregnancy.

You explain to Mr. and Mrs. M.K. both the danger to Mrs. M.K. and the potential hazard to the fetus, who, if born at this stage, might have some chance of survival. The parents are agreed that every effort should be made to insure a viable baby, so an emergency unit for caesarean section is readied as you prepare for the DC cardioversion. At this point, as you are watching the monitor of Mrs. M.K.'s EKG, you see a ventricular fibrillation pattern develop.

* * * * * * * *

1) Would you electrically defibrillate Mrs. M.K.?

2) Would you do an emergency caesarean section to remove the infant before extreme lack of oxygen has compromised its survival chances?

Think about these questions, then proceed with the rest of Case 24.
* * * * * * * *

Before a decision is reached as to defibrillation, Mrs. M.K. spontaneously converts to her previous rhythm of atrial fibrillation. At this point, rather shaken up, you obtain further consultation from an obstetrician. He is of the opinion that a C-section could well be fatal for Mrs. M.K. because of the sudden load placed on the circulatory system; whereas a normal delivery, which spreads the stress out over a longer period, should be tolerated well.

Meanwhile, an obstetrical consultant has been administering test doses of oxytocin (a hormone stimulating contraction of the uterus) and finds that even a slight uterine contraction seems to produce significant slowing of heart rate and lowered blood pressure in the fetus. This obstetrician states that the infant will not survive a normal vaginal delivery; however, if the pregnancy is continued one more week, the infant would clearly survive a C-section. You now have to decide whether to recommend a caesarean section which will most likely kill the mother, or await spontaneous onset of normal labor and most likely lose the baby.

What is the most appropriate manner of reaching this decision? What would be your recommendation?

In Case 24 you have a situation which is often talked about in medical-ethics discussions, but which in real life seldom occurs in such pure form—a situation in which you have to choose between the lives of two individuals. Quality-of-life criteria are hard to apply to the situation of comparing two individuals; and, in addition, data about either individual is hard to come by here.

Presumably you must talk this over with the parents. If Mrs. M.K. says that she wants to live, who is to speak for the baby's point of view? On the contrary, if Mrs. M.K. says that she wants the baby to live even if it means her own life, is she expressing her real feelings, or rather some idea of what society expects of a mother, i.e., to be self-sacrificing for her child? And if Mr. M.K. says that he wants the baby, does he have a right to make a martyr of his wife?

Case 24 is based on a real case. In the end, the physicians decided to await spontaneous labor—apparently because it is more of an established medical tradition to sacrifice the infant to save the mother, and also because the quality of life the infant would face growing up without its mother was judged to be low enough to justify this. As it turned out, this was another happy-ending case. The second obstetrician's prediction was wrong and the child survived.

---

## CASE 25

The year is 1978; Michigan's brain-death statute has been in effect for three years, and a law to allow mercy killing in terminally ill patients at their request or that of the next of kin was passed by the legislature last session. None of this is of much help to you as you try to figure out what to do with Mr. Lewis. Mr. Lewis has been in a coma and maintained on a respirator for 26 days, ever since the auto crash in which his wife was killed. For three weeks you still had some hope that the 58-year-old patient might be brought back to consciousness; now you have pretty much given up, but the state of his reflexes and movements are too equivocal to allow you to pronounce him dead by the Harvard criteria. You have told Mr. Lewis' two grown children that there seems as if there is nothing to be gained, and if no dramatic change for the better occurs within 24 to 48 hours, you will disconnect the respirator.

This morning you have a visitor in the form of a lawyer for the Great Atlantic and Pacific Life Insurance Company. He tells you (which you had not been aware) that Mr. Lewis is protected by a six-figure insurance policy which pays double indemnity in cases of accidental death. However, to qualify under that clause of the policy, the death must take place within 30 days of the accident.

The lawyer says that his company has developed a fear that you are plotting in concert with Mr. Lewis' children to turn off the respirator inside the magic 30-day limit, "despite the fact that he is obviously still alive." In order to guard itself against this course, the company has authorized him to inform you that you will be sued for the amount of the insurance policy should the respirator be turned off, in the absence of clear signs of death, within the 30 day period.

No sooner has this gentleman left than you are visited by the attorney newly retained by the Lewis children. He reminds you that proper regard for the best interests of your patient's family would require that the respirator be turned off immediately, "since he is obviously already dead. Anyway, he should have a right to death with dignity, without all sorts of tubes stuck in him." In case you need encouragement to consider these interests more closely, the lawyer notes that should you cause the family to lose the double-indemnity sum, they plan to sue you for that amount.

After finishing the half-full bottle of bourbon in the bottom drawer of your desk, what do you do then?

314    We have no intention of offering an answer to this rather futuristic case. It was included to point out that no medical decision, especially one that is a matter of life and death, takes place in a social vacuum. Death to the public at large means not only respirators, defibrillation, and autopsies, but also funerals, mourning, insurance policies, wills, and many other things. Considerations of these other matters are bound to intrude themselves into medical decisions, often in highly inconvenient ways. Sometimes these considerations will be ethically relevant, as in the injunction of certain orthodox religions that the body must be whole at the time of burial; in other cases these considerations are merely static in the decision-making system. It is far from easy to tell the two apart in all cases.

315    This concludes the series of sample cases to illustrate quality-of-life decisions. These cases should have shown that "quality of life" is a complex concept which may seem to mean different things in different cases. They should also have shown that no matter how much we might value philosophical consistency as an ideal, and search for criteria that would apply to all cases, the temptation is very strong to treat each case according to its own peculiar features and within its particular emotional context. However much we might reject the consequences of a strict sanctity-of-life view, we might occasionally be envious of the person who has spared himself so many difficult decisions by adhering to it.

316    Your final charge before leaving this topic is to review in your own mind the concept of "quality of life," as we have explicated it by means of the sample cases. Have you been able to pull out some consistently applicable criteria? Or have you found yourself, like most of the present-day medical profession, reduced to making ad hoc decisions for each individual case, without much regard toward universalizability?

When anyone is so brash as Joseph Fletcher was to suggest 15 criteria for personhood, it is easy for us to respond by picking holes in his theory. But if we are agreed that some such set of criteria is needed, the question is: can we do any better? Refer again to Fletcher's original list in Appendix III. Can you do any better? Do you accept Fletcher's own conclusion, that the criterion of cerebral function really summarizes the entire matter? Or do you think that some of his other criteria, or some not on his list, must be added in? Try to set up your own list; you will have plenty of opportunity to use and refine it as quality-of-life considerations come up in subsequent chapters.

Ch. 7 ⬇ 317

# 7. Determination of Ethical Participation

In Chapter 4, it was concluded that so long as the "Contractual Model" is accepted, we must acknowledge the right of the patient to participate in ethical decisions which affect his life. This leaves unanswered two important questions which we shall now take up. First, in those cases where the patient is incompetent to assume this responsibility, who ought to participate for him? Second, are there cases in which others besides the patient have so much at stake that they have a right to participation also?

317

This question of ethical participation is obviously an important one. Ironically, it can at times become too important. In ethics, we must be most interested in the decision itself—the basis on which it is justified, and the criteria by which it is to be applied. Being human, we often, without realizing it, search for some means to escape the responsibility of confronting the decision directly. Too often, a handy way out is to start worrying about "who should decide?" instead of "what decision should be made?" We can then get into detailed considerations of who should be consulted, when, how, in what order, etc., and conveniently let our minds drift from the basic issues.

318

The worst form of the preoccupation with "who" instead of "what" is the "Let's form a committee" syndrome, which has been much too prevalent in the areas of allocation of scarce resources and of human experimentation. It is pleasant to discuss how many members the committee should have and how they should be chosen in order to represent all the different interest groups. You then feel that you have done your duty, while the committee itself is stuck with the dirty work; and if the committee just muddles through instead of developing ethically sound criteria and procedures, you can't be blamed.

319

However, our discussion of the "Contractual Model" and paternalism should make it clear why we cannot avoid the "who" question. The unconscious paternalism that infects nearly all members of the medical profession leads one easily to forget that there are many decisions which are not the doctor's to make; and that there are many others for which the doctor must play the role of information source rather than true participant. While avoiding getting too hung up on "who?", the ethical physician must continually be asking himself "who?" lest he deprive a patient of his ethical rights.

320

REVIEW
"CONTRACT" | 110

Here, however, we might re-emphasize some important characteristics of the "what"—the decision that is to be made. First, recall that the decision is made in a state of relative ignorance, which can be reduced but never eliminated. Even if, in principle, we could gather all the data that is relevant to the decision—which we cannot—the time for the decision would still be long past after we had done so.

321

REVIEW
UNCERTAINTY | 35

322    Second, recall that any ethical judgment is based in part on predictions concerning the future—the consequences of the alternative actions. While these future predictions are only one ingredient in the decision-making process, they are essential; if they are faulty, the decisions will be flawed as a result.

323    Because of these two aspects of decision-making, we can conclude a third: some of our decisions will be based on the best information we can collect at the time, and will still turn out to be wrong. Looking at the matter in retrospect, we cannot conclude that the decision-making procedure was faulty just because a wrong answer was obtained; and we cannot conclude that the right procedure was chosen just because an ethically valid action was the result. The best we can do is test out the various alternative procedures, pick the one which has the most potential for choosing valid actions, and then work on applying it to the best of our ability, learning from the mistakes as we go.

324    The other ingredient needed for ethical decisions, of course, is the set of values against which the consequences are to be weighed. Combining this fact with the three points just mentioned, we come to a general conclusion: *If we can assume that the set of values is shared by a group of people, the best decision-maker among that group will be the one with the most realistic and most accurate view of the future.*

325    Right away we can see we are headed for trouble here, because we have to start with two things that we have a great deal of difficulty in measuring. First of all, generally people in the same subculture share the same basic set of values; but in the same token, each person has a set of values which differs somewhat from that of any other person. How can we tell if two individuals share the same values in any instance, and how can we be sure that the values which are of particular relevance to the medical decision to be made? Likewise, since the future has not yet happened, how can we tell who has the best view of it? While we can eliminate those whose views are based on mere intuition or fantasy, we will still be left with those whose views are carefully reasoned out and still disagree on important points.

326    This explains why we must suspect the idea that the physician should be the major decision-maker. His view of the future is likely to be the best among the parties involved, as regards the strictly medical events. His view may also be very good regarding future occurrences in the feelings and psychological status of the patient. But it is stretching things a bit far to contend that the physician shares the same set of values as the patient, especially since in many cases the physician may be of a different socio-economic group and of a different subculture from the patient. It is also stretching things a bit to contend that where the values are not shared, the physician's values are "better" than the patient's in any objective sense.

We can now start dealing with the "who" question, since we have just begun by casting suspicion on the notion that the physician, as a rule, ought to be the primary decision-maker. The next party we might want to consider is society. It is generally agreed that society has a stake in many if not in all of the kinds of decisions we have been discussing. However, society (whatever that is) certainly cannot participate directly in any decision-making (although, of course, it participates indirectly by shaping our values). We are then left with sticky questions about which individual or social institution can speak in place of society for any given case.

327

Regardless of who speaks for it, it seems clear that society does have a stake. All individuals are part of society, and stand to suffer if society as a whole suffers. Thus we can say in principle that if a person does something that is not in the best interests of society, he himself, along with everyone else, will eventually suffer the consequences. However, even if we recognize this to be the case in the long run and in the broader view, we cannot exclude the possibility, and indeed the probability, that there will be specific conflicts of interest in specific instances, where, according to our best analysis, the best interests of the person, both short- and long-range, can best be served by doing something that seems to be at variance with societally legitimate dictates.

328

When faced with such a conflict, our general tendency is to go along with the individual, on the grounds that society can stand a small insult better than the individual can stand a large one. (This assumes a particular sort of relationship between the individual and society, which we will describe in more detail in Chapters 17 and 18.) However, we cannot accept this as a rule. As we saw in the section on professional confidentiality in Chapter 4, there were several instances which seemed to call for maintaining a confidence even where society could benefit from disclosure, and other instances where a disclosure seemed ethically valid despite the patient's own interests. We cannot treat individual-society conflicts as simple cases, therefore, and must proceed by carefully investigating the consequences of each particular case. The identification of such an apparent conflict should serve as a red flag to warn us that we are going to get into trouble if we try to solve the matter simply by habit or by inclination.

329

How about other individuals in the decision-making process? We have already established the rights of the patient under the doctor-patient "contract" so long as the patient is competent. In Chapter 4, we recognized several categories of incompetent patients, whom we could exclude from decision-making without violation of the "contract." These were:

330

1) *the unconscious patient*
2) *the conscious but irrational patient*
3) *the child patient, below the age of understanding*

For those instances in which we want to consider abortion as possibly being in the best interests of the person-to-be, rather than abortion strictly on behalf of the mother or of society, we can add:

4) *the unborn patient*

331    For societal and legal purposes, we recognize by convention persons who can speak for patients in all these categories—the spouse or next of kin in the first two, the parents in the second two. (These conventions are not absolute. For example, in human experimentation, the question has arisen of whether parents can consent for their children to take part in an experiment from which the children get no therapeutic benefit. There is a growing sentiment that parents "have no right to make martyrs of their children," and that only the court can give consent for the child in such a case. Courts have also ruled that Jehovah's Witness parents cannot refuse blood transfusions for their children.)

Are these customary representatives adequate also from a medical-ethical viewpoint, or must we seek another way of obtaining a proxy decision?

332    We assume that when a patient makes his own decision, he is acting for his own best interests, and in accordance with his own set of values (assuming the decision to be well-thought-out and rational). When we see an individual make a rational decision to do what we feel to be contrary to his best interests, what we are saying is that if we were in that situation, that would be contrary to our own values; so this other person must have some different values from our own in order to make that decision. Our disagreement cannot be taken as evidence that the action was not in his best interests. The only one who can say that is the person himself, if in the future he looks back upon the decision and sees that it was faulty in the light of new information.

333    So what we seem to need is an individual who has the same personality and set of values as our incompetent patient, but who is conscious, rational, above the age of comprehension, and born. Clearly this individual is a hypothetical fantasy. How closely can he be approached by the parties alluded to by societal convention?

334    First take the case of parents. While many of the laws and conventions of society reinforce the notion that parents know better what is in their child's best interests than anyone else, psychological investigation of the family relationship fails to bear this out in any general way. Why do parents have children? The strictly altruistic, and ethically ideal, motive, of wishing to give life to and assist in the nurture of a unique individual with his own needs and values, is most often combined with or totally replaced by self-centered motives. While we may not be so crass as to want children in order to have more hands to work and make money for the family, we might very well subconsciously want children because of the emotional gratification—reinforcement of a virile or feminine self-image. We might also subconsciously seek to direct the child's life in order to compensate for deeply felt unmet needs or ambitions of our own, instead of allowing the child to choose a course consistent with his own individuality.

Now consider the next of kin, say in a passive euthanasia case such as those described in the last chapter. When a person is near death, a very common emotional reaction of the immediate family is to feel guilty about the real or imagined things that they should have done for the person and now cannot. As a means of assuaging this guilt, they might well become suddenly over-solicitous and over-protective. Possibly having secretly wished for the death of their parent or spouse over the past few years, they are now led by their guilt and emotional confusion to demand shrilly that all possible means be used to keep the person alive. None of these motives bear any relation to the question of whether the person himself would be better off alive or dead.

335

This train of argument may well be bothering you. If these societally designated proxies can't make the decision in the patient's best interests, who can? The doctor? Or do you have to get a court order in every such case?

336

Clearly the court solution is impractical, and one might well object that having the doctor decide is paternalistic. After all, medicine is practiced in a social context, and it is arrogant of doctors to imagine that they are independent of usual social constraints. So if these designated proxies are good enough for the rest of society, they ought to be good enough for us, without the need for us to ask them prying questions to determine their competence. This approach eliminates the problem—except in the all-too-frequent cases where the next of kin ducks the responsibility completely and leaves it back on the doctor's shoulders.

No matter how much we might want to avoid paternalism, though, there is a second danger which we cannot ignore. That is the danger (alluded to above in Case 12) of forgetting who the patient is.

337

The doctor can communicate with the parent or spouse, while he either cannot communicate at all, or can do so only at an unsatisfactory level, with the incompetent patient. When the doctor does what is satisfying to the parent or spouse, they can verbally express their appreciation, while the patient cannot demonstrate any gratitude. There is, therefore, the obvious danger that the doctor will come (unconsciously, of course) to prize the satisfaction of the parent or spouse above the presumed best interests of the patient. There is no problem where the interests of the two parties do not conflict. But as we just saw, there is no guarantee that this will be the case.

REVIEW ↑
CASE 12 ⋮ 192

The concern which lies at the base of all this is the duty of the physician to consider the interests of the patient as an individual as his primary concern. As we noted in Chapter 4, there are times when societal responsibilities may outweigh this duty. Future physicians will be called upon increasingly to temper their actions with a greater awareness of society's needs and priorities. But if medicine as a profession ever began to put the consideration for the individual in a secondary position, it would cease to be the institution it is supposed to be now, and would become something completely different.

338

339    If the doctor wishes to follow this duty to the individual patient, it would seem that the duty does not cease just because the patient is unable to communicate his own perception of his best interests. The next of kin may in fact be well suited to speak for the patient. Even if this is not the case, the next of kin is a valuable source of data about the patient's values and desires—or, in the case of the unborn patient, about the quality of life that the person-to-be might expect to experience. Therefore the doctor should never hesitate to consult with the next of kin; and, if satisfied with the results, willingly yield to his decision. But the doctor, to protect his patient, must listen critically and be alert for any signs that might indicate a conflict of interests.

340    All this discussion has led to the following general conclusions about rights of participation.

*1)    The primary decision-making responsibility rests with the patient, so long as he is competent.*

*2)    When the patient is incompetent, the socially designated next of kin and other close relatives should be allowed to speak for the patient.*

*3)    If the physician has reason to doubt whether the individuals in No. 2 are representing the patient's best interests, he may choose other individuals to involve in the decision process, or as a last resort may make the decision himself; however, he assumes the responsibility for demonstrating that his doubts were based on reasonable evidence.*

*4)    Any of the individuals named above, except the doctor, may opt out of the decision process by being unable to decide or by refusing to take responsibility. In such a case the doctor must seek the opinion of an alternative patient representative (such as a court order or a more distant relative) if there is time, or make the decision himself if there is not. The doctor cannot opt out of the process.*

*5)    As a general rule, all the individuals named must act within the usual constraints imposed by society. Where these constraints have become so rigid as to constitute a conflict between society's best interests and the patient's best interests, the case must be decided individually by careful consideration of the consequences.*

341    The criteria just listed, if followed, will help insure that the doctor has included the appropriate participants in the decision process from the ethical standpoint. He has another task as far as his legal responsibility goes; the list above does not address this other responsibility. In some cases his legal duties can be fulfilled by doing less than what the ethical rules would suggest; an example was Case 12 where the doctor is legally covered by the mother's informed consent, but is ethically required to obtain informed consent (or at least to inform) the minor child as well. In other cases, where the physician is wary of a lawsuit, he may want to do more than the ethical guidelines would require in order to protect himself. An example is a case where the patient is senile and where his mental status might be open to question, but appears to the doctor to be competent. If the doctor fears that some relatives might later disagree with the therapy given, he might want to get some other relatives to give consent in addition to obtaining it from the patient.

REVIEW    ↑
LAW vs ETHICS ¦ 67–68

We can now start to apply these guidelines to cases, and we can start with a simple and a common one. 342

---

CASE 26

343

Mrs. L.K., a 74-year-old widow, has been your patient for 15 years. Recently she has been getting confused and forgetful, but she is aware of her surroundings and you would hesitate to label her mentally incompetent.

Some recent symptoms of Mrs. L.K.'s have worried you enough to put her in the hospital and run some tests. You are now quite certain that she has a metastasizing carcinoma and that she probably has six months to a year to live. You really cannot offer her any realistic hope of palliation by chemotherapy or radiation.

Before discussing your findings with Mrs. L.K., you reveal the bad news to her two children. They are immediate and unanimous in their response: "Don't tell Momma she is going to die. Tell her these are just non specific symptoms of old age. Let her live out the rest of her days in peace."

What do you do with the information you have?

---

While you are always free to disagree, you should have no trouble guessing what we are going to say about this case. Mrs. L.K. is not incompetent. She came to you as a patient and your doctor-patient "Contract" is with her. Her impending death is morally relevant information to her; maybe there is something she very much wants to do before she dies. At any rate, even if you "don't tell Momma" (and if Momma doesn't know already), her children, in their concern about keeping up the concealment, will soon communicate to her without words that something is being kept from her. The likely result will be resentment and concern rather than "peace." 344

At any rate, all the above suggests that the children have no right of participation in this instance. Since you had no intention of following their advice if they suggested concealment, you might have avoided ill feelings by not suggesting that they can make the decision. Rather, you might start out with, "Your mother has to be told this in the near future. I want your opinions on what would be the best way and the best time to do this."

Going back to our discussion of what makes a good decision-maker, we have, in effect, faulted the children in Case 26 on both counts. By rushing to speak for a person who is still able to think and to communicate, they have raised doubts about the extent to which they actually share the values of the person. And they have shown themselves as having a faulty view of the future by assuming that "peace" will automatically result from an attempt to conceal important information. It is clear that their own emotional responses have interfered with their ability to be good ethical decision-makers. 345

346    The second question in this chapter refers to the case of a competent patient in which other individuals have a significant stake in the outcome and, hence, a right to participation in the decision. The key word here is significant. In some sense, all of society has some stake in the outcome of any medical decision. However, since we tend to regard medicine as having primary obligation toward the patient as individual, we usually demand proof of a very substantial interest before we will allow another party to overrule the patient's wishes.

347    Refer back to Case 18 in Chapter 6, where the court ordered a transfusion for a Jehovah's Witness mother in the interests of her 7-month-old child. We dodged the ethical questions in the following discussion. We must first ask if an individual has the moral right to desert his family through suicide; and then, if the person has already determined to do so, whether the physician is morally justified in either aiding him or opposing him.

To the court, however, the case was clear. The 7-month-old daughter had such a significant stake in the outcome that she had not only a right of participation (by proxy), but also the right to summarily overrule the mother.

348    In medical ethics, the one case where the right of another's participation is most clearly upheld is sterilization of a married individual. It is almost universally agreed that the consent of the spouse as well as the patient is ethically required.

Note that an analogous right does not extend to abortion. If the motive for abortion is the presumed best interest of the fetus, then the father does not necessarily have a final say. If the motive is the "right of the mother to control over her own body," then the father has no right to make a woman carry and bear his child against her will.

349    Many cases, however, are not so clearcut. The physician may find a large cast of characters surrounding the patient's bed, producing mutually contradictory statements, and each demanding to have his say. The physician then has to sort out those who have a legitimate stake in the matter from those who merely have useful data to offer and from those who have no business being around at all.

## CASE 27

The four-day-old infant was being maintained on a respirator due to severe respiratory deficiency. While there had not been time for chromosomal analysis by karyotype, all evidence pointed to a diagnosis of Trisomy 18, a genetic disorder leading to severe mental retardation, growth failure, and numerous anatomical abnormalities. While there have been scattered reports of patients with the anomaly living to adulthood, 87% die within the first year of life.

A conference is being held to decide what to do with the infant.

The CHIEF OF PEDIATRICS reported several conversations with the father, who had said, "If you cannot guarantee that my child will be normal, I don't want you to do anything for it." The chief said that he shared the sympathies of the father and had told him, "I promise to do everything in my power to see that your wishes are carried out."

A PSYCHIATRIST also had several conversations with the father, and feels that the father is presently in a state of acute denial; however, if the respirator were turned off at the father's initiative, later guilt feelings could create psychiatric problems for him. He also noted that parents who bring a retarded child home only to have it die later might well suffer guilt over that also.

The PSYCHIATRIC SOCIAL WORKER contradicted the psychiatrist and states that she feels that the family would be put under extreme stress if the infant were brought home.

At this point, the NURSE who has been most directly responsible for the care of the infant interrupted with an obvious sense of outrage. She insisted that the infant had every right to live and could not be allowed to die by the hand of man. In fact, if necessary, she said she was willing to try to adopt the infant and care for it herself.

A PEDIATRIC RESIDENT called attention to a patient of his own, who has a slight respiratory difficulty but cannot be put on a respirator because the Trisomy 18 infant is using the last available machine. Without the respirator, the other infant, who is otherwise healthy, may run a 50% risk of some brain damage.

Who should decide? What should the decision be?

(Adapted from: Case 107, Columbia University Program in Medical Ethics, courtesy Robert M. Veatch)

---

Note on Case 27: Did you notice that no mention was made of the infant's mother anywhere in the case history? When this case was presented to 200 nurses in a New York hospital, fewer than a dozen noticed this point.

For the remainder of the discussion, assume that there was some pressing reason why the mother could not be available to register an opinion. Also, assume that the father's view represents the view of both parents.

352     The question of "who should decide" was raised when this case was printed in <u>Medical World News</u> (Sept. 12, 1972). A compilation of the responses by readers:

  46—the child's physician
  41—"the parents" or "the father"
   4— the physician plus the parent(s)
   2—the physician plus the psychiatrist
   1—a committee of professionals and laymen
   1—the hospital administrator
   1—a clergyman
   1—a medical panel
   1—the parents plus the health workers
   1—"none of the above"

353     These tabulations indicate two things—first, why the idea of making ethical decisions by majority vote is so poorly received in general; and second, the fact that very few nurses and psychiatric social workers read <u>Medical World News</u>.

        In deciding who should decide in one particular case, how much is one's opinion swayed by the course of action preferred by the various parties—that is, how likely is one to choose as decision-maker one of those who agrees with one's own choice of solution? If the professional titles of the various characters had been listed without reference to their views on the case, how might the tabulated results have been different?

354     Another interesting feature of the <u>Medical World News</u> poll was the wide range of weights given to both the chief's promise and the father's wishes. Responses ranged from the position that a great weight should be put on them, to the position that they should be ignored. On the chief's promise, comments included: "It's not binding; it's thoughtfully vague." "A promise is a promise." "It's meaningless reassurance." "It was a mistake." "A rash promise, and he should admit it."

355     Anyway, let's get out of medical sociology and move on to medical ethics. By analogy to several of the cases raised in Chapter 6, we have a quality-of-life decision to make here which relates to our motivations in the present situation. Either the goal should be to do what is in the hypothetical best interests of the child, in which case we have to analyze which of the parties is best able to speak for those. Or we may eliminate the child by noting that he is a "nonperson" by some set of quality-of-life criteria, so that the emotional needs of the family unit then become our primary concern. This does not necessarily mean that the parents should make the decision, since there is evidence on the table that the father may not be in an emotional state to know his own long-term best interests.

Notice that in this case there might not be a conflict between the best interests of the child and the emotional needs of the family. If the latter would best be served by allowing the child to die, it might also be that the quality of life to be anticipated by this child is low enough to justify passive euthanasia on the basis of the child's own interests.

356

There is, however, a clear conflict between the ethical duties assumed by two members of the health care team—the chief's promise to the father vs. the nurse's perceived obligation to uphold her own sanctity-of-life imperative. Recall that at the end of Chapter 4 we pointed out the artificiality of viewing the doctor-patient relationship as simply a one-to-one situation. We noted that in the future, the decisions to be made would increasingly be assumed by a health care team instead of the solo physician. Here is a working example of the problems that can arise.

357

Did the nurse's outburst sound to you to be ridiculous, or naive, or irrelevant? If so, note the following passages from the Code of Ethics for nurses:

358

"The nurse's primary commitment is to the patient's care and safety. She must be alert to take appropriate action regarding any instances of incompetent, unethical, or illegal practice by any member of the health care team, or any action on the part of others that is prejudicial to the patient's best interests."

And:

"The nurse's respect for the worth and dignity of the individual human being extends throughout the entire life cycle, from birth to death..."

Even if we must respect the basis for the nurse's ethical concern, however, we are forced to regard her proposed solution as ethically naive. Is she going to adopt and care for every mentally retarded child that is not wanted by the parents?

359

The conflict is such that no matter what is done with the infant, either the doctor or the nurse will be placed in a position of having to violate what he or she feels is the proper ethical duty. (Even if a compromise between their two positions were possible, it might not coincide with the best interests of either the infant or the family.) Does this mean that one or the other is being forced to lose his own moral integrity? If we say that the moral integrity of individual members of the health care team are of secondary concern as opposed to the needs of the patient, are we in danger of slipping into the "Engineering Model" of the health-team-patient relationship? And if the moral integrity of the health professionals must be protected, how can this be done if the team is still obligated to act in unison?

360

361      We can dodge these difficult questions for this instance simply by having all team members agree that the parents are best qualified to speak on behalf of the infant, and that the team will abide by the parents' decision. The questions do not disappear, however, for we can easily imagine a similar case in which the parents were either unable or unwilling to make any decision on their own.

362      We have considered the case in which the competent patient is called upon to share some of the decision-making responsibility because another individual has a significant interest in the outcome. There is another side to the coin. Are there some cases in which a competent patient may be deprived of part or all of his usual decision-making responsibility, because of some peculiar features of the case itself? One type of case that has been proposed as an example is the sticky situation presented by a possible self-fulfilling prophecy. Case 28 illustrates a way in which this problem might arise.

---

## CASE 28

363      Mrs. A.B., a 41-year-old mother of two, has become pregnant again. Because at her age there is a higher risk of her having a child with Down's syndrome, you, as her physician, have suggested amniocentesis—withdrawal of an amniotic fluid sample from around the fetus to obtain a few fetal cells which can then be analyzed to see if they contain the normal 46 chromosomes, or the 47 that would be indicative of Down's syndrome or another genetic anomaly.

      Mrs. A.B., a high school teacher, wants to have this child, but she has indicated to you that she wants to consider an abortion if the child has Down's syndrome. There is not much time to decide since the pregnancy is in the 18th week before the results come back.

      The report of the karyotyping shows that the fetus has no extra chromosome of the G group and thus is free of Down's syndrome. But the fetus is not "normal." Instead of the usual XX chromosomes of the female or XY of the male, the fetus' sex chromosomes are of the XYY composition.

      You are familiar with the research on the XYY genotype and that it is inconclusive. Studies of the inmates of institutions for those who have committed violent and antisocial acts indicate that persons with the XYY genotype are found among these groups more frequently than would be expected by chance—giving rise to theories that XYY individuals are more prone to violent or antisocial behavior. At the same time it has been shown that there are many XYY individuals who lead perfectly normal lives with no indications of sociopathology. There are no physical or mental abnormalities of significance which have been directly tied to the XYY genotype.

      What do you tell Mrs. A.B. about the results of the karyotype?
Is she entitled to participate in the decision of whether to abort or not?

      (Adapted from: Hastings Center Report, February, 1972)

This case is what Robert Veatch calls a "condition of doubt" situation—the doctor "has to decide not only which facts to communicate, but what the facts actually are....Some day there may be more evidence, but the decision is demanded today." This condition of doubt has a direct bearing on the ethical decision.

364

A person could argue against telling Mrs. A.B. about the extra Y chromosome as follows: From a technical view, your "contract" with Mrs. A.B. was to tell her whether or not the child has Down's syndrome, so you are not obligated to pass on any further information you learn coincidentally. Furthermore, if you consider Mrs. A.B. as your patient, you would be doing harm by generating a considerable amount of anxiety about the future for her child—an anxiety for which you do not have any hard data that could ease it.

365

If you broaden your view of the "patient" to include the entire family structure, the case is even more compelling. Suppose you tell Mrs. A.B. and she elects to have the baby. From then on, she will be unable to avoid thinking of the possible fate, and will always be searching every aspect of the child's behavior, looking for the slightest clue toward any personality disorder. She might be led to go overboard either as a strict disciplinarian or in showering affection on the child, in hopes of preventing later problems. Is there any situation more likely to produce a child with a behavior disorder, even if no tendency toward it existed at the start? This is the problem of the self-fulfilling prophecy, where the attempts to avoid something end up producing it.

366

Or suppose you tell and Mrs. A.B. then decides to abort. The chances are good, based on present statistics, that you will be aborting a "normal" fetus with no sociopathic tendencies.

(To be fair, we have to add that if you do not tell, Mrs. A.B. might still learn of the XYY later. Then her anxiety at that time will be further compounded by her knowledge of your concealment.)

Before considering the arguments on the other side, note what the self-fulfilling prophecy argument boils down to. It is saying that Mrs. A.B. has no right of participation because this right would demand information in order to be exercised; and the possession of this information would mean that Mrs. A.B., in spite of herself, would be very likely to produce the undesirable outcome through her own actions. This might sound like a rather extreme position. However, it serves to remind us that the participants in these sorts of ethical decisions are not spectators on the sidelines. They are active parties in what will follow the decision, and they are changed as persons by the act of participating in the decision. (Call this the Heisenberg uncertainty principle of medical ethics if you will.) The change brought about by the decision process itself ought to be taken into consideration when figuring the consequences of an ethical action.

367

368    Now the arguments in favor of telling. If we go back to our basic premise we have to ask one question: is the decision to abort or not to abort an ethically relevant one for Mrs. A.B., and is the information about the XYY genotype a piece of information that could figure significantly in the decision? We pretty much have to answer "yes" on both counts. It then follows that we are obligated to tell Mrs. A.B. and, within the confines of our own ignorance, give her what assistance we can in helping her to understand the implications and in helping her to deal with her natural anxiety.

    Note that, since the natural confusion of the information is very high, Mrs. A.B.'s decision to abort or not may very easily be swayed by the way we present the information or even by the tone of voice. This is one situation in which whether we say "the glass is half empty" or "the glass is half full" may make a very significant difference. How would you handle this problem?

369    It is also possible to approach Mrs. A.B.'s case from a different angle, that of societal values over the consideration for the individual. Given especially that Mrs. A.B. already has two children and would have been willing to abort this fetus anyway had it had Down's syndrome, we might argue that society already has enough problems without taking the chance, however small, of another murderer or rapist being born. This argument might lead us to say to Mrs. A.B., "The tests show that the chromosomes of the child are abnormal" (or even, "The tests show that the child has an extra chromosome"), knowing full well that she will then elect to abort. In this way you fulfill your societal obligation without "really" lying to your patient.

    How do you feel about this line of reasoning?

370    This is beginning to get a bit confusing, so perhaps it would be well to go back to the ethical decision-making method and state more clearly what moves we have been making. (This is analogous to the old rule on how to run laboratory equipment: "When all else fails, read the directions.") Back in Chapters 4 and 5, we evolved an ethical rule which could be stated as: "The doctor ought to inform the patient and allow the patient to make the decision in any matter which is of ethical significance to the patient, unless the patient himself has given indication that he does not wish to be told." (For shorthand, we'll state this rule as, "Inform...")

MAY SKIP
TO CH. 8 ↓385

371    A consequence of this ethical rule is that Mrs. A.B. ought to be told about the XYY karyotype. But it's telling Mrs. A.B. that seems to bother us. If in fact this consequence is contrary to some important value that we hold, this would be an indication that the rule is invalid as stated and is in need of revision. But so far we just know we are bothered; we have not determined what value has been challenged and in what way.

Two proposals have been put forward. One is the condition-of-doubt label.
This assumes that we place a low value on confusion and anxiety, and hence
are unwilling to produce it in a patient. We have refined this view to hold that
anxiety is unavoidable when the facts are unpleasant, and that the patient's
right as decision-maker overrules the value judgment in a normal case. However,
in a case in which the facts are confused (thereby rendering the patient less
capable of exercising his right effectively), the negative value placed on anxiety
assumes primary importance. Therefore, we ought to change the rule to,
"Inform...unless there is a significant amount of inherent doubt in the data,
and the patient is likely to suffer considerable anxiety as a result."

372

The other proposal is that of the self-fulfilling prophecy, which holds that
by telling the mother, we will have two bad consequences: 1) the raising of
a messed-up kid, and 2) the misery of the mother who is producing the messed-
up kid but cannot help herself (in both cases assuming that she did not elect
abortion; if she did, that would be a different bad consequence). The values
in play here are obvious; few of us positively value misery and messed-up kids.
This proposal, then, would have us modify the rule to: "Inform...unless doing
so would set into motion a situation, outside the conscious control of the
patient, which would produce misery for the patient or for another participant."

373

Before we decide to make one (or both) of these modifications of our
rule, we have to decide whether it is really a bad thing to tell Mrs. A.B. If it
is, then we still have to determine the consequences of adopting either of the
alternative rules. If, however, it is not, then we can maintain our original rule.

374

We have already listed many of the good and bad consequences of telling
Mrs. A.B. The problem is complicated by two uncertainties: whether Mrs. A.B.
will get an abortion, and whether XYY individuals do really have a genetic
tendency toward violent behavior.

We can construct a table to consider all these possibilities and classify the
consequences accordingly. For this we will assume 1) that in telling you do
as much as possible to avoid swaying Mrs. A.B. toward either choice; and 2)
that if you do not tell Mrs. A.B. there is a 100% chance that she will go ahead
and have the child. We will also assume for the moment that not telling Mrs.A.B.,
and instead making up something to tell her that will persuade her to have an
abortion, is farther than we are prepared to go. These assumptions result in
Table 2.

375

We have set up a matrix like the example of Bayesian decision-theory in
Chapter 2; in theory, we can now plug in numerical values for the probabilities
and desirabilites of each of the squares, and obtain a preference ranking.
However, we have so little data on which to base the numerical values that the
result of this procedure would probably be what the computer programmers
call "garbage in, garbage out"; we would be using numbers to cover up our
ignorance. Therefore, let's keep the matrix but instead try a qualitative approach.

376

377

REVEIW
"BAYESIAN"
THEORY    |86—97

Table 2

|  | Causal connection between XYY and sociopathic behavior | No causal connection between XYY and sociopathic behavior |
|---|---|---|
| Tell Mrs. A.B. and she decides to have abortion | 1. You told the truth. Mrs. A.B. got her right to participate. Mrs. A.B. is made anxious. Society is spared possibility of birth of sociopath. Mrs. A.B. has no baby. | 4. You told the truth. Mrs. A.B. was given right to participate. She is made anxious. She has no baby. Society has one less mouth to feed, but also loses "normal" productive member. |
| Tell Mrs. A.B. and she decides not to abort | 2. You told the truth. Mrs. A.B. was given right to participate. She is made anxious. She has a baby which may be normal or sociopathic, with societal consequences as above. | 5. You told the truth. Mrs. A.B. was given right to participate. She is made anxious. She has "normal" baby which she then may make abnormal by self-fulfilling prophecy mechanism. |
| Don't tell Mrs. A.B. | 3. You told a lie. Mrs. A.B. denied her right to participate. She is not made anxious. She has her child, with same risks and consequences as above. | 6. You told a lie. Mrs. A.B. denied her right of participation. She is not made anxious. She has "normal" baby and presumably will raise it normally. |

Note: In Squares 1, 2, and 3 the risk of the individual being a sociopath is related to how many XYY individuals develop that way (we know not all of them do) and how amenable the trait is to environmental correction. In Squares 4, 5, and 6 it must be remembered that the "normal" baby might still develop into a sociopath, by mechanisms other than the XYY genotype. The risk of this would be equal to the percentage of sociopaths in a randomly selected population.

We can start out by making some assumptions. First, presumably you are prepared to tell a lie if it can be shown that this will benefit Mrs. A.B. (If you accept the rule, "Never tell a lie," and admit no exceptions, you are not following our ethical method.) So whether you tell a lie or the truth must be of lesser consequence to you than the outcome for Mrs. A.B.; we can assign a zero value to your truth-telling, as being ethically neutral.

Next, note that we cannot predict in advance whether Mrs. A.B. will place a high value or a low value on her right of participation, until she is actually put on the spot. We also cannot know whether she is the sort who handles anxiety in stride or who tends to fly off the handle. However, it would be very inconsistent with everything we have said up to this point about the doctor-patient "contract" if we did not place a higher positive value on participation than the negative value on anxiety. After all, the anxiety can be lessened by judicious handling and emotional support by the physician; deprivation of rights cannot be so easily made up. So we can assign a moral value of "++" to granting the right, and "——" to withholding it without consent, while we assign a value of "—" to creating anxiety by telling Mrs. A.B. and "+" to preventing anxiety by not telling.

We can now assign arbitrary values to the other consequences. Call the consequence of aborting the child, from the mother's view, a —— while having the baby is ++. If society is spared the risk of the birth of a sociopath, we cannot call this more than + because one individual more or less cannot matter that much. The non-birth of a "normal" individual might otherwise be seen as —, but since we are having a population problem, we might want to call that 0 instead. If the baby is born and there is a risk of it becoming a sociopath, we know that the risk is less than 100%, and it is most probably significantly less than 50%. Under those circumstances the bad effects on society cannot be more than —, while for the mother, this would be a severe personal tragedy, so for her it would be ——. Because we have argued that the self-fulfilling prophecy is preventable, given that the mother is warned and that you or another doctor give good follow-up care, we can label this consequence a —, instead of making it worse. If we know the mother will raise the child normally, call this +.

Table 3 shows all these weighted-desirability values inserted into the appropriate squares in the table. Also in each square is the sum of the consequences in that square; the sum for each row of squares is shown at the right.

Table 3 gives us the following preference ranking:

     Tell followed by no abortion
     Don't tell
     Tell followed by abortion

However, assuming that we try to tell Mrs. A.B. in a way least likely to sway her opinion one way or the other, we cannot know in advance, if we tell her, which course of action she will choose. Therefore, we have to add the desirabilities for the two "tell" rows together. This gives us the new preference ranking:

     Tell

     Don't tell

382    We conclude, based on the values that we have placed on the various items, that we are better off telling Mrs. A.B. Therefore, our original rule can stand up; we need take into account neither the condition-of-doubt objection nor the self-fulfilling-prophecy objection in the rule itself (although we want to use both as warnings to ourselves to remind us of our responsibility).

If you disagree with our conclusion, you can go back and change some of the value assignments to make the sums come out in your favor. One way to do this is to put less weight on the right of participation; but, as we noted, this can be seen as the equivalent of putting a low-priority judgment on the entire doctor-patient "contract" as we described it in Chapter 4. Therefore, you should be willing to accept the various consequences, including paternalism, possible increase in patient mistrust, and all the others mentioned in that chapter.

383    We have devoted this much space to Case 28 not because it had a great deal to do with the topic of this chapter, but more because it gave us a good chance to illustrate some of the ethical decision-making methods we described in Chapter 2. However, consideration of this case has shown us that we want to be very careful before we decide that a competent patient is to be deprived of participation in a medical decision which has important ethical implications for him or her. Some significant reasons, such as condition of doubt and the self-fulfilling prophecy, can be given for denying participation, but in the final analysis these can generally be shown to be of insufficient weight to overturn the doctor-patient "contract."

384    With this, then, we can conclude our discussion of ethical participation. However, this problem will arise frequently in other cases as we go on to discuss specific issues in medical ethics. As we go on to these, you might want to refer back to the guidelines we listed earlier in this chapter, to see how they apply to the new cases.

Ch. 8 ▼ 385

Table 3

| | Causal connection between XYY and sociopathic behavior | No causal connection between XYY and sociopathic behavior | Sum |
|---|---|---|---|
| Tell Mrs. A.B. and she decides to have abortion | 0<br>++<br>−      [0]<br>+<br>−− | 0<br>++<br>−      [−]<br>−−<br>0 | − |
| Tell Mrs. A.B. and she decides not to have abortion | 0<br>++<br>−<br>++      [0]<br>−<br>−− | 0<br>++<br>−<br>++      [++]<br>− | ++ |
| Don't tell Mrs. A.B. | 0<br>−−<br>+<br>++      [−−]<br>−<br>−− | 0<br>−−<br>+<br>++      [++]<br>+ | 0 |

# 8. Specific Issues in Medical Ethics

We have now completed our discussion of the four key issues in medical ethics as outlined in Chapter 3. If you have been an active participant in this discussion, you now have in your possession at least the beginning of a conceptual understanding that will allow you to grapple effectively with any medical-ethical decision—an understanding that will allow you to come up with a thoughtful and rationally justifiable answer in the face of uncertainty and limited data, and in the face of the awareness that "right" answers may not be available.

385

However, while the conceptual understanding is the key to making any further progress, it ought to be fleshed out considerably, both with actual practice in making various types of ethical decisions, and with the data that are needed to understand particular ethical issues. On the latter point, recall from Chapter 2 how empirical data enters into the ethical decision-making process.

386

For example, abortion is now a timely medical-ethical issue because a woman must go to a physician to get an abortion. With the advent of "morning-after pills" which are now being tested, a woman will be able to have an abortion by herself, with the drug store being the only necessary resource. While abortion will not thus cease to be a medical-ethical issue, the practical power of making the decision will have passed out of the physician's hands. The existence of such a pill is the sort of data that one needs to approach such issues in a sensible manner.

We will attempt to provide both the practice with sample cases and some of the basic data for eight general areas of important issues in medical ethics. We will, however, try not to lose sight of the basic issues that we have already covered, and will try to show how these issues apply to each of these eight areas. Below is a short summary for each.

387

The problem of BEHAVIOR CONTROL cuts across all four areas that we have discussed. Perhaps most basic is the question: to what extent is our concept of our "quality of life" dependent upon freedom from obvious restrictions on our ability to make voluntary and self-aware decisions; and in what way would our self-perceived quality of life be altered if we no longer had control over our own actions or thoughts? Also, our whole understanding of the doctor-patient "contract" and of the meaning of informed consent must be modified when we take into account the fact that behavior-control techniques are already being used in medicine.

388

BEGINS ON 401

CONTROL OF REPRODUCTION has always been an emotionally charged issue, since we are making very significant quality-of-life decisions—both with regard to a child-to-be when we decide whether or not he is to be conceived; and with regard to the parent when we decide whether or not she shall bear a child. Also, this is another area where rights of participation have tended to be unclear: does society, either in its own right or as spokesman for the interests of the unborn, have anything to say, and if so, how is it to be heard?

389

BEGINS ON 478

390       HUMAN EXPERIMENTATION has also been an emotional issue for medical researchers, looking back as they do upon the vast progress made by medical science in this century. This has not prevented thoughtful investigators from raising tough questions—how is the doctor-patient relationship altered if the doctor is also an experimenter? And how can informed consent be meaningfully applied where there is so much uncertainty involved, as when the investigator himself does not know whether patient X is getting the experimental drug or a placebo? And can there ever be voluntary informed consent in the cases of minors or prisoners, both of which groups now make up significant pools of experimental subjects?

BEGINS ON 540

391       We have already shown that ALLOCATION OF SCARCE RESOURCES is, to some degree, an element of any ethical decision. The most significant resource-allocation problems, however, have to do with scarce societal resources such as money, technically sophisticated equipment, and trained personnel. Since society has a stake, what is its right of participation in these medical decisions—and what is the mode by which it is to be represented, since "society" is only an abstraction? How does the doctor-patient relationship change as the doctor is brought increasingly under resource-allocation constraints?

BEGINS ON 608

392       EUTHANASIA AND ALLOWING TO DIE have already been alluded to under the discussion of quality of life. The problem now before the public and the medical profession is: if quality of life decisions are to be made, and we are going to accept the physician saying that a certain patient may be better off dead than alive, how far are we willing to let the physician go in implementing this decision; and what sort of safeguards are we going to demand?

BEGINS ON 659

393       Another area in which societal interests have threatened to come into conflict with individual freedoms is that of MASS SCREENING PROGRAMS, such as genetic screening to locate carriers of sickle cell genes in the black community. What sort of voluntary consent is to be required for such programs? Has this sort of program turned society or some agent of it into the "doctor" in the doctor-patient relationship—and if so, how has the "contract" been rewritten as a result? How much governmental knowledge of our medical status as individuals is consistent with our ideas of quality of life?

BEGINS ON 717

Medical people have always made value judgments about which hereditary traits are good and which are bad, but until the development of recent technology, there was no way to attempt to implement any of these judgments. The issue of GENETIC ENGINEERING is analogous to euthanasia, in that the question arises of how far we will allow medical scientists to put their quality-of-life judgments into actual practice. Only here, the judgment affects not just one individual, but entire generations of unborn individuals—possibly the entire species. We saw how difficult it was to decide what constituted "informed consent" on behalf of a fetus in utero. Who can give "informed consent" on behalf of posterity?

BEGINS ON 765

Among the societal constraints that have the capacity to put significant strain upon the "Contractual Model" of the doctor-patient relationship are certain aspects of ORGANIZED MEDICINE AND MEDICAL ECONOMICS. While the physician may (wrongly) feel that he is not responsible for what society as a whole or what the government tells him he has to do, he is less able to cop out when the offending party is his own profession. If certain aspects of the medical profession itself, present or future, constitute part of the problem, at what point is the doctor ethically justified in refusing to participate? We stated that the doctor is released from his "contract" with the patient if following the patient's requests would entail an act which the doctor finds morally abhorrent. What is the nature of the individual practitioner's "contract" with his profession?

BEGINS ON 841

After dealing with these eight issues, we will conclude with two chapters on important basic concepts. The first is the question of how one defines "health" and "disease", and in particular the role of value judgments in this most basic area of medicine. If it is shown that our definitions of "health" and "disease" are based as much upon values as upon empirical knowledge, then the idea of medicine as an inherently ethically related enterprise will become still more clear.

The last chapter will provide a brief introduction to the very important and emerging concept of "bioethics." While the world of science and technology has traditionally been seen as separate and distinct from the realm of human values—a fiction which, for reasons already explained, we have used above for purposes of illustration—"bioethics" attempts to bridge this gap, by demonstrating how such contemporary problems as the destruction of the environment and the widespread sense of cultural rootlessness arise directly from the perpetuation of the science-values dichotomy.

BEGINS ON 895

397    To have been theoretically correct, we actually ought to have started out with the basic principles of "bioethics," since these relate the consequences of human values to man's biological survival. We would then have gone from these general principles to medical ethics as an applied case. However, in order to keep this book within reasonable size limitations, it will be possible only to give some very brief comments on bioethics. As in all other cases, the related readings listed in the reference section will provide adequate resources to fill the gaps.

398    Having skimmed the remainder of the table of contents, it remains to put into perspective the material that has not been included in this book. In general, the primary gap has been left in the area which we have alluded to several times as "medical sociology."

It may not have been clear why we drew such a firm distinction between medical ethics and medical sociology. In the earlier chapters, the first order of business was to outline an ethical method, and to prove that one exists. Since there is so much fuzzy thinking in actual practice about what ethics is all about, it seemed important at the time to clarify this by pointing out some things medical ethics is not. In Chapter 2 we took pains, for example, to point out that medical ethics is not the Hippocratic Oath, nor is it the law. One other thing it is not is medical sociology, which falls into the category of the empirical data that must be plugged into the ethical problem-solving method.

REVIEW ↑
DATA ┆ 38

399    Making use of this sort of distinction for conceptual clarification, however, is justified only so long as we remember that in actual practice, the distinction must break down. No one, doctors least of all, can be isolated from their social backgrounds. The values which are at the heart of the ethical decision-making process will be determined in large part by social context; and social context will lead one to emphasize some pieces of empirical data and to ignore others. Since medicine and the health professions form a rather distinct and autonomous subculture, it is clear that ethical decisions in medicine cannot be treated in isolation from these considerations. We have called attention to medical-socio-logical concepts where they have been particularly relevant—for example, the question of how widespread is the belief that fully informed consent will scare patients away from needed treatment.

400    The material that is being omitted from this book, which is often included in other books on medical ethics, involves issues such as the proper role of the doctor as an agent for various social institutions, such as military doctors, prison doctors, and psychiatrists called upon to help commit individuals to institutions involuntarily. Also of importance are matters such as the power of the drug industry and the implications of the fee-for-service system, which are touched upon in Chapter 16 but which could be discussed in much greater depth. These topics are being omitted largely because the sorts of ethical decisions they entail are very similar to those described in this unit; the problem is not deciding what is ethical so much as it is acquiring the freedom of action to follow one's ethical judgments. The interested reader will find chapters devoted to all these problems in the books edited by Torrey and by Visscher, which are listed under the "Medical Ethics—General" heading in the references. Also see the suggested reading list for Chapter 16.                    Ch. 9 ↓ 401

# 9. Behavior Control

Presumably all of us, to some degree or other, control our own behavior. Behavior control becomes a matter of medical ethics either when the means utilized to control one's own behavior fall into the category which we term "artificial," or else when one person undertakes to control the behavior of another. These may be accomplished by a number of techniques.

401

Possibly the oldest form of behavior modification by artificial means was the use of psychoactive drugs. Alcohol may have been the oldest such substance in general use; of course the number of compounds available for such purposes has increased considerably in recent years. This category must include commonly abused street drugs, drugs used in psychiatry such as tranquilizers and anti-depressants, and substances such as alcohol, coffee, and tea which in the public mind are usually not classified as drugs at all.

402

A second group of behavior control techniques could be classed as "persuasion," in which there is no physical-chemical contact between the controller and controlee. Psychotherapy fits into this category, as do the newer methods of behavior modification and operant conditioning; we also have to include mass control techniques such as propaganda and advertising. Sometimes these are used in combination with other techniques. For example, the drug succinyl-choline in certain doses gives the subject a very unpleasant sensation of drowning. This has been used in behavior modification, to negatively condition persons such as alcoholics by attempting to associate the unpleasant sensation with the unwanted behavior.

403

A third and particularly controversial technique is psychosurgery, which is distinguished from neurosurgery in that the brain to be operated on in the former has no identifiable pathological lesion. The first such technique was lobotomy, pioneered in the 1930's, which fell into disuse when it became obvious that the result was usually an almost complete blunting of the victim's emotions and higher functions. Psychosurgery is now on the rise with new techniques that are claimed to be more specific than the old lobotomy. A new development is the implantation into specific brain areas of micro-electrodes, which can then be electrically stimulated at will.

404

All the techniques mentioned have been shown to be effective in producing changes in behavior—how precisely, we shall come to later. The next question is what motives a person might have for wishing to control the behavior of another person by these means. We might distinguish three general types of motives.

405

1) Therapeutic: the assumption is made here that the control is being offered to correct some defect which the person to be controlled recognizes as such, or would recognize if he were rational. The therapist is acting as an agent of the patient; this is merely an extension of behavioral self-control.

2) Societal: it is assumed that certain types of behaviors are detrimental to society and thus to the good of all the individuals that make up society. Behavior control may be used to prevent or correct these behaviors.

**405 cont.**  3)  Manipulative: person A controls the behavior of person B without regard for person B's best interests, because the result is beneficial in some way to A.

**406**    Before examining the ethics of each of these motives, we might note that often elements of all three are operating in any given case. Since (as in the case of abortion) the line of argument used to justify the act will be partly determined by the motive, it is easy to see how this mixture of motives leads to lack of clarity in ethical debates on this subject. For example, one of the most slippery concepts in use today is the idea of "rehabilitation" of criminals, in which the motives of therapeutics and of benefit to society are combined in a tangled and sometimes self-contradictory manner. Also, in any instance where one person (such as the doctor) is in control of either the "therapy" or the "social benefit," the problem of manipulation is almost bound to arise, even if only to a slight degree.

**407**    We might now wish to attach ethical values to the three motives—saying for example, that the manipulative is to be condemned; that the societal is to be condoned in certain special instances, but that we ought to have stringent safeguards to prevent its misuse; and that in most instances, with minor safeguards, the therapeutic is all right.

   However, this argument is premature, unless we show that there is some viable alternative to the use of the behavior control techniques which we wish to prohibit. As we saw in Chapter 2, there can be no ethical decision if there is no real choice among alternatives. One line of argument, put forth most ably by the psychologist B.F. Skinner, calls for increased use of behavior control techniques precisely because this choice is not a real one in this instance.

**408**    Anyone arguing why behavior control is wrong is most likely to fall back on arguments appealing to the freedom of the individual to make choices, or to the dignity of the individual human being. Skinner retorts that in fact, concepts such as "freedom" and "dignity" are empty and outmoded. Just like primitive man might invent a rain god to explain a natural phenomenon of which he has no real understanding, we have invented "freedom" and "dignity" as pseudo-explanations of human conduct whose motives are hidden from us. Freedom and dignity are concepts not of reality but of ignorance.

**409**    By following the "freedom and dignity" ethics (Skinner says) we withhold praise from a person who does something for some obvious motive, such as money, while praising someone who does the same thing for "the good of humanity" or some other "altruistic" motive. If we really looked into the matter, Skinner contends, we would find that the second person was also acting out of a motive, such as some psychological force in his character, and was just as powerless to disobey that motive as was the first person. Therefore neither person has done anything intrinsically worthy of praise or blame, and the concepts of "freedom" and "dignity" apply in neither case.

In Skinner's behaviorist view, all behavior is conditioned——we do what we have been positively reinforced to do and avoid what we have been negatively reinforced. If the language of "freedom" and "dignity" has any use, it is because many of us have been conditioned to those words, so that they reinforce our acting in socially useful ways. But they lose this usefulness if they lead us to praise or blame people, or to question motives, instead of seeing that behavior modification through conditioning is the only effective way to go.

410

Once we see the emptiness of the freedom-and-dignity way of looking at things, Skinner argues, we come to realize that our behavior is always being controlled or shaped by forces outside of our power. Society condones this, as with advertising and Madison Avenue techniques. In some places society even places a very high value on it, such as the behavior modification and control that we call "going to school."

411

Even though we control others' behavior and others control ours, the whole system is very inefficient, precisely because we try to deny what we are really doing by hiding behind the freedom-and-dignity concepts. The real challenge, Skinner says, is to replace these ineffectual techniques with scientifically proven methods. In particular, we must look into the matter of behavior counter-control. If these things are done, the "good guys" will be able to control behavior to achieve the greatest social good and individual happiness; and they will also be able to prevent the "bad guys" (who are now threatening to run the show) from taking over the behavior control system for their own manipulative ends.

412

Skinner's views can be (and have been) attacked on a number of philosophical grounds. However, at present they represent one of the most formidable obstacles that an argument opposed to the more widespread use of behavior control must overcome. They also illustrate a point that we have alluded to earlier—that the kinds of ethical decisions one makes are closely tied up with one's personal view of the future. Clearly Skinner is envisioning a Utopia that has many features which we might not want to include in our view of the future world; and this is the basis for much of the debate.

413

What has been said against Skinner's arguments? The best critics of Skinner generally agree that the environment plays a large part in shaping our behavior and our values, but object that Skinner's views place too much emphasis on externally observable behavior while neglecting the internal workings of the mind.

414

What proof can be offered that these internal workings exist? One line of thought, on philosophical lines, is related to the views of existentialism. Simply put, this denies that free will is something that either exists within us or does not. Rather, freedom is something we achieve through our own actions—we become free through the process of making choices.

415    Rhinelander launches a more direct philosophical attack by showing where we might catch the Skinnerian attributing his behaviorist model to others but not to himself. For instance, by Skinner's theory, it would be incorrect to say that one is a behaviorist because one believes that it is true; that is a motive and assumes one has the freedom to choose what to believe. One must simply say that the behaviorist has been positively reinforced by behaviorist theory. But we might well expect to find the behaviorist wanting to insist on more than that, which he cannot do without denying his theory.

416    Another view, somewhat less abstract, is offered by Platt, who seeks a compromise position between the two extremes of the "freedom" and "dignity" ideas and Skinner's total rejection of them. Platt does this basically by preferring the phrase "self-control" to the idea of "free will." *This recognizes the existence of an individual, internally experienced "self," which is what the humanistic critics of Skinner are anxious to maintain; on the other hand, by omitting the word "free," it reminds us of Skinner's point that the behavior of the "self" is determined in large share by environmental factors.*

417    Platt also adds a note to remind us that "largely determined by environmental factors" does not mean "completely determined" in the sense of allowing accurate predictions of all behaviors from outside observations. Because of the complexity of the brain structure and because of the random nature of mental processes, there will always be a level of uncertainty in our knowledge of the workings of the mind. Thus, at least some of the "privacy" that the humanists want to protect seems to be safe.

418    We should also note that Skinner has given a practical warning in his emphasis on counter-control. Behavior control can work; and if we assume that various evil people may at some time want to use it against us, our only defense is to know enough about the techniques of behavior control to be able to detect this—or, even better, to be able to use morally acceptable means of control to reform those evil people. Therefore, in this as in many other areas of experimental biology, we might want to encourage basic research in behavior control, even while we are opposing behavior control as applied technology.

419    We have now examined the motives for employing behavior control. According to our ethical method, this discussion has only set the stage for the major task, which is to determine the consequences of behavior control— in particular, the side effects that are not part of the intended consequences and which may not be immediately evident. In keeping with our views of the future, we also want to inquire particularly into the long-range side effects for society.

The specific side effects of each individual drug or psychosurgical procedure would have to be listed separately; however, some general observations are possible. While psychology and neurophysiology have hardly scratched the surface when it comes to understanding the mind and the sources of behavior, it does seem to be a legitimate conclusion that mental functions are complexly integrated, and involve feedback circuits among a large number of subcomponents of the system. *Just as killing off a species of insect, or drying up a pond, can eventually disrupt an entire ecosystem, the alteration of one of the mental subcomponents by chemical or physical means must eventually have an impact upon many other, seemingly unrelated mental functions.*

It is of interest that the scientific justification offered, implicitly or explicitly, for modern psychosurgery is the idea that specific emotions or behaviors, such as rage or pleasure, are located in specific areas of the brain. It is ironic that at the same time when the neurophysiological theories of brain function are becomingly increasingly complex, the psychosurgery researchers are going back to this less sophisticated view.

This account of the complexity of the mind leads to the conclusion that, while we might have to do research to determine the unwanted side effects of any particular technique, these unwanted side effects will almost certainly exist. It might also suggest that the ethical problems will be greater where the number and magnitude of these side effects are greater. (One could also argue the other way: we were able to mobilize medical opinion against lobotomy in the 1940's precisely because the effects were so grossly observable. The newer methods are more dangerous and more open to misuse precisely because they are more subtle.)

The side effects we are particularly concerned about might be described as "lessening of consciousness" or "lessening of choice." These occur with lobotomies or the use of tranquilizing drugs, which seek to eliminate the particular unwanted behavior either by lessening the subject's power to perform a whole series of behaviors; or else by making him less aware of a variety of external stimuli, some of which had acted to trigger the unwanted behavior.

It should be noted, however, that some experts, who agree that the lobotomy procedure of the 1940's and 1950's had too many adverse side effects to be used justifiably, nevertheless feel that the emotional and political reaction to these old techniques has gotten in the way of recognition of genuine advances in the form of the new techniques, which produce much smaller and more specific lesions. In reviewing the current literature, Sweet cites in particular one study in Australia, which performed a limited psychosurgery technique called cingulotomy on 48 patients, all of whom had been treated unsuccessfully for severe depression, with medical therapy, for at least five years. Sweet quotes the investigators as reporting that 88% had "remission of all symptoms and ability to work at the pre-illness level or better," with "no instances of impairment of social awareness or deterioration in ethico-moral behavior after operation." *

*Reprinted, by permission. From the New England Journal of Medicine 289:1117, 1973.

**423**    Sweet also questions the universal assumption that any psychosurgery is an irreversible procedure: "Although it is true that new neurons do not replace the ones destroyed, those that remain possess extraordinary capacity to re-establish new connections or take over functions that they did not have before."

Sweet concludes his survey by noting that the results of limited psychosurgery in a number of English and Australian studies, on patients who have not responded to other therapy, are good enough so that new controlled, randomized studies ought to be carried out in the U.S. Thus, he feels that psychosurgery might well be employed ethically in at least one class of patients—those unresponsive to all other therapy. However, the physiologic rationale that he offers for why limited psychosurgery "works" is essentially no more sophisticated than the one given above—the equation of specific brain areas with specific mental functions.

**424**    If we conclude from all this that there is still a significant possibility of behavior-control techniques of this type producing undesirable side effects, we ought to bring in the quality-of-life argument. By most lists of criteria, one is less of a "person" if he has a lowered range of alternatives and if he is less able to respond to environmental stimuli. These are among the behavioral side effects commonly claimed as the result of psychosurgery, and certainly as the result of the use of the major tranquilizing drugs. Focusing on the consequences for the individual patient, then, one would have to weigh these adverse possibilities against the patient's present quality of life in a mental institution. (Sweet contends that many of the candidates for psychosurgery are presently, in fact, compulsively and repetitively over-responding to internal instead of external stimuli, so these sorts of "side effects" might be exactly what is required.)

**425**    If one focuses on some of the possible longer-range consequences, one may use a biological analogy, and anticipate some of the points we will discuss under bioethics in Chapter 18. If we look just at the survival value of different behaviors in the natural world, we are drawn to the conclusion that variability and adaptability are two qualities which give a species an increased chance for survival. If it turns out that behavior control techniques tend to limit the individual's adaptability, and tend to produce uniformity of behavior by blunting individual differences, we might be fearful that such techniques might decrease the survival capacity of man as a species. (However, how widespread must the use of such techniques become before this would occur?) We might argue as an alternative that we ought to try to solve our problems by creating new, more sophisticated behaviors, rather than seeking to eliminate or mask existing behaviors in hopes that the problem will go away.

**426**    Note that usually behavior control is not aimed at behavior alone; behavior is not "bad" unless it occurs in a particular context or setting. The problem is not bad behavior, but rather behavior that is inappropriate for the environment in which it occurs.

*Therefore, as relates to quality of life, one of the central questions on behavior control is: Do we want to live in a future where these conflicts are resolved by changing persons' inner selves, or one where they are resolved by changing the outer environment? If our answer (as we would expect) is some of each, the question then becomes how much of each and in what situations.* We can see arguments of this sort today. Those who would rather manipulate environments than people urge eliminating poverty as a solution to the problem of crime, while those who prefer a different future want to throw the criminals in prison.

Take another, more extreme argument against behavior control. This would say that the possible tyrannical uses of these techniques outweighs any good that we might derive from them; and that if we allow even the so-called harmless uses now, we are just opening the door to future abuses.

This argument ought to look familiar; we called it the "domino theory" when we examined it in the context of sanctity of life. We saw there that it made the error of assuming that the entire decision, for now and ever after, was being made in one sweep; and of denying that there would be many times in the future when we could step in and say, "Okay, we have now gone far enough." (One author, tongue presumably in cheek, stated this in the form of a rule: "Never do anything for the first time.")

REVIEW
"DOMINO THEORY" 227

However, there may be reasons to give the "domino" argument more weight in the matter of behavior control than we assigned to it before in different contexts. That is because it is the nature of <u>some</u> sorts of behavior control techniques to diminish one's capabilities for making choices in the future. While in the matter of legalizing abortion, there is nothing to prevent us from stepping in later if someone wants to start shooting elderly patients in nursing homes; if we allow our behavior to be controlled now, we might be rendered unable to object in the future if abuses are planned.

We might, therefore, not dismiss the domino argument so easily here. At any rate, it should serve to remind us that we must be particularly sensitive to long-range consequences.

## CASE 29

R.J. is a 33-year-old man who has been diagnosed as having temporal lobe epilepsy, which occasionally causes him to exhibit involuntarily violent behavior when he has an epileptic seizure. On two occasions he has physically assaulted members of his family, and he is very concerned about what he might do in the future. You are aware that this sort of problem has been traced to specific organic lesions in the brain. So far your attempts to treat him by drugs have been of limited success. You are considering referring R.J. to a neurosurgeon who has had some success in treating such cases. You have explained to R.J. what would be involved in such surgery, and he has indicated his desire to go ahead.

However, when you chanced to mention this case to your minister, he raised objections to such neurosurgery on moral grounds. He contended that the essence of man was free choice, and that it was immoral to surgically tamper with a man's brain so that he would act in the way we wanted.

What do you do in Mr. R.J.'s case?

430      First question: Is this a psychosurgery case? Recall that we defined psychosurgery as surgical intervention into the brain in the absence of demonstrable organic pathology. While we have not made sections of Mr. R.J.'s brain for histological examination, we have presumptive evidence to believe that if the diagnosis of epilepsy is correct, such pathology is likely to be present. Therefore, the label of "neurosurgery" is justified.

     Second question: Which of the three motives is operative here? The case was written so that the cards were heavily stacked toward the therapeutic motive. We have the patient's voluntary and presumably informed consent. As primary physician, you are not even going to get any fee for the surgery, while you would get a fee if you continued to treat Mr. R.J. medically.

     The answers to these questions show why Mr. R.J.'s case presents fewer ethical problems than many other cases we could envision.

431      How do you evaluate the minister's argument? It is not too hard to overcome because it represents a mockery of the facts of the case. Mr. R.J.'s problem is precisely the lack of free choice. When he has a seizure, he commits violence whether he wants to or not. With the surgery, if performed correctly, there is at least hope that he will no longer have these seizures, though he will still be capable of violent acts if provoked for other reasons.

     This argument ought to reinforce the notion that control of behavior and free ethical choices are by no means contradictory notions. If we could not control our own behavior, how could we act ethically? We would never know if our bodies would implement the ethical judgment we had made, or whether our bodies would, of their own accord, do exactly the opposite.

432      All of our discussion of Case 29 assumes that there is such a thing as temporal lobe epilepsy and that it has been correctly diagnosed in this case. Opponents of psychosurgery have charged that this diagnosis is abused in such cases—that such a diagnosis is made where no organic lesion has in fact been identified, in order to justify the surgery. This debate has become so polarized that two authors, Breggin and Mark, have described the case of the same patient in radically different terms. Mark describes a patient with symptoms similar to those in Case 29, and states that after surgery he returned to essentially normal function. Breggin states that he is familiar with that case and that the man actually ended up back in a mental hospital in much worsened condition. You will have to read the arguments of Mark and Breggin and take your pick (see references for this chapter).

## CASE 30

As public health physician employed by the metropolitan school system, you are aware that there is a disorder in children known as hyperkinesis, which produces "hyperactivity" beyond the conscious control of the child. Such children are unable to pay attention for any length of time and thus do poorly in school, out of proportion to their actual intelligence. Because there has been no organic lesion identified although the disease is presumed to have an organic basis, the condition is also referred to as "minimal brain dysfunction."

You also know that amphetamines, which are called "speed" because they tend to produce increased activity and alertness in people who use them, have a paradoxical effect on hyperkinetic youngsters—the drugs slow them down and allow them to sit still and pay attention. One such drug commonly used is methylphenidate, manufactured under the trade name of Ritalin.

Your school nurses want you to write a blanket prescription for Ritalin for any children found to need it by the teachers. They argue that the teacher sees the child all day and thus is best qualified to judge those children who would benefit from the drug.

What do you do?

---

This case represents more than a strictly medical decision—it asks one to determine a matter of public policy as regards a technique of behavioral control. How ought one to approach such a determination? You might wish to begin by taking a specific proposal and examining it according to questions such as:

1) What are the criteria for the "disease" that you are treating? Who has determined these criteria?

2) Who is going to assess the individual subjects based on these criteria to see which have the disease? Are they competent to do so?

3) Who is going to apply the treatment to the subjects thus selected? Are they competent to do so?

4) What is the goal of the treatment? Who is going to assess the subjects to see whether this goal has been accomplished?

5) What are the other consequences of the treatment? In particular, what are the social consequences for the subjects who have now been labelled as having this disease?

Taking the proposal as put down in Case 30, we see that no mention is made of the criteria for determining hyperkinesis. In fact, the diagnosis requires careful psychological evaluation, to rule out other possible causes such as emotional disturbance. We see that the teachers are going to judge which children are "hyperactive" so that the nurses can give out the Ritalin, and that no provision has been made for followup on individual cases.

436    When a plan of this sort was put into effect in Omaha several years ago, it was found in a later survey that 30% of the school children were receiving Ritalin. Simply by statistics, it is impossible that that many children were actually suffering from hyperkinesis in the strict medical sense. In retrospect, it was clear that the teachers were simply displaying a low tolerance for the normal activity levels and low attention span of youngsters in the elementary school age group, and were using their own exasperation with their chaotic classrooms as the criteria to determine use of the drug. The result was that 30% of the school children were being made to ingest a psychoactive drug, and possibly were receiving significant training for later life—if you have a problem, reach for a bottle of pills to solve it.

437    It is interesting to ask what happened to the medical profession in Omaha during all this business, especially since doctors are traditionally very jealous about their power over the prescribing of drugs. We might also wonder what happened to the parents during all this. It may well have been that the idea that their child was receiving a medicine to help him do better in school was satisfying enough to the parents. This brings back the point about the social context in which behavior occurs. We live in a society that is still dominated by the so-called "protestant ethic," which among other things places very high value upon socially useful work. Thus, we might be expected to be much more tolerant of the use of behavior control when it serves the purpose of promoting this kind of "socially useful" behavior. Although caffeine is demonstrably a drug and has a number of known harmful side effects, we hear no social condemnation of the morning cup of coffee that allows us to wake up enough to trudge to work. (It is now being suggested that a cup of coffee or two for the hyperkinetic child may replace Ritalin as the standard approved therapy!)

438    As far as amphetamines go, it is interesting to review the situations in which these drugs are "medically indicated" and "medically not indicated." The former category involves only two conditions: hyperkinesis, and narcolepsy (in which the victim is subject to falling asleep spontaneously at inopportune moments). Uses of amphetamines not sanctioned by the medical establishment include street users who want to get "spaced out", and use as "diet pills" because of their (temporary) effect of curbing appetite.
       While there are medical justifications for this categorization, it is at least curious that the distinctions correspond almost precisely to the values of the "protestant ethic." Narcoleptics and hyperkinetic kids can't work effectively, so it is all right to use drugs on them to correct this. Obesity, on the other hand, does not preclude useful work, and besides the fat person ought to have enough will power to eat less without using a "crutch." And it is clear that the person who is high on speed is not being socially useful at all and ought to be condemned.

439    Final note on Case 30: One critic suggested that as long as you were going to use some sort of drug to solve the problem, it would have made much more sense to give tranquilizers to the teachers.

## CASE 31

You are the same school physician. After kicking the nurse, who wants to dispense Ritalin, out of your office, you pick up the latest medical journal and read that a new drug has just reached the market. Its chemical name is 3', 5'-cyclic I.Q., and it is being marketed under the trade name of Precocitabs. Its effect on children is to increase the measurable I.Q. by 15 to 20 points as well as improving performance on school exams, intellectual problems, and all sorts of other mental tasks.

While the drug has not yet been tested in pregnant women, clinical trials involving 4000 children over a two-year period have turned up no significant side effects from the drug.

Would you want to prescribe this drug for all the children in your school system? None of them? Some of them?

---

While so far we have emphasized the use of behavior control techniques to get rid of bad behavior, there is certainly another side to the coin. Such techniques could conceivably be used to promote "good" behavior. We would then be stuck with coming up with some consensus on what "good" is. Those who believe that abuses of behavior control can best be prevented by keeping the number and types of allowed intervention to a minimum are particularly dismayed by these proposed "good" uses.

How does your judgment on this case compare with your judgment in the Ritalin case (remember the five questions)? If there is a difference, is it rationally justifiable? Is it possible to make ethical judgments on "psychoactive drugs" across the board?

---

## CASE 32

You are a clinical psychologist specializing in behavior modification through operant conditioning techniques. A middle-aged woman, Mrs. B.K., comes to you seeking treatment. She states that she suffers from feelings of anxiety and depression, and freely relates these to the fact that her husband is continually involved in affairs with other women. However, Mrs. B.K. is devoted to her family and enjoys the security of marriage, so even though she has decided that her husband will never change, she considers divorce out of the question. She wants you to help desensitize her so that she will not have this emotional response to her husband's affairs.

Do you accept Mrs. B.K. for therapy or not, assuming that you have the techniques required to bring about the desired goal?

---

Let's examine both sides of this case. If you agree to treat Mrs. B.K., you seem to be coming down on the side of those who would prefer to alter the individual's inner self, when one could conceivably alter the environment instead. (Or you could argue that the environment is, for all practical purposes, unalterable, since the husband is not willing to seek therapy.) Is this the same as saying that the problem is not in the family relationship, or in the husband, but rather within Mrs. B.K. herself? And if you are not saying this, then why treat Mrs. B.K. instead of the place where the problem actually exists?

444     On the other hand, suppose you decide not to treat (as did the therapist in the original case), on the grounds that you would only be helping Mrs. B.K. to ignore a very real problem in her environment. You might argue that her desires not to be upset by her husband's tomcatting and her desires for the security of marriage are incompatible, and the sooner she comes to the realization that she can't have her cake and eat it too, the better off she will be.

However, is this a fair statement of the real situation in which Mrs. B.K. finds herself? Is she all that unaware of what her problem is and what alternatives are open to her? Since she has made this particular choice, isn't it a bit paternalistic of you to decide that you know what is in her best interests better than she does?

If you are not going to treat Mrs. B.K., you would seem at least to have an obligation to steer her to someone else who can help her with her problem, be it internal or environmental. What advice are you going to give her on this score?

445     If, instead of coming for behavior modification, Mrs. B.K. went to a psychiatrist with a request for a tranquilizer, you might propose a compromise. You might ask to prescribe the tranquilizer as an immediate step and to help gain the confidence of the patient; then, in followup visits, you could enter into discussion of the real problem and try to assess how Mrs. B.K. might best solve it.

The only thing wrong with this course is that once the immediate needs are met by the symptomatic treatment, the patient's motivation to grapple with the underlying problem will be greatly diminished. Thus, your compromise could easily turn into a cop-out, with the patient joining the growing army of chronic tranquilizer users. Of course, you could avoid this by exercising diligence and good clinical judgment.

## CASE 33

446     A 22-year-old black law student comes to you saying that he thinks he could use the help of a psychotherapist. He states that his problem is constant anxiety, which he attributes to the pressures of competing with his mostly white classmates who have had a better academic preparation than he was able to get at his all-black college. So far he has kept up with his studies, but has lately been worried that the anxiety and the pressure were interfering with his academic performance. He thinks he could do better if he could relax more.

In the course of your routine questioning, you elicit the information that he is a practicing homosexual and has been for several years. He contends that he is comfortable with his sexuality and that he has had no anxiety or guilt related to any of his homosexual encounters or relationships.

Do you:
1)  Try to treat him for his homosexuality, since that is the most likely cause of his anxiety?          447

2)  Treat the anxiety alone, accepting his reasoning that it arises from academic pressure?          448

Are you justified in the assumption that the homosexuality is more likely 447
to be the source of anxiety than the academic pressure? As the case is written, what is the evidence to support this? Or are you making the assumption that all homosexuals are anxious and guilty as a result of their sexual preferences?

Even if the question just preceding is answered in the affirmative, recall that the student did not ask you to treat his homosexuality; he stated that he saw no reason to alter his sexual habits. Is it overly paternalistic to attempt to change a behavior which the patient does not want to change? (More pragmatically—what are your chances of succeeding?)

↓ 448

---

448

In recent years psychiatrists have been sharply divided on the issue of whether homosexuality is "abnormal" in its own right, or if at least some homosexuals can be well-adjusted (provided society gets off their backs). At any rate, you seem justified in deciding to treat what the patient came to you complaining of, and of accepting an obvious source of anxiety without creating a more obscure one on your own.

Don't forget that if your attempts to treat the anxiety on the basis of the academic-pressure assumption fail, you can always re-evaluate the situation with the patient to determine whether the homosexuality might be a problem after all.

↓

449

In the actual case, the psychotherapist decided the treatment should be directed immediately at the homosexuality. This led one commentator to note that the poor patient went to the doctor with one problem (anxiety) and came away with two (anxiety plus the "problem" of homosexuality). Furthermore, he was especially bad off in that both his problems have a very poor prognosis— the anxiety because the doctor is refusing to treat it; and the homosexuality because psychotherapy has a very bad track record in treating this disorder. Presumably, patients do not go to doctors in order to have their problems multiplied and rendered incurable.

↓

450

Incidentally, can one make any ethical generalizations about psychotherapy as related to behavior modification? Obviously psychotherapy can succeed only if the patient accepts the authority of, and opens himself up to, the therapist. This could be seen as an advantage, since these are unlikely to occur where there is not genuine voluntary consent. Behavior modification enthusiasts, on the other hand, attack psychotherapy on the grounds that it represents an unwarranted invasion of privacy; through their own techniques, they claim, the same or better results can be achieved in a shorter time without any of this paternalistic prying.

This leads to the old question about treating the "symptoms" rather than the "root causes" of mental disorders. The question certainly has important ethical implications, since the amount of invasion of privacy or loss of self-esteem to which you might be willing to subject a patient has to be weighed against the likelihood of a successful outcome with that sort of therapy. This debate is so complex, however, that it can better be presented within the context of a psychiatry course.

↓

451     The symptom vs. cause argument leads to a more basic question. You may have noticed that the list of three motives which began this chapter made no mention of "mental illness," although some such concept has been alluded to in several places since. Just what do we mean by "mental illness"? The answer to this question is of great importance if we are going to distinguish the situations where the therapeutic motive is acting from the purely societal or manipulative cases. It is also of prime importance as the answer to the first model questions we presented for deciding public policy with regard to behavior control therapies.

452     One view, which has become popular in psychiatry with the advent of recent biochemical discoveries relating to brain function, holds that mental illnesses are discreet entities, for each of which a distinct pathological—biochemical lesion has been or someday will be found. The finding of this specific lesion for each specific illness will then lead to the discovery of specific treatment modes, which will probably emphasize chemical means to correct the biochemical imbalances. If certain aspects of psychiatry do not meet these specifications, it is assumed that this is because all the facts are not yet known.

453     The extreme opposite view holds that there is no such thing as mental "illness." Rather, there are problems of communication and disorders of human relations; these are considered more or less tolerable by other people depending on a number of social factors such as socioeconomic class.
        When, because of the social and cultural context, the disorder is viewed as being particularly intolerable, the responsible person is labelled with the mythical label of "mentally ill." This is not a descriptive term; rather it is a political move to justify the things that we wish to do to the person. These may include both good things like offering sympathy and removing the responsibilities of job so that the person can be treated; and the nasty things like locking the person up in an institution and taking away his civil rights.

454     It seems clear to everyone but the psychiatrists who support these two extreme views that the answer lies in a bit of both. There may well be a spectrum of mental disorders, ranging from the almost purely "organic" to the ones for which no pathological lesion has been or probably will be identified. As a matter of fact, we have to broaden this spectrum to blur over the distinction between "physical" and "mental" illness, since many diseases of other parts of the body affect the brain functions, and many mind disorders show themselves as, or lead to, problems in other organs. Given the many intricate interconnections between the "mind" and "body," it would be rather surprising if it were any other way.

455     When it comes to formal definitions, one might suspect that the whole problem is related to immediately seeking to define the disease, while the state of health is presumably what we are really interested in. Can we do better by trying to define "mental health"?
        Try out this rather complicated definition, paraphrased from one offered by Robert Neville:  Mental health consists of maximizing the various mental capacities, in a balanced manner, so that it is possible both to have inner understanding and peace, and to achieve relevant and discerning fulfillment with respect to the outer environment. (From a presentation to the Workshop on Medical Ethics, Berkeley, Cal., July 1973)

We'll leave it to you, if you wish, to decide what is meant by each specific item in the definition. For now, notice two points. First, this definition repeats our earlier observation that mental health must be assessed with respect to the outer environment in which the behavior is to occur. But in addition, it adds mention of "inner understanding and peace"—in effect adding on an inner environment as well, and demanding that the healthy mind will be in harmony with both environments. It is precisely this "inner world" which is denied by the behaviorist followers of B.F. Skinner and others, who would hold that the externally observable behavior expresses the whole realm of mental function. If one denies the existence of the inner environment, it is not hard to see how Skinner can discard the concepts of "freedom" and "dignity" so easily.

Second, note that this definition has stacked the deck against those types of behavior control that act by a general blunting of emotion or intellect. According to the definition, a person is rendered less mentally healthy by any such means. We noted before, in the discussion on "primum non nocere," that medicine has accepted the principle of making a person sicker in order to make him well later, such as surgery. However, in order for this to apply, there must be reasonable assurances that the sickness will be only temporary, and most of the behavior-control therapies fail to offer this assurance.

REVIEW
"PRIMUM . . ." | 308—309

So far behavior-control techniques have been attacked on the grounds that they are consciousness-limiting, and the impression may have been given that all or most behavior control techniques fall into this category. Of those drugs used outside of the doctor-patient relationship, alcohol and the opiates do seem to fit this description; but the hallucinogenic drugs seem to be a different case entirely. At least in the view of their advocates, such drugs are used precisely for their mind-expanding capability; in fact, some say, they may even make the user more mentally healthy. (Is this somewhat analogous to the high-I.Q. pill hypothesized in Case 31?)

Several justifications for the expansion of consciousness by chemical means can be advanced. One is an alternative-religion model, in which Utopia is viewed as an esthetic experience in the present instead of an ascetic afterlife yet to come. Another rejects the possibility of using drugs to achieve a single cohesive world-view, but rather makes reference to the desirability of variability and pluralism, and sees drug experiences as additions to the variety of one's life.

While several objections can be cited to these views, this seems to be another instance of disagreement based on different views of the future. One states that drug use does not lead to real mind-expansion, but only gives an escapist a superficial impression of doing so; and it is really the escapism rather than the supposed mind-expansion that the user seeks. It is hard to see how such a statement can be proved or disproved on empirical grounds; it may boil down to differences in taste and life style. Besides, people are capable of using just about anything as an escapist device, if escape is what they want.

Another objection points to the deleterious side effects of drugs such as marijuana and LSD as reasons not to engage in their use. Again, potential risks must be weighed against potential benefits, and it is clear that the risks must be very great to outweigh the benefits proposed by the alternative-religion or the pluralism-of-experience models, so long as one actually values those outcomes highly. Besides, even the "protestant ethic" has social consequences that could be termed adverse side effects; the side effects always seem to be minimal if one places a high value on the hoped-for outcome.

460      In summary, it must be acknowledged that one can frame an adequate ethical foundation for the use of psychoactive drugs for the purpose of expanding consciousness.

As noted, this is not a central issue to medical ethics since these drugs are generally obtained and used without the services of a physician. The most important medical-ethical issues concern the position the medical profession is to take on the social policies relating to the use of drugs, and whether there is an obligation to educate the public at large on the possible side effects, or lack of them, arising from drug use.

461      Related to this public obligation is the work of some groups of investigators who openly admit that they view marijuana as a great evil and want to see it outlawed. They have on occasion announced their research results before news conferences, claiming that they have evidence to show (e.g.) that marijuana increases the incidence of infection by altering the white blood cells. When the research subsequently appears in scientific journals, their original claims are often found to be overstated considerably. Responsible researchers might well ask what the long-range consequences of this sort of policy will be on public trust in statements of the medical profession.

462      Before ending the discussion, we might say a bit more about the problem of labeling, which was mentioned in the last of the five public-policy questions. Going back to the views on mental illness, one of the social reasons for diagnosing a person as having a "mental illness" is so that that person can assume what sociologists call the "sick role" and accept treatment. A little reflection should reveal the numerous social consequences that befall a person once it becomes known to others that a diagnosis of mental illness has been made; the case of the Democratic vice-presidential candidacy in 1972 was a particularly dramatic illustration. *It is not hard to see that in certain cases, the probable future stigmatization might well outweigh the present benefits of undergoing formal treatment. At any rate, the physician will be very careful about what he calls the condition he is treating.*

463      The labeling problem (like the problem of how to treat a dying patient) is one in which the ethical components are rather elementary; the real problem, initially, was one of awareness that the problem existed. As soon as psychiatrists in general realized that these consequences did occur, and that they had it in their power to do something about it, their ethical obligations were rather speedily agreed upon. (However, conflicts between roles can still arise; review Case 7 in Chapter 4 for a specific example.)

REVIEW ↑
CASE 7 ¦ 138

Further warning on the labeling question is provided by a much-publicized 464 study of Rosenhan. His group of pseudo-patients presented themselves at psychiatric facilities in California complaining of symptoms specifically chosen as typical of no known psychiatric entity. They were immediately diagnosed as schizophrenic and admitted, and a few had quite some trouble getting out again. While it would be unjust to psychiatry to overgeneralize these results, clearly it is possible to overestimate the true validity of diagnoses related to mental disturbances.

---

## CASE 34

On this fine day in 1978, Mr. T.S., aged 31, has been incarcerated in a 465 state mental hospital for five years. He previously served two short jail terms for aggressive behavior. On his third arrest, a court psychiatrist adjudged T.S. to be suffering from a personality disorder and recommended institutionalization for observation and treatment. The period of institutionalization has been extended since T.S. contended that he was being imprisoned for political reasons and demanded immediate release. He has had several incidents of aggressive and violent behavior toward the staff.

T.S.'s name comes up when a newly developed psychosurgery technique completes the experimental trial period and is approved for therapeutic use. The procedure involves implantation of electrodes into various subcortical areas of the brain. Sensor electrodes are able to detect the discharges that characterize the onset of an aggressive wave. A transducer then directs a microcurrent to other electrodes which stimulate areas that produce a state of passivity until the aggressive wave is past. When the patient has calmed down, the system is turned off. Evidence to date indicates that the surgery is reversible; if the electrodes are removed later, the patient will revert to his pre-operative state.

Since T.S.'s parents are his legal guardians, they are approached by a staff psychiatrist and told that if they consent to the surgery and it is successful, T.S. will be released and the "problem" will not recur. Of course, to assure this he must maintain the electrode system and its connections (the transducer is a miniaturized gadget that is worn like a hearing aid), but this would be a condition for his continued freedom. The psychiatrist tells the parents that if they refuse consent, the hospital will be happy to release their son whenever he responds to conventional therapy; but five years of that treatment has not made much of a dent, and the prognosis in that case is considered poor.

The parents are thoroughly confused by all this and turn to you, the family doctor, for advice. What do you tell them?

(Adapted from a case prepared by Steven Posar)

466    Let's start on Case 34 according to the procedure suggested before: first, what motives are operating? There seem to be two equally attractive possibilities, depending on how generous one wishes to be in one's views on human nature. We might argue that the psychiatric staff wants to help T.S. (who is too screwed up to want to help himself), are frustrated by their lack of success with conventional therapy, and have convinced themselves that the psychosurgery may well be the answer they are seeking. Since the treatment is directed at specific centers in the brain and works only intermittently, and since the operation is reversible, their ethical qualms have been laid to rest—in their view, this is not one of the consciousness-blunting situations.

However, they need consent for the procedure to help T.S., and it so happens that they are practicing in a situation where they wield power over T.S.'s freedom. It is tempting to use this power as an additional lever to pry loose the consent they seek—and they have succumbed to the temptation. In sum, their motives are therapeutic in the main, but they have muddied the waters by throwing in a bit of social-good and/or manipulative behavior.

467    We might also argue that it does not just "so happen" that these psychiatrists are in a position of power—that social role pervades their entire thinking processes. They are paid agents of the social institutions, and it is to the institutions that they owe primary allegiance. Their patient is society, not T.S.

Clearly it is in society's interest neither to allow T.S. to roam the streets in his present state, nor to support him at public expense while he beats up the staff. This psychosurgery neatly solves both problems and thus becomes an important social good; possible deleterious consequences to T.S., if any, may be ignored. However, since society still requires some form of consent for such a procedure, and since this consent may best be obtained by emphasizing the benefits to T.S. personally, it would be cosmetically prudent to emphasize the therapeutic aspects of the psychosurgery. In conclusion, this argument holds the motive of pursuit of social good to be primary; a small dab of the therapeutic motive has been added for flavoring.

(Note that this argument takes a narrow view of "social good." Is it in the long-range best interests of society to ignore the needs of its individual members, or vice versa?)

REVIEW SOCIETY
vs. INDIVIDUAL    328

468    Since even people who are attempting to honestly and openly tell us their motives may not be sure themselves what their motives are, it seems that we are unlikely to reveal the "real" motives simply by questioning the parties.

Why do we want to know motives anyway—the ethical decision-making process does not call for them as essential ingredients. The problem is that the ethical process works only when the frankness with which consequences are listed and weighed is at a maximum. When a person puts forth a justification, we may be led to wonder whether these are his genuine reasons, or whether he has put together, consciously or not, the kind of rationalization that he thinks will most likely appeal to us. Determining motives is a useful preliminary step to clear the air. In this case we have only besmogged the air by so doing, so we must proceed by formal consideration of the consequences.

One might wish to question whether such surgery would really be "reversible," given what we know about the complexity of the brain. Wouldn't any such procedure, no matter how small the electrodes, produce some residual permanent damage to brain cells, even though it might be too subtle to measure? The answer is probably yes; we might generalize that any physical or chemical intervention into the brain is irreversible to some degree. However, this applies to externally located stimuli also; experience is irreversible. If I have an adorable 3-year-old child and I see it run over and killed by a drunken driver before my eyes, that is an irreversible experience, and the residual damage from that is likely to be significantly greater than from the psychosurgery proposed for Mr. T.S. Thus, we cannot build a case against the surgery on the grounds of irreversibility, unless we are prepared to apply it across the board against all forms of conventional therapy as well.

This brings us to probably the most significant question about the consequences of the proposed psychosurgery: what it is that constitutes aggression. How the kind of life T.S. would lead with the electrodes measures up against a list of quality-of-life criteria depends strongly on this. (By the way, note that the sanctity-of-life view that provided such a simple answer on problems of allowing to die has nothing to offer here toward reaching a solution.) If it should turn out that the impulses suppressed by the electrodes are restricted simply to those which produce actual violent behavior directed toward the body of some other person, or of T.S. himself, then the quality of life T.S. can enjoy might well be improved by the surgery.

On the other hand, psychologists are not completely clear to what extent so-called aggressive impulses are responsible for actions that we tend to regard as socially useful and personally fulfilling. Suppose T.S. gets a job after his discharge and decides he wants to work extremely hard in order to get a promotion; would his sensors interpret this as an aggressive impulse and turn on his passivity switch until the thoughts went away? Or suppose T.S. falls in love and, one fine moonlit night, starts to express his passionate desires through word or deed. Would his "electronic conscience" immediately put an end to the performance?

Note that these considerations apply both to the therapeutic motive and to a narrowly defined social-good motive; in the latter case, we might decide that in our complex and competitive society, an individual who had no aggressive tendencies whatever is a social liability rather than a gain. Two other considerations, however, apply more directly to the therapeutic motive, or to the social-good motive if we define it in broad enough terms.

473    First, would the electrodes suppress the aggressive behavior only and allow T.S. to retain the awareness that he had had an aggressive impulse; or would the system wipe out both the impulse and all awareness of it? If the former, we might suggest having the surgery as a therapeutic trial: T.S. could go out in the world and see what it would be like to live without acting out his aggressive feelings. If he liked it, all well and good. But he would also have the basis to make an informed choice that he preferred the "freedom" and "dignity" of being able to express himself through his actions; if that were the case, he could have the electrodes removed and go back into the institution. But if the electrodes cut out awareness, he would in effect never know that things were different; he could not compare his life after surgery to his previous life. In that case the psychosurgery would be a consciousness-blunting procedure, and would diminish T.S.'s activities as a moral free agent.

474    Second, would the electrodes be activated by the desire of Mr. T.S. to have them removed—that is, if he had a thought that he should have the operation reversed, would the electrodes act to suppress this thought as aggressive? If so, then the procedure clearly has become an irreversible one, even if he would revert back to his "normal" state if the electrodes were to be removed. Again, in this instance, the result of the procedure would have been to limit T.S.'s range of choices, and thus to make him less human in a moral sense.

475    Once we obtain the answers to these questions, we might restate the assumptions upon which we have been basing our inquiry. The major ones might be:

1)    *In a case such as this, the long-range interests of the individual and of society coincide; i.e., it is not in the best interests of society to allow individuals to suffer a lessening in their quality of life.*

2)    *While we might not have decided on a definitive list of quality-of-life criteria, our list does include, as a high-priority item, the requirement that a "person" have an awareness of himself and that a "person" be able to make free choices in a moral sense.*

These assumptions, plus the answers to the questions, would point the way to a decision, in our own minds, of what would be in Mr. T.S.'s best interests. If his parents overruled this decision, whether we would be justified in ignoring their position would have to be decided along the lines of the determination of ethical participation as described in Chapter 7.

Presumably, if we were in 1978 when this psychosurgery had concluded 476 its experimental stages, we would have answers to the questions that we raised. Right now, we have no answers, because experiments with electrodes of this type have been largely (though not entirely) restricted to animals.

This case points up a major problem with all the behavior control issues— our relative lack of knowledge about how the human mind works. It may be that the acquisition of some of this knowledge in the future will help to clarify our ethical decision-making—allowing us to ask the key questions more precisely, where now we tend to get bogged down in side issues. One thing we can predict, however, is that the number of ethical problems related to behavior control will not be diminished by new knowledge. We have had ample demonstration that new knowledge and new technology create new ethical dilemmas even as they make the old ones obsolete.

Before leaving the subject of behavior control, you might want to review 477 Case 15 (Chapter 5), in which part of the question was the effect of behavior-control techniques, and mental illness, on the patient's ability to give informed consent. You might also want to look ahead to Case 38 (Chapter 11) to see what happens when behavior-control techniques take place within the setting of medical experimentation on human subjects. Ch. 10 478

# 10. Control of Reproduction

This chapter will be concerned with the topics of contraception, sterilization and abortion. There is considerable overlap between these topics and those treated in Chapter 15, "Genetic Engineering." The distinctions made here must be arbitrary to some extent, because of the mutual interaction of genetics and environment (rather than either alone) which produces the individual human being. As a rough guide, we will discuss in this chapter the question, "Under what circumstances should an individual, or this individual, be conceived or born?" We shall postpone until Chapter 15 the question, "What ought to be the genetic makeup of this individual?"

478

One of the factors lending major importance to the control of reproduction is the age-old human desire to experience sexual intercourse without having to deal with the consequences of pregnancy. There is nothing new or novel about this; contraceptive techniques and potions are described in ancient Egyptian papyri. What is new is the technology that allows "recreation without procreation" to be accomplished with reliability and with minimal discomfort and inconvenience.

479

Another factor which is a very new issue, however, is the desire to control reproduction in order to slow the rate of population growth. While it was predicted as early as 1800 that population would eventually outstrip food supply, only recently has the immediacy of the population explosion stimulated social planners to advocate widespread and drastic action. The most significant ethical issues are raised by the contention, which is becoming increasingly common, that voluntary measures alone will be insufficient to meet the crisis.

480

The techniques for control of reproduction are generally put into three categories. Contraception prevents the union of sperm and egg that results in the fertilized zygote. Abortion removes the zygote-embryo-fetus from the mother's uterus and kills it before it is independently viable. Sterilization renders a person incapable of producing gametes and thus unable to conceive children in the future.

481

It should be noted that there are gray areas in this categorization, most importantly between contraception and abortion. The intrauterine device, or IUD, is generally dispensed and classed as a contraceptive. However, while its precise mode of action is unknown, the best guess is that it acts by preventing the implantation of the fertilized zygote into the uterine wall. Thus, the IUD actually induces an abortion within the first week of pregnancy; since the mother discharges the zygote with her normal menstrual period, she is not aware of ever having been "pregnant." The same applies to the "morning after pill" which is now available for limited use in several forms.

482

483     Another technique which is presently controversial but growing in usage is that of pre-menstrual extraction. A woman who has a late menstrual period can have her period induced in the physician's office by means of mechanical suction of the uterine lining with a thin, flexible rubber tube. If the period is late due to pregnancy, the still very tiny fertilized zygote will be removed along with the other material. However, this cannot be labeled an abortion since no tests were done to determine if the woman was pregnant. If enough doctors are willing to carry out such a procedure, the later abortion in its present form may become unnecessary in many instances. The ethical problems of abortion would still be present, but they would have their emotional impact blunted by the fact that the physician cannot <u>know</u> that he is removing a living embryo.

484     Keeping these unclear distinctions in mind, we shall first deal with contraception and sterilization, since these topics can be outlined briefly as regards their ethical implications. Next we shall come back to abortion, and shall supplement the discussion of it under "Quality of Life" (Chapter 6) with some additional material.

485     Contraception has pretty much ceased to be a medical-ethical problem except for certain issues related to religion and to distribution of health care. First of all, very few would attempt to carry their contentions for the fetus as far as the germ cells prior to conception, and contend that the prevention of the union of egg and sperm constitutes the killing of a human being. While most of the objections to various forms of contraception have come from religious groups, notably the Roman Catholic church, the Planned Parenthood Association takes pains to point out that <u>some</u> form of birth control is approved by all major religions. (While it is true that the "rhythm method" is the only alternative to abstinence available to pious Catholics, the "rhythm method" is nevertheless fairly reliable when the menstrual cycle is determined by regular checks of body temperature.) Furthermore, most religions are beginning to temper the Biblical injunction to "be fruitful and multiply" with a realization that parents have an obligation not to have more children than they can care for adequately.

486     The religious objections to contraceptive techniques of one sort or another are generally based either on an assumption that such techniques are "unnatural" and therefore sinful to use, or on the more extreme view that sex itself is sinful unless procreation is intended. (Catholic consciences have stretched this latter view to allow periodic abstinence in the form of the rhythm method, instead of demanding total abstinence as a strict interpretation of the view would demand.) While the correctness of these two views might be argued by theologians, it is clear that, as a sociological fact, the public at large do not adhere to these ideas, at least in the U.S. If the majority of the public have rejected these notions, it seems hardly the place of the medical profession to try to reinstate these notions, so long as there is no medical-ethical objection to contraception independent of religious views. The medical question is then one of matching the right technique with the right patient, and taking proper regard for the side effects of the technique being used.

If we assume at this point that those people whose religious values allow contraception will go to a doctor to request it while those opposed to contraception will stay away, the only ethical problem remaining is the case of a physician whose own religious views stand in opposition to certain contraceptive techniques which the patient requests. According to our discussion of the "Contractual Model" in Chapter 4, this physician cannot be made to provide information or treatment of this nature if he would violate his own moral principles by doing so. That is, if he feels that the use of such contraceptive devices is sinful, and he feels that to lead others (the patient) into sin is itself sinful, he would be allowed not to provide the treatment.

REVIEW
"CONTRACT" 110

While up till now we have tended to be uncritical of this "escape clause" in the doctor's side of the contract, we might note two instances in which it would be ethically questionable for the physician to make use of the "escape clause" in a case regarding contraception. The first would be where the physician only offers to the patient those contraceptive techniques which conform with the doctor's own standards, and neglects to mention the existence of alternatives. Recall that the "Contractual Model" would suggest that, where no strong medical contraindications exist to any of the contraceptive techniques, the patient should be told about all the alternatives and allowed to choose the one that best suits his own values. While many educated people are familiar with the entire range of contraceptive devices simply from reading newspaper articles, many less well informed patients will remain ignorant of alternative methods if, for example, a Roman Catholic physician describes the rhythm method as the only form of birth control available.

The second questionable practice exists where the patient population is limited in its choice of physicians—a situation that applies to most of the patients in the U.S. who are members of the lower socio-economic classes. A physician who, for religious reasons, believes that abstinence is the only acceptable method of birth control presents no problem in an affluent suburb where several other doctors are readily available. This same physician, if he were practicing in an inner city clinic where he was the sole source of medical care for a certain population, would be guilty of depriving that population of routine medical care if he persisted in allowing his religious views to influence his practice.

Given these two examples, it might seem appropriate to amend the "escape clause" to the following: *The doctor is not obligated to enter into a course of treatment that the patient requests if to do so would violate the doctor's own moral values, EXCEPT where that doctor represents the patient's only entry into the medical care system, and to deny the treatment would be to deprive the patient of routine and acceptable medical care.* That is, where there is no alternative available for the patient, the obligation to provide medical service takes precedence over the physician's right to protect his own moral sense, where his values conflict with those of the patient.

491    This exception will not sit too well with physicians with a strong religious orientation. After all, if I feel that the birth control pill is sinful, and a patient comes to me requesting contraception, and I tell her that the pill is an alternative technique which I will not prescribe but which other doctors will, and she subsequently goes to Dr. X and gets a prescription for pills—haven't I contributed to her sin just as much as if I had prescribed the pills myself, and am I not just as responsible in the eyes of God?

        The counter argument would be that this is one of the risks a person takes when he enters a profession which is obligated to provide a service. The religious physician who cannot accept this kind of moral compromise seems to have two choices: he may go into a speciality such as radiology where such moral conflicts are least likely to arise; or he may work in the political sphere to increase both the number of practitioners and the level of education of the public, so that in the future patients with different religious values need not come to him.

492    One other problem with contraception, which is somewhat related to the religious objection, is worth noting—providing contraceptives for minors. It is a view commonly held by many members of society that giving contraceptive devices or information to minors is wrong because it will encourage illicit, premarital sexual activity. (Another objection, a holdover from our Puritan heritage, holds that pregnancy is God's "punishment" for the "sin" of sex. Many people have this as their major objection to providing contraceptives for minors, even if they will not admit it openly.)

493    Since doctors are members of society, a number of doctors will hold this view and so will be unwilling to provide contraceptives to minors. This societal view has also led to laws prohibiting physicians from providing contraceptives to minors, so that even those physicians who feel that the consequences of an unwanted pregnancy outweighs any real or imaginary increase in promiscuity may be inhibited from acting according to their conviction. Such a physician, faced with a minor requesting contraceptives, will have to face the ethical dilemma of refusing the request or breaking the law.

494    Fortunately, a more enlightened attitude is making some headway. One aspect of this is the idea of the "emancipated minor," which holds that if a minor is "mature" enough to come to the physician and request contraceptives, they are "mature" enough to have them—at any rate, they have already made the decision on their sexual activity, and the doctor's refusal will likely not change it. Some states have passed laws that will allow a physician to dispense contraceptives to "emancipated minors" without the necessity of parental consent, since it is the fear of having to tell their parents which leads many teenagers, under the old law, to engage in sexual intercourse without benefit of contraception.

Another newer attitude is that all aspects of human reproduction and sexuality, including contraception, should be taught in the public schools. In some states, this requires repeal of laws which forbid this. (In one recent case, a mother was prosecuted for "contributing to the delinquency of a minor" for bringing her teenage daughter to a lecture in which population control was discussed!) Repeal of such laws must overcome the opposition of those segments of the public mentioned above. In Michigan in 1973, the state medical society supported the repeal of such a law, but its efforts were overshadowed by the vocal public "moralists." This is an area in which it would seem that the physician in his community could do much to increase popular awareness and information on the issues. The decision of the individual as to how much involvement in such political activity is appropriate is of the sort that we will discuss in Chapter 16.

495

From an ethical viewpoint, sterilization is irreversible contraception, and the same types of ethical considerations apply. (It should be noted that it is possible to reconnect the cut ends of the male vas or the female oviduct and restore function in a variable percentage of cases of surgical sterilization. However, there is always a significant failure rate, and so most authorities hold that the patient should be told to consider the operation of sterilization irreversible, at the time that he or she is making up his mind whether to have the operation.)

496

Thus, if we neglect the problem of the physician with religious objections, the ethical problem of sterilization boils down to the problem of informed consent; or, in the case of an incompetent person, the question of who is qualified to give proxy consent. This latter problem has become prominent recently with renewed attempts to sterilize patients in mental institutions. Some civil-rights proponents have apparently taken the position that sterilization carried out on a person who cannot give voluntary informed consent is intrinsically wrong, since such "treatment" cannot be construed as doing anything to further the health of the individual.

497

One argument in favor of sterilization of mental patients by proxy consent bases its appeal on the idea that such patients will be unable to care for their children in any adequate fashion. The only problem with this is that according to whatever criteria of "adequate" parenthood you might choose, a large number of parents outside of mental institutions would be found unfit, and ethical consistency would demand their sterilization as well (unless they submit to "parenthood training" or some such thing). While we shall return to the question of what to do about "incompetent parenthood" briefly in Chapter 15, we might note now that the idea of sterilization for it would be exceedingly unpopular.

498

499      An argument which sounds a little better would restrict sterilization to those patients in whom the mental illness is known to have a significant hereditary component. One could say that if the patient were rational, she would herself desire to be sterilized to avoid passing on the trait to her offspring. Do you think that this is consistent with the criteria for proxy consent we listed in Chapter 7, if the appropriate legal guardian agreed to this? Or do you regard this argument as a contrived rationalization?

500      In discussing informed consent in Chapter 5, we noted the utility of considering "informed" and "consent" as separable components, and we also noted that "consent" by itself implies that the consent was given freely and voluntarily. The problem of voluntary consent will be particularly important in discussing sterilization, and later on in human experimentation.

REVIEW CONSENT ↑ 168

501      Suppose (as certain politicians apparently would like to have happen) that a black mother on welfare with six children is told that if she does not come to the clinic to be sterilized, her checks will be discontinued. If the mother shows up at the clinic and signs the "informed consent" form, we can assume that she is "informed" in that she knows what sterilization will mean for her. But it would take a large stretch of the imagination to call this "voluntary" consent. Here the coercion is being applied not by the physician actually doing the procedure, but by external agencies or circumstances.

502      The problem of what we might call "informed non-consent" becomes a central one as the pressures to limit population growth spawn new social programs which seek to make people accept contraception or sterilization by the use of positive or negative reinforcements. Note that while the threat of punishment if sterilization is not agreed to is a clear case of coercion, the offer of a significant reward to a poor person also raises the question of just how "voluntary" the consent might be—review Case 3 in Chapter 4.

     Note that we have not said that "informed non-consent" is wrong necessarily. The person who goes to court to pay for a traffic ticket submits just as involuntarily as the black woman threatened with loss of her welfare checks. If society as a whole should decide that the population problem has reached a crisis stage, it would seem appropriate for society to force individuals to accept sterilization. Our ethical concerns in such a case would be that the burden is imposed equally over the entire child-bearing population.

The important point to remember about this is that the doctor who performs the sterilizations under those circumstances is operating outside of the doctor-patient relationship as we have defined it. He is a paid agent of society, and has no special interest in the individual. Therefore, if he has to justify his actions, he must appeal to societal needs rather than to the doctor-patient "contract." This is similar to the observation made in Chapter 9, that the psychiatrist who "treats" a psychopath in order to make him less a danger to society has no business justifying his acts by the therapeutic motive.

There is nothing intrinsically wrong with a doctor operating outside of the doctor-patient relationship as outlined here. We have already noted that the nature of this relationship might well change anyway as societal needs become more pressing. The ethical obligation is simply to call a spade a spade; else the ethical decision-making method cannot be applied.

REVIEW SOCIAL
vs.
THERAPEUTIC MOTIVES | 466—467

There is one other problem with sterilization that sometimes is mentioned in ethical contexts—should the husband or the wife be sterilized? This might be strictly a medical decision based on the side effects of the male and the female operations, with the psychological side effects included. (One writer on the subject contends that females should be sterilized because men undergoing vasectomies are much more likely to suffer psychological sequelae due to supposed loss of masculinity; if so, he neglects to mention that this is a treatable, if not a preventable, side effect.) The only reason this is not strictly a medical decision is because a number of physicians, indoctrinated in the male-oriented system that is the medical establishment today, allow their personal and irrational values to interfere with their clinical judgment. Since we have already shown that this kind of unexamined insertion of values into medical judgments is inconsistent with the ethical decision-making method, this problem is one of medical sociology more than one of medical ethics.

Since the ethical considerations regarding contraception and sterilization apply in general to all the various techniques used, we will not bother to list all available kinds of contraceptives and all methods of sterilization. Articles which do list these are given in the references.

Artificial insemination is another reproductive issue which is ethically problematic mainly in connection with particular religious views. Artificial insemination with the husband's sperm, or AIH, used in cases such as when the sperm count is low and several ejaculates must be pooled together, tends to be less of concern than insemination with donor sperm (AID) in cases where the husband is completely sterile. However, both AIH and AID are forbidden by the Catholic Church.

In a few cases where the wife has become pregnant by AID without her husband's knowledge (do you feel that performing such a procedure would be sound or ethical medical practice?), the husband has subsequently filed for divorce on the grounds of adultery; such suits have generally been unsuccessful. We will pass over the notion that AID is adultery, along with some other purely religious objections (which are listed in Nelson) such as the one that artificial insemination is sinful because masturbation is required to collect the specimen.

508    As we suggested with contraception, patients holding such religious objections presumably will not seek the procedure, and physicians with such objections may refuse to do the procedure themselves. Of more concern is the couple seeking to have artificial insemination performed, but where one or both of them is ambivalent and may have psychological reactions which may act to the detriment of the child. Prominent among these reactions might be feelings of loss of masculinity by the husband, and resentment of "another man's sperm" inside his wife. As with any such procedure, these possible reactions should guide the physician in his interview with the couple and in his discussion of informed consent.

509    Another problem might be a couple in which only one has the religious or emotional objections. Typically the wife might want the baby while the husband is adamant. The ethical issue here is more one of an intra-marital dispute rather than artificial insemination per se. We should note that the so-called "right of a woman to control of her own body" (which we shall encounter under abortion) might not apply in a case where the husband is liable for future child support.

510    Finally, we might touch upon two consequentialist-type objections to artificial insemination: first, that it violates the nature of the marriage bond by separating procreation from the bond of sexual intercourse; and second, that by a domino-type reaction, acceptance of it will justify all sorts of further technological changes in procreation up to "test tube babies." The first objection amounts to saying that physical sex is really the key feature of the marriage union, which sounds strange coming from religious authorities; one suspects that this is just a disguised version of the old argument that anything "unnatural" is unethical (an argument used in the 19th century to oppose anesthesia during childbirth). The "domino theory" argument can best be dealt with in Chapter 15, with regard to objections raised by Paul Ramsey.
       We will now turn our attention for the remainder of this chapter to abortion.

511    In Chapter 6, we argued that the ideal way to treat abortion is by means of a set of quality-of-life criteria that may be consistently applied across the entire spectrum of the human existence, from conception to death. Thus, problems of abortion, allowing to die, and euthanasia, as well as other problems, would be decided by applying these criteria. We saw, however, that these ideal criteria do not exist; so that in practice, abortion is treated as a separate issue. Therefore, we will now consider some of the strategies proposed for dealing with abortion as an issue by itself.

In the absence of a quality-of-life approach which would allow us to look at any human being, at any time in its development, and declare whether it is a "person," it would seem that we are stuck with having to designate a point in time in the development of a human being, after which the developing life is worthy of our protection. While quality-of-life criteria have a tendency to appear arbitrary, point-in-time decisions are prone to appear even more arbitrary.

512

One such approach is put forth by Paul Ramsey, a theological ethicist. He agrees that we need a consistent approach which will handle problems of death as well as problems before birth, but he rejects the entire quality-of-life concept. He says that there should be a time in development, before which a potential human life (while still worthy of great respect) may be destroyed, but after which it immediately becomes equal with all other human lives and is deserving of our full protection.

As to when this time occurs, Ramsey acknowledges some good arguments in favor of placing it at conception, but notes that the fertilized egg may not be an "individual" in that it may subsequently divide to form identical twins. (Since the soul cannot split, this has led some theologians to questions when the soul enters the body.) Therefore the time Ramsey decides upon is very early in embryological development after which splitting of the embryo is not likely to occur; this is well before the time most abortions are performed.

513

Ramsey (who is Protestant) denies that this all-or-none view of his is a sanctity of life approach; he calls it instead an "equality of life" proposal. However, it is not hard to see that if a sanctity-of-life advocate agreed with Ramsey on when "life" begins, the practical consequences of Ramsey's view would be pretty much indistinguishable from those of the sanctity-of-life view.

514

As a matter of policy, most Roman Catholics who follow the sanctity-of-life approach place the critical time at conception. This leads to problems, especially with regard to the "gray area" between contraception and abortion. A Roman Catholic physician of the liberal wing, Viola, says with regard to the IUD: "A significant number of fertilized ova (some estimate one in three) never implant in the uterus under normal conditions. If in fact these are lost souls, the Church should be consistent and make efforts to administer baptism to them. This problem is extended further to the 10 percent of developing fetuses which abort [spontaneously] after implantation and have been relegated to a theological limbo." *

515

At the other end of the point-in-time spectrum are those like philosopher Michael Tooley, who would draw the line at that point when the nervous system is fully developed——near one year of age. The supporting argument is that fully human capabilities cannot exist otherwise. Note that this argument holds promise for the consistent quality-of-life notion sought in Chapter 6—— it applies to "brain death" as well as to abortion. But most people would reject it because it would justify not only abortion but infanticide as well.

516

*From M.V. Viola, "Abortion: A Catholic View." In: Ethical Issues in Medicine, ed. E.F. Torrey. Boston, Little, Brown, 1968.

517    Engelhardt offers a similar argument, based on the notion that only rational, self-aware beings can have value in themselves and thus have rights. His position derives from the deontological ethics of Kant (see Appendix I). But he notes that while things other than ends-in-themselves may not have rights in that sense, they may still have very high value and be worth protecting. Thus, while infants are not "persons" in the strict sense of being rationally self-aware, good child-raising practices demand that we treat them as if they were persons. While not persons in Engelhardt's strict sense, infants occupy the social role of persons and as such have very high social value. Thus Engelhardt would allow abortion up to around the point of viability, but would prohibit infanticide.

518    It is important to note that Engelhardt's argument is rather more sophisticated than many we have so far dealt with——indeed we cannot do justice to it in a short space. For one thing, it is not strictly a point-in-time argument, since Engelhardt avoids setting a specific point. For another, it is a sanctity of life argument in that a self-aware rational being is seen as having value in and of itself; but it is not an "absolute sanctity of life" argument such as we criticized in Chapter 6; for example, Engelhardt's view is not inconsistent with euthanasia.

519    Since until recently abortion was outlawed in most states except to save the life of the mother, the issue of abortion was very much a legal one; and one of the major medical-ethical issues was that of whether the physician was justified in breaking the law in order to perform abortions. This situation changed dramatically with the U.S. Supreme Court decisions of 1973, which ruled that two typical state abortion statutes were unconstitutional. In proposing the proper legal approach to abortion, the Court also made use of a point-in-time argument, but did so differently from Ramsey and the Catholics.

520    The Supreme Court began by recognizing two rights—that of the state to protect the life of a human being, including an unborn fetus; and the right of a woman (under the 14th amendment to the Constitution) to determine what she will do with her own body. The point-in-time problem then becomes one of deciding at what stages these rights become important.

521    The Court concluded that during the first trimester of pregnancy the woman's right was primary, and the state had no right to intervene. At any time after the first trimester, the Court stated that the state might intervene for the purpose of preserving the life and health of the mother (e.g., by requiring that abortions be carried out only by certain specified techniques, or in certain facilities). After the fetus becomes viable, however, presumably around the 28th week of fetal development, the Court said that the states may (not should) pass laws to prohibit abortion, except in those cases where, in the judgment of a physician, the mother's life or health was at stake. While declining to define "health," the Court suggested that it had psychological and social factors in mind in addition to purely organic considerations.

This Supreme Court decision has itself been attacked with charges of arbitrariness. For one thing, even the most liberal abortion law (New York) allows abortion until the 24th week, and many gynecologists contend that the proper limit for safety is the 20th week. However, the Court's guidelines would presumably allow abortions well beyond the New York limit. It has also been noted that while the Court places great weight on the right of the woman to decide what to do with her own body, it says that the physician and not the woman shall make the decisions regarding "life and health" that occur in later pregnancy.

522

We can summarize the three major approaches to the issue of abortion in Figure 3. You should be able to examine all of them critically in order to decide which of them, or which combination of elements of them, you wish to apply.

523

Having listed several alternative strategies for dealing with the problem of abortion, we can now do as we did with the problem of death in Chapter 6, and list the reasons we might have for performing an abortion. This provides an indication of where we must start with the job of ethical justification.

524

1) To end the life of an infant with a known or highly probable genetic or congenital deformity
2) To end the life of an infant who, we predict, will suffer from a bad home environment if we allow him to be born
3) To remove a pregnancy which the mother does not want for financial or other reasons
4) To eliminate an additional birth in the interests of population control
5) To save the life of the mother where this is threatened by the pregnancy

These reasons are listed in approximate order so that (1) gives the greatest weight to the presumed interests of the fetus while (5) gives the least weight. Note that in (1) and (2), our motive might very well be primarily to save the individual-to-be from suffering, although the family stands to benefit from the abortion also. We might thus distinguish (1) and (2) by calling them "prenatal euthanasia" as opposed to merely abortion.

525

It is interesting that (1) as a motive is often forgotten in the popular debate on abortion. It should be remembered that in order to diagnose a genetic abnormality such as Down's syndrome by the technique of amniocentesis, the test can be done no earlier than the 12th week and the results are often not available until four weeks later. Those who would propose the 12th week, for example, as the last week in which abortion will be allowed, may be forgetting that their proposal would eliminate the possibility of abortion for reason (1).

From previous discussions, we can see that a quality-of-life approach would allow abortions for all five reasons, in certain circumstances. A strict sanctity-of-life view, on the other hand, would allow only reason (5). It should be noted that with modern life-saving technology, the instance in which a pregnancy is a genuine threat to the life of the mother is very rare nowadays. (For an exception, see Case 24 in Chapter 6.)

526

527

# Figure 3

## Alternative Approaches to Abortion

### I. Quality of Life

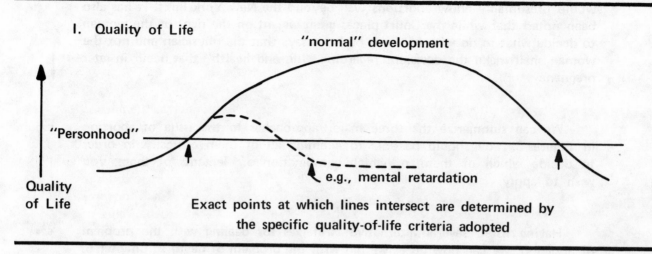

"normal" development

"Personhood"

Quality of Life

e.g., mental retardation

Exact points at which lines intersect are determined by the specific quality-of-life criteria adopted

### II. All-or-none Views

A "life"

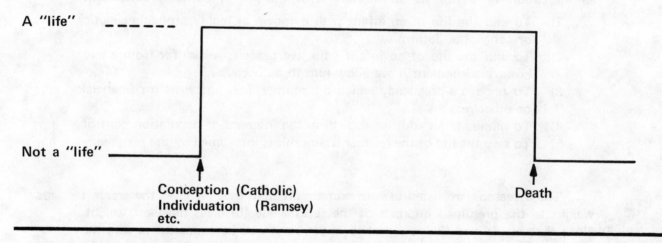

Not a "life"

Conception (Catholic)
Individuation (Ramsey)
etc.

Death

### III. U.S. Supreme Court

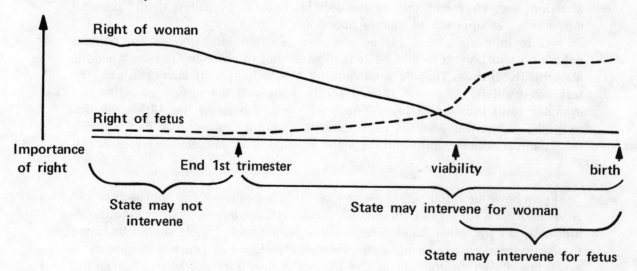

Right of woman

Right of fetus

Importance of right

End 1st trimester

viability

birth

State may not intervene

State may intervene for woman

State may intervene for fetus

150

Suppose now that one has adopted a quality-of-life approach to the abortion issue. One can then easily accept abortion for reasons (1) and (2) since these appeal directly to the quality of life that the person-to-be is likely to experience. One can also easily accept (5) where there is direct conflict between two lives. If, as is likely, it is agreed that overpopulation leads to a lessened quality of life for all, and sociological evidence indicates that abortion is the most effective way of dealing with the problem, one might then accept (4) as well. It seems, however, that there may well be a snag at (3).

528

By most quality-of-life standards, a fetus would not be a "person." However, even though the standards do not say so, one instinctively wants to regard a non-"person" with potential to become a "person" directly in a different light than one would consider a non-"person" who can never become a "person." Thus, one is led to put some value on the fetus "person-to-be," but how much value? Can the value be overruled by the simple expressed desire of the mother ("abortion on demand")? Or must one demand evidence for some severe dislocation in the life of the mother or the family before the value of the fetus is overruled? And if one wants to demand the latter, how can one do so without adopting a frankly paternalistic approach, and deciding for the woman whether she should have a baby or not? Clearly, in a situation that demands a complex ranking of values, no pat answer is possible. A quality-of-life advocate might well decide that he may perform an abortion (3), but he will probably be much less comfortable about it than with an abortion (1) or (2).

529

One ethicist who has approached the abortion issue from a consequentialist viewpoint is Bok. Because she refuses to engage in definitions of "personhood," an activity which she feels has pernicious consequences, her arguments have to do with reasons for performing abortion such as in our list above, and under what circumstances these are strong enough to outweigh the usual and beneficial social reasons to protect life.

530

For one thing, Bok feels that the reasons for protecting life grow relatively stronger as the time of viability approaches; thus she sees early abortions as being ethically preferable to late ones. Also, abortion done by techniques which simply separate the fetus from the mother ("cessation of life support") are preferable to techniques which directly damage the fetus. (Unfortunately, the former may have more medical morbidity associated with them than do the latter.) Other crucial variables are whether the pregnancy was voluntary or not, and whether the mother's reasons for wanting to end it are significant or merely capricious.

531

Unfortunately Bok does not make quite clear whether she is addressing her argument toward the pregnant woman or toward the doctor, as to who should reason along those lines. If she intends the doctor to do so, is she more consistent with the "Contractual" or the "Priestly" model of the doctor-patient relationship? Furthermore, does our analysis of active vs. passive euthanasia in Chapter 6 have any bearing on Bok's argument on preferable abortion techniques? How do you assess her other points?

**532**     Do you think that Bok is correct in assuming that she can give good answers to the abortion question while avoiding the problem of trying to define "personhood"? If not, can you clearly state the flaw in her reasoning?

**533**     Of course, this line of ethical justification would be incomplete without consideration of the long-range consequences of adopting a policy of unrestricted abortion. Two places which now provide abortions readily at low cost, on demand, are Japan and Hungary; in both countries the abortion rate is greater than the birth rate. It is clear that in those circumstances the women have adopted abortion as a means of birth control, and have preferred it, for the most part, above other available means of contraception.

**534**     If one considers fetuses as "persons," these data seem reprehensible, since fetuses are being killed where the same effect could have been achieved had the women put themselves to a little more trouble and used the standard contraceptive techniques. If one does not consider fetuses as "persons," and places a relatively lower value on them as "persons-to-be," then the most significant question is the medical one: in terms of harmful side effects, are the women better off undergoing abortions intermittently or using contraceptives such as the pill or IUD on a regular basis?

**535**     Two sociological conclusions might be suggested by the experience in the two countries mentioned. One is that if abortion is readily available, the majority of the population do not consider it morally wrong, even in Hungary with its centuries of Catholic tradition. The other is a counter-argument to the "domino theory" arguments of the Catholics and Ramsey, that abortion-on-demand will necessarily lead to a weakening of the restrictions against infanticide. No such tendency toward infanticide has been observed; clearly the populace can accept abortion while still maintaining a clear distinction.

**536**     Those who have been following the popular debate on abortion laws over the past several years may be disappointed that we have passed so quickly over the major "pro" and "con" arguments on this issue. This has been done for a reason. The entire debate on abortion has been marked both by an extreme polarization of views, and by the relative inability of disputants on both sides to separate the true facts of the case and the relevant value judgments from their own emotional feelings. The result has been a plethora of statements on both sides which can most charitably be described as silly.

**537**     On the anti-abortion side, one has found the Catholic establishment adhering to a strict sanctity-of-life view on abortion, and spending millions of dollars on propaganda campaigns to champion the rights of fetuses, while continuing to endorse warfare and capital punishment. One has also seen individual speakers stating that an exception to the prohibition on abortion can be made in pregnancy resulting from rape—as if the resulting fetus is less of a "person." This last argument strongly suggests that in the minds of many, pregnancy was considered as punishment for the woman who engaged in intercourse without "precautions," to allow her to get an abortion would be allowing her to escape her "just desserts." On the other hand, since the rape victim had no choice, mercy could be shown in her case. Somehow the supposed rights of the fetus got lost under all that Puritan self-righteousness.

Meanwhile, on the pro-abortion side, one could read statements such as, "Bear in mind that...the [Catholic] Church did not equate abortion and murder till 1869." (Mendel did not get around to publishing his laws of inheritance until the 1860's; are the laws therefore less valid?) Or one might hear the argument that anti-abortion laws were wrong because the rich had the resources to evade them and get abortions while the poor were forced to go to incompetent and unsafe illegal abortionists. A comparable argument in the 1850's might have stated that the government should buy slaves and give them free to the poor Southern farmers, so that they could enjoy equality with the rich landowners.

538

If the complete rundown of the pro and con arguments on abortion had been included in this unit, it would have been for the purpose of illustrating how an ethical debate should NOT be conducted. Since we have been giving examples of common ethical "errors" all through this unit, further illustration was considered unnecessary. As usual, any deficiencies can be corrected by consulting the works in the reference section.

539

Since no new cases were included in this chapter, you might wish to review the following cases, all of which deal with control of reproduction: Case 2 and Case 3 in Chapter 4; Case 13 in Chapter 5; Case 22 and Case 24 in Chapter 6; and Case 28 in Chapter 7.

Ch. 11 ↓ 540

# 11. Human Experimentation

Until very recently, the fantastic advances made by medical science and technology in the last century—many of which relied heavily on experiments carried out with human beings as subjects—were generally accepted as an unqualified and unquestioned good. However, the modern, complex problems associated with "progress" have stimulated views which cast science and technology in the role of villain rather than savior. While these views have been extended to include much of medical practice, it has naturally been the practice of experimentation on human beings that has aroused the most criticism and suspicion. It is within this emotional atmosphere that a discussion of the ethics of human experimentation must take place.

540

To start this chapter, we will depart from the usual format and insert a historical digression. This is appropriate because a few events have had a particular impact upon the ethical thinking in this area. Also, there might be a lesson in the problem of "belated awareness," in the fact that problematic research had been going on for so long before anyone called attention to the basic ethical issues——issues which today seem obvious.

541

The first major dent in the idea that medical science could only be "good" came with the close of World War II, when the experiments conducted by Nazi doctors upon the concentration camp inmates were revealed to the world. Following the traditional route, the medical profession sought to prevent a recurrence of those horrors by establishing a code of ethics for research on humans. The first such code was the Nuremburg Code of 1949; an updated version is the widely cited Declaration of Helsinki of 1964 (Appendix IV).

542

Despite all this, the general view within the medical profession was that unethical experimentation was only carried out by Nazis or similar degenerates, and so the problem was almost non-existent in a humane country such as the U.S. Thus, an article by Henry Beecher, a respected researcher in anesthesiology, landed like a bombshell when it was published in 1966. Not only did Beecher contend that as many as 12% of the studies being conducted by experienced researchers were unethical, but he gave specific examples of unethical research direct from the scientific journals (with names omitted). Beecher stated: "During ten years of study of these matters it has become apparent that thoughtlessness and carelessness, not a willful disregard of the patient's rights, account for most of the cases encountered."

It is instructive to look at some typical examples cited by Beecher.*

543

*Reprinted, by permission. From the New England Journal of Medicine 274:1354, 1966.

544    "Example 3.   This involved a study of the relapse rate in typhoid fever treated in two ways. In an earlier study by the present investigators chloramphenicol had been recognized as an effective treatment for typhoid fever, being attended by half the mortality rate that was experienced when this agent was not used. Others had made the same observation, indicating that to withhold this effective remedy can be a life-or-death decision. The present study was carried out to determine the relapse rate under the two methods of treatment; of 408 charity patients, 251 were treated with chloramphenicol, of whom 20, or 7.97%, died. Symptomatic treatment was given, but chloramphenicol was withheld, in 157, of whom 36, or 22.9% died. According to the data presented, 23 patients died in the course of this study who would not have been expected to succumb if they had received specific therapy."

545    "Example 12. This investigation was carried out to examine the possible effect of vagal [nerve] stimulation on cardiac arrest. Having been impressed with the number of reports of cardiac arrests that seemed to follow vagal stimulation, [the researchers] tested the effects of intrathoracic vagal stimulation during 30 of their surgical procedures, concluding, from these observations in patients under satisfactory anesthesia, that cardiac irregularities and cardiac arrest due to vagovagal reflex were less common than had previously been supposed."

In the kinds of surgery during which this experiment was carried out, the vagal stimulation was in no way necessary for the success of the therapeutic procedure. No mention of informed consent was made.

546    "Example 17.   Live cancer cells were injected into 22 human subjects as part of a study of immunity to cancer. According to a recent review, the subjects (hospitalized patients) were merely told that they would be receiving "some cells"...the word cancer was entirely omitted..."

While Beecher mentioned no names, this same case was treated in more detail by Katz in his book, Experimentation with Human Beings. The case illustrates the attitudes of at least a few medical scientists toward ethical questions and the rights of patient-subjects.

547    In the early 1960's a certain Dr. S. was conducting experiments to determine natural immunity to cancer. For this purpose, he had been injecting patients at his hospital, as well as prisoner "volunteers," with cancer cells, to see how effectively their bodies would reject the foreign tissue. There was at least some evidence that such injections might result in metastasis with a malignant tumor being formed in the patient's body. Despite this, Dr. S. wanted to do new experiments, in which the response of chronically ill patients (who supposedly had decreased immune response) would be compared with his healthy patients. For this he needed subjects who were chronically ill with diseases other than cancer, and he had no such patients at the two hospitals where he was working.

Dr. S. therefore wrote to a physician at J.C.D. Hospital to get permission    548
to use patients there for his research. He said in his letter: "You asked me if
I obtained [written] permission from our patients before doing these studies.
We do not do so at M. or J.E. hospitals since we regard this as a routine study,
much less dramatic and hazardous than other routine procedures such as bone
marrow aspiration and lumbar puncture. We do get signed permits from our
volunteers at the Ohio State Penitentiary but this is because of the law-oriented
personality of these men, rather than for medical reasons."*Dr. S. somehow
forgot to mention that at least one of these "routine" procedures done previously had produced what seemed to be metastatic cancer.

Dr. S. got permission to use patients at J.C.D. Hospital in New York, and    549
carried out the experiment described by Beecher as "Example 17." However,
some of the staff physicians who were involved in the study—and who, unlike
Dr. S., had some responsibility for the medical care of the chronically ill
patients—raised some objections to the way the research was being conducted.
The final result, after a number of months, was that a case against Dr. S. was
brought before the New York State Board of Regents, which is responsible
for licensing physicians in the state.

At the Board hearings, one doctor testified: "The patient was not told    550
that the injection would contain cancer cells. The reason for this was that we
did not wish to stir up any unnecessary anxiety, disturbances, or phobias in
our patients. There was no need to tell the patients that the injected material
contained cancer cells because it was of no consequence to the patient."
The patients were asked to sign a consent form before entering the experiment,
but the information about the true nature of the experiment was withheld.

In a news interview during the hearings, one reporter (who was apparently    551
familiar with the ethical decision-making "short cut" we described in Chapter 2)
asked Dr. S. if he would be willing to accept an injection of cancer cells into
his own bloodstream. Dr. S. said he would not, because "there are relatively
few trained cancer researchers, and it seems stupid to take even that little
risk."
      REVIEW
      "SHORT CUT"   43

How did this study stand under the then-current (1963) codes of ethics    552
for human experimentation? You can see that it violates several parts of
Section III of the Declaration of Helsinki, which was adopted in 1964. It also
was in violation of the then-current U.S. Public Health Service policy. It was
not in violation of the current A.M.A. code of ethics; these merely required
that the experiment be conducted by skilled medical investigators, be based
on animal experimentation, and be conducted with the voluntary consent
of the patient (not necessarily informed). In 1966 the A.M.A. updated its code
to conform more with the Declaration of Helsinki.
      REVIEW
      CODES   65

*From J. Katz, with A.M. Capron and E.S. Glass, Experimentation with Human Beings.
New York, Russell Sage Foundation, 1972. Pp. 663-664.

553     While the provisions of these codes apparently had not been impressed on Dr. S., the Board of Regents was apparently in agreement with them: Dr. S. and a colleague were censured for unethical experimentation. This ruling was not unanimously accepted by the medical profession, as shown by a letter from a physician to the New York Herald Tribune, Jan. 26, 1964:

"Here, then, we have a wide possibility: if there is such a thing as a biological mechanism as a defense against cancer, then it may be possible to stimulate it either before cancer strikes or perhaps even later when cancer has taken hold. This is the question Dr. S. is trying to pursue. It would be a shame if a squabble over who told what to whom should destroy a thrilling lead in cancer research."

554     As for the views of Dr. S's colleagues in the research sphere, these views were made known rather plainly. The American Association for Cancer Research elected Dr. S. as its vice-president in 1968, and as its president in 1969.

Since that time, the public awareness on the ethics of experimentation has been increasing, culminating with the outcry over the exposure of the U.S. Public Health Tuskegee syphilis study, in which there was evidence that several hundred black males, over a 25-year period, had been deprived of treatment for their disease even after it had become known that penicillin was a highly effective anti-syphilitic agent. Given this public mood, it is likely that a scientific body would think twice before bestowing public praise on Dr. S. today.

555     We have now seen the kinds of research that has caused the ethical questions to be raised, and the kinds of attitudes that caused the practices to come about in the first place. However, we would not want to lose sight of the fact that these criticisms certainly do not apply to all human experimentation. For instance, the human experiments around 1900 that proved that yellow fever is transmitted by mosquitoes, which used soldier volunteers as subjects, was a good example both of concern about informed consent and concern about the continuing welfare of the subjects.

556     The problem, then, is to separate the ethical from the unethical research, and since much research is financed by government funds, many legislative and administrative bodies are currently considering policy measures. One recent policy is the proposal of a committee of the National Institutes of Health, some of whose provisions we shall have a closer look at later. For now, we shall turn to an examination of some of the features of human experimentation which create ethical problems.

557     To start, we should distinguish, as the Declaration of Helsinki does, two types of experimental situations. In a therapeutic trial, the subject has the disease for which the experimental treatment is being intended, and thus could possibly benefit from the results. (Remember that in a controlled therapeutic study, such as the one with typhoid fever in Beecher's example 3, a particular patient might not actually be receiving the treatment.) In a non-therapeutic study, such as the experiments of Dr. S., no benefit for the subjects is foreseen; the benefit, if any, will fall to future patients and to society at large.

Next, we shall consider one approach to determining the ethics of an experiment. Recall the praise the Herald Tribune letter-writer had for the potential of the line of research Dr. S. was pursuing. The implication was clear that if good results came out of the experiment, it would have been worth while, and "squabbles over who told what to whom" would be irrelevant. On the other side of the coin, a speaker at a symposium on the controversial Willowbrook experiment, in which retarded children in a state home were inoculated with hepatitis virus in hopes of eventually developing a vaccine, stated that the experiment was unethical in part because no vaccine had been discovered. (This speaker was premature; the researchers have since published reports of an experimental vaccine.)

558

Are the results of an experiment the legitimate guide to whether an experiment is ethical or not? *Recall that the purpose of ethical decision-making is not to allow us to decide whether to praise or blame other people for what they have done in the past. If ethics is to be of any use, it must be a guide for what we ought to do now.* We can't wait for the results to come in to decide if an experiment we propose is unethical—we must predict as best we can the possible consequences, and compare these with our values. What are the consequences of doing an experiment such as Dr. S. did without informed consent, in terms of the future trust of the public in the medical profession? Would people go to doctors if they felt that they could never know if they were being treated or if they were being experimented upon? How do these risks compare with the slight advantage in terms of convenience of getting subjects by not informing them? Those are the ethical questions.

559

REVIEW RETRO— SPECTIVE ETHICS 155

While an act is ethical or unethical at the time it is performed, and does not become one or the other later by virtue of hindsight, nevertheless the ethical method makes clear that the intended outcomes of the experiment, and their likelihood of achievement, are among the consequences that must be fed into the ethical equation. Specifically, the potential benefits to be gained, both by the individual and by society as a whole, must be weighed against the risks of untoward side effects to the individual. This is what is referred to by the common term, "risk-benefit ratio."

560

For example, the NIH guidelines say of experimentation in children: "The investigator must...stipulate either that the risk to the subjects will be insignificant, or that although some risk exists, the potential benefit is significant and far outweighs that risk." We speak of a favorable risk-benefit ratio when these conditions apply, and an unfavorable ratio when they do not.

561

However, both risks and benefits are uncertain, and uncertainty about probabilities poses an ethical problem of increased complexity. Therefore, some of the ethical dilemmas of human experimentation grow directly out of the modern concepts of proper experimental design.

562     Modern medical experiments, whenever possible, make use of two major devices to reduce experimental bias to a minimum. One is the controlled study— a treatment is never evaluated by itself, but is compared with the effects either of no treatment, or, if another treatment exists, of that other treatment. This requires that the subjects be divided into two groups. However, as we touched upon briefly in Chapter 4, the mere knowledge by the patient or doctor of what treatment is being given may, through the "placebo effect," influence the outcome. Therefore, the second device used is the double-blind study—neither the patients nor the investigators are to know until the experiment is over who was receiving what treatment.

563     In a therapeutic situation, the ethical question arises of whether a controlled, double-blind study can be undertaken at all. If the two groups are being given drug A and drug B, both of which are known to be somewhat effective against the disease, in order to learn which is better, then the experiment presents minimal ethical problems in that regard. But suppose that you have a new drug which you strongly suspect (but have no proof) is effective against a disease for which there is now no treatment? Is it ethical to deprive half of your sick subjects of this potentially healing drug? And if it is, how would you go about obtaining informed consent for this controlled study?

564     The dilemma, of course, originates in the uncertainty. If you knew that your drug was effective, you would not be doing the experiment. And the history of medicine is full of highly touted remedies which, upon later scientific investigation, turned out to be worse than the disease. Right now it looks as if the randomly selected and unknown control subjects are the unlucky ones. If, on the other hand, the drug later turns out to have a highly fatal and unanticipated side effect, the control group will have been the lucky ones. Thus one could just as well argue that it would be unethical not to have a control group, in order to give at least 50% of the patients the chance to escape any unforeseen side effects.

565     Possibly a more telling argument is as follows. Presumably, people consent to being experimental subjects at least in part because they foresee some possible benefit to society. Any experiment involves some risk to the subject, however slight. Therefore, you have a tradeoff: societal benefit vs. subject risk. Since subject risk is an unknown factor, and assuming you have already minimized the known risks as much as possible, do you not then have an ethical obligation to do everything you can to increase societal benefit, in order to make the whole thing worthwhile? And increasing societal benefit entails making the results as useful and as unequivocal as possible—by use of the most precise and unbiased experimental technique. Therefore, we could conclude that unless the risk to the control group was much greater than to the experimental group, it would be unethical to do an experiment which falls short of the best possible design: the controlled, double-blind study.

However, it may be in some cases that in choosing the optimal experimental design to generate good data, not enough alternatives are explored. Weinstein has criticized the notion that only trials in which subjects are randomly assigned to the experimental and control groups are statistically valid. Randomization as a strategy has both strong and weak points, and in some experiments patient self-selection would work as well. Weinstein also encourages more use of adaptive designs: instead of waiting for all the data to tabulate results, one feeds in the data as the experiment is proceeding; so that if one of the two therapies starts to show clear superiority, the minimum number of subjects will have been exposed to the inferior treatment.

## CASE 35

You are the chief investigator of the Veterans Administration Cooperative Study Group on Antihypertensive Agents. This group was formed because, while it was known that a number of drugs were effective in reducing the blood pressure of people with essential hypertension, there has been considerable dispute as to whether just reducing the blood pressure is effective in preventing the sequelae of hypertension—heart attack, stroke, etc. To decide this question, it was felt that a controlled study was needed. In order to get several hundred patients in both the experimental and control groups, a number of hospitals have been enlisted in the study. The study is planned to last for 5½ years and you have received funding for this period.

The experiment began in 1963. You are now reviewing some interim reports of data collected after the subjects have been in the study for an average of 16 months. In this particular group, the patients were those who had a systolic blood pressure between 115 and 129 mmHg at the beginning.

In the experimental group, which has been receiving antihypertensive medication, there has been one stroke and one instance of drug toxicity. The latter resolved itself without permanent damage when the drug combination was readjusted.

In the control group, which has been getting placebos instead of active drugs, four patients have died as a result of conditions attributable to their high blood pressure. An additional 10 patients have developed signs of more severe hypertension and have been removed from the study for treatment. There have also been two heart attacks, two cases of congestive heart failure, and one stroke.

Your statisticians assure you that the differences so far between the control and experimental groups are statistically significant.

What do you do now?

What you did do, as a matter of fact, was to discontinue the study. The group felt that the continuation of the study beyond this point would provide no information more convincing than what was already available, and that under such circumstances it would be unethical to go on depriving the control subjects of what you now know is effective treatment. (In the group with blood pressure less than 115 mmHg, the results were more equivocal, and that study was allowed to go the full 5½ years; the end results confirmed the effectiveness of antihypertensive treatment in that group also.)

569     While many ethical problems of experimentation are related to the experimental design, a more basic question has to do with the whole purpose of experimentation, and what it means for the doctor-patient relationship. Recall that in past chapters we have seen that the fact that the person treating you is a physician does not mean that you are his "patient," in the sense of the doctor-patient "contract." If you are a child, the real patient may be your mother. If you are a prisoner in a mental institution, the real patient may be the institution or society itself.

    Who is the "patient" in an experimental situation? That is, who gets the supposed benefit? We have already noted the benefits for future patients in particular and for society in general. The investigator himself is benefitted by the prestige and by being able to obtain future grants to do more research. In a therapeutic trial, the subject may or may not benefit; in a non-therapeutic trial he almost certainly will not benefit, other than in the strictly spiritual sense of having done a good deed for society.

REVIEW
"CONTRACT"  110

570     In a non-therapeutic trial, therefore, it seems a gross misuse of words to call the subject the investigator's "patient." The therapeutic trial seems to have some elements of the doctor-patient relationship, but other elements foreign to it. Suppose a patient in the experimental group develops some previously unobserved symptom which might be a side effect of the drug. As a doctor, the researcher's first obligation would be to stop the drug. As a researcher, however, he is strongly tempted to continue the drug in order to get new data about this unexpected discovery. There seems to be a strong conflict of interest here. While in other experimental situations the conflict might be much less, it seems that, by the very nature of experimentation, the conflict can never be completely eliminated.

571     *Awareness of this problem has led many authorities to the conclusion that the investigator-subject relationship is inherently different from the doctor-patient relationship; and to place a person into an experiment where he is solely under the care of the investigator is to deprive the person of medical attention. If the patient's own doctor cannot continue his care during the experiment, the investigating group must include a medically competent "patient advocate" distinct from the investigator, who has the power to remove the person from the experiment as soon as it appears to him that continuation would be detrimental to the patient's health. An institution cannot receive a research grant from the Public Health Service unless it has made provision for safeguarding the rights of the individual subjects in this manner; and other funding agencies are establishing similar policies.*

We should note that this distinction which is so clear to ethicists may well be unclear to the patient-subject, as John Fletcher has reported from interviews with experimental subjects. When a person walks up to the bed wearing a white coat and asking them how they feel today, the patients immediately tend to regard him as "their doctor" and often do not perceive that he has interests in the matter very different from those of the usual doctor-patient encounter. This problem is especially prominent when, as often happens, a non-therapeutic trial is "piggybacked" on a therapeutic one, and patients already enrolled in the therapeutic study are asked to be subjects for the additional experiment as well. Patients may mistakenly confuse the two studies and feel that if they refuse to join in the non-therapeutic one, they will be excluded from treatment.

This problem of patient misunderstandings has important implications for the next facet of the experimentation issue—informed consent.

## CASE 36

You are the director of a community hospital in Lansing. You are approached by a Michigan State University faculty member with the following request.

He is doing research on the laboratory diagnosis of certain infectious diseases, and wants to know how the reactions of blood serum from the general population compare with reactions of serum of individuals with known infectious disease, as far as his new tests are concerned. He requests permission to ask your pathologist for the serum that is left over from the tests that have been run on blood from hospitalized patients. Generally slightly more blood is drawn from the patient than is required, to guard against spoiling a test, and any excess is just discarded into the sink.

You ask whether he intends to pool the serum or to keep it in individual samples. He says that he intends to keep the samples separate so that, if he should turn up a very abnormal result, he could check the hospital records on that patient to see if any information there might explain the abnormal test.

Would you approve of this request?

In your consideration of this request, did you think about the presence or lack of provision to obtain informed consent?

At first glance, this seems silly. What difference does it make to a patient if you use some of his serum that is already drawn and which would otherwise end up in the sewer anyway?

However, remember what was said in Chapter 5—that what is "routine" to you as an expert may not be at all routine from the patient's viewpoint. Suppose you do turn up an abnormal test, and want to look into the patient's record to explain it. Does the patient want people who are not directly involved in his medical care snooping into his files? And even if you don't look into the record, many patients might well have had some disease in the past which they do not want others to know about, but which you could detect with your tests. Don't you have an obligation to get the patient's consent before you take a chance on invading his privacy in this manner? (Review the hospital patient's "Bill of Rights" in Appendix II.)

575      In Case 36, once the idea of informed consent occurs to you, it is not hard to figure out what you would say to the patient in order to obtain his informed consent. But go back to the situation of the double-blind therapeutic trial. The full, morally relevant information is as follows: You are suffering from a disease for which there is now no good treatment; we have a treatment that might help you but we cannot be sure; we do not know the risks and the true risks might be very significant, even worse than your disease; if you agree to enter the study you will be randomly assigned to one of two groups; you have a 50—50 chance of receiving a placebo therapy instead of the real treatment; neither you nor we will know which group you are in; if, at any point, your life or health seems to be endangered by the experiment, we will remove you from the study and give you any treatment necessary. Are you ethically obligated to tell all of this to the patient, or only some of it? If you tell all of it, how many people will agree to take part in the experiment? If, as a result of a full disclosure, you have too few subjects to get good results, are you meeting your obligation to society and to medical science?

576      *Presumably the answer to this problem is clear. If "informed consent" is to mean what it says, then a full disclosure of all the relevant information—including admission of uncertainty where it exists, and revealing any alternative sources of treatment that may be available—would seem to be an absolute requirement.* If this procedure leads to too few subjects, this will have societal implications which we will turn to later.

      Now throw another monkey wrench into the works. So far we have been talking about voluntary informed consent—recall the distinction between voluntary and involuntary consent we made in Chapter 10. However, two of the most prolific sources of subjects for medical experimentation have, up to now, been prisons and institutions for the mentally incompetent. We ought to raise some hard questions about the ability of such individuals to give voluntary consent.

REVIEW CONSENT    |    500—502

577      On the question of informed consent, Beecher is quite dogmatic: "Ordinary patients will not knowingly risk their health or their life for the sake of 'science.' Every experienced clinical investigator knows this. When such risks are taken and a considerable number of patients are involved, it may be assumed that informed consent has not been obtained in all cases."*Or else, presumably, that it was obtained under some sort of duress.

      On the issue of prisoner subjects, one extreme point of view states that, in the worst-run prison experiments, the authorities threaten the prisoners with various punishments unless they "volunteer," and often do this behind the back of the researcher. In the best-run trials, the prisoners are either led to believe or allowed to believe that their participation will possibly lead to an earlier parole. In either case, the consent is obtained under a form of duress, and cannot be considered voluntary. Therefore all experiments of a non-therapeutic nature involving prisoners is unethical.

*Reprinted, by permission. From the New England Journal of Medicine 274:1354, 1966.

It could be said that no one can ever give consent without being under some form of duress, internal or external. The question therefore boils down to how much duress is tolerable before the consent becomes truly involuntary. For example, we might conclude that a prisoner can give voluntary consent, if he is fully informed, even if the idea of an earlier parole is held out to him. After all, if the risk of the experiment is great, a rational prisoner would decide that an extra year in jail is preferable so long as he emerges in one piece; and if the risk is smaller, who is better qualified than the prisoner to weigh the size of the risk against a longer period of freedom? On the other hand, we might conclude that the threat of being beaten by the guards would be a clearly unacceptable amount of duress.

Another interesting counterview is that a truly repentant prisoner might regret his crime against society and might sincerely wish to try to make amends through some degree of personal sacrifice. Right now, he can do so by volunteering for an experiment. This argument would hold that it would be unethical to deprive him of this opportunity by deciding to discontinue such experiments in the future. (This argument might sound good coming from a prison chaplain. If it came from a researcher, we might suspect some conflict of interest.)

Much of the debate on this issue has taken the form of a simplistic debate of "experiment on prisoners" vs. "don't experiment on prisoners." A more creative attitude, which shows the value of listing alternatives and of specifying the conditions in ethical statements, is shown in the proposed NIH guidelines. The importance of voluntary consent is emphasized, and several reasons are listed as to why a prisoner might be under more coercion than a free person: he might volunteer for the money; he might anticipate earlier parole; he might be just bored and volunteer for a change; or the food and shelter in the prison may be substandard, whereas better food and beds will be provided to the experimental subjects.

This does not mean, however, that informed consent cannot be obtained from prisoners, the NIH concludes; it just means that one must have additional safeguards here (as well as with mentally incompetent persons and with children). First, the NIH proposes that a prison must be accredited before research can be done there, and accreditation should require adequate food and shelter, the presence of adequate daily activity to dispel unusual boredom, and the opportunity to earn money in other ways besides research. Thus, the factors most likely to interfere with truly voluntary consent are kept to a minimum. In addition, the NIH suggests formation of a "Protection Committee" to provide "supplementary judgment"—that is, someone besides the prisoner himself ought to decide that the risk-benefit ratio is indeed favorable. This is in addition to the ethical review committee that must oversee any experiment involving human subjects under Federal funding. Finally, NIH states that the rate of pay and the possibility of early parole for research subjects must be commensurate with the opportunities available to the prisoner through other work or activities.

581    Another factor that might be termed duress has been observed to arise from illness itself, not from incarceration. John Fletcher and others have reported that experimental subjects sometimes seem to have a high level of the guilt that is part of the "sick role" in our society—the guilt that comes from perceiving oneself as a burden on others without being able to perform a socially useful function in return. Participating in an experiment for the good of society is an excellent way of assuaging this guilt, and a researcher, deliberately or not, may play upon these guilt feelings (which are often unrecognized by the patient himself, and therefore more easily manipulated) in order to obtain a consent that might otherwise not have been offered.

582    Another serious problem has arisen regarding experimentation in children, where proxy consent has to be obtained from the parents. In general, therapeutic trials in children have not posed much more of a problem than in adults. The situation gets sticky in non-therapeutic studies, especially in testing new drugs.

The drug problem arises from the current guidelines of the Food and Drug Administration. Reacting (some say overreacting) to past disasters such as the use of thalidomide in pregnant women before it was known that deformed children would result, the FDA has enacted stringent requirements which must be met before a new drug can be approved for use.

583    After extensive animal experimentation, the FDA requires three phases of human experimentation. First, the drug must be tested in a small group of healthy individuals to determine what its toxic levels are, how it is handled biochemically in the body, the nature of its side effects, etc. By necessity, this requires non-therapeutic experimentation. The last two phases are therapeutic trials on first a small, then a large, patient population.

Since it is a biological fact that children, in terms of their body physiology and biochemistry, are not just smaller versions of adults, and drugs may have very different effects in human beings of different ages, the FDA will not allow a drug to be used in an age group unless it has been tested in that age group. Therefore, a new drug cannot be used in children unless non-therapeutic as well as therapeutic trials are carried out in children.

584    Certain cases of this nature have come to court, and in these instances the courts have tended to make an exception to the general rule that parents are best qualified to speak for their children. The trend in these court decisions is to hold that while an adult is free to take risks himself if he so desires, he has no right to accept the same risks for his child, if there is no way the child can benefit—"You can be a martyr yourself but you can't make a martyr out of your child." If a child is to be allowed to be a non-therapeutic subject at all, some courts have found, only the court, not the parents, is competent to give consent for him or her. This approach has arisen from a number of cases where it appeared that parents had been offered financial or other inducements to allow their children to be used in a study.

The other side of the argument relates to the distribution of the benefits 585
of new medical research. That is, if it is unethical to apply the FDA drug
guidelines to one class of people, and you do not change the FDA guidelines,
then, as a consequence, that class is effectively deprived of any possible health
benefits that might result from the discovery of new drugs. Some have spoken
emotionally of pediatric patients being turned into "therapeutic orphans" if
these kinds of ethical considerations are applied too slavishly. Others have
turned their attentions to the FDA guidelines and asked whether experiments
could not be designed so as to combine the first two phases of drug testing.
If toxicity levels and side effects could be determined by testing in sick children,
the need for non-therapeutic studies would be sharply reduced.

The proposed NIH guidelines make several points about experimentation 586
on children. First, as noted above, a favorable risk-benefit ratio is required, and
determining this means determining the risks. Therefore, the NIH states that
if the experiment can be done on animals or on adults, and all the necessary
information obtained that way, it ought not be done on children. If the experiment cannot be done on adults or animals in order to determine the estimated
level of risk, then it cannot be determined whether a favorable ratio exists,
and the experiment ought not be done on children. If the risks can be estimated
from animal or adult experiments, but additional information is still needed
before therapeutic application can be made, then experimentation on children
may be considered. An exception is allowed in therapeutic trials where the
child is in grave danger already from his illness, and the illness cannot be
treated by other means.

As we noted, some courts have apparently been fearful of parents volun- 587
teering their children for experiments in exchange for money or other benefits.
NIH seems more worried about turning orphanages and juvenile detention
facilities into tempting sources for experimental material. Therefore, the guidelines call for consent of both parents, and forbid research on children without
parents or who are detained by a court order in an institution. The guidelines
also call for a Protection Committee, as with the prisoner experiments. Furthermore, if the child is above the common law "age of discretion" of 7 years,
his own consent should be obtained.

588       Two of the pediatric patients in your practice are sisters, aged 5 years and 18 months, who suffer from hyperargininemia. This hereditary disease, in which cells cannot produce the enzyme arginase, leads to high levels of the amino acid arginine in the blood and spinal fluid, and, over a period of time, to severe mental retardation as a result. The older sister is already severely affected and the younger seems to be developing the same way.

      You are approached by a scientist who wants to inject Shope papilloma virus into the children. Rabbit experiments have suggested that injection of this virus leads to increased levels of arginase and hence decreased blood levels of arginine. It is hypothesized that the virus carries a gene for its own kind of arginase, and once the viral genes get into the cell, the cell can make this kind of arginase.

      The scientist has since observed that 35% of lab workers exposed to papilloma virus have lowered serum arginine levels, without showing any signs of disease. Thus, he concludes, there are grounds for believing that injecting the virus into the sisters could lower their arginine levels without harmful side effects. At any rate, he says, considering their quality of life as severely retarded individuals if nothing is done, the experiment is worth a try.

      On further questioning he acknowledges that some other experiments suggest that instead of having its own gene, the virus merely stimulates the cell to make more arginase from its own genes. This undermines the rationale for the treatment in the case of these sisters, where no cellular gene is present to start with. Also, he admits that many viruses previously thought to be harmless are now thought to cause serious disease after remaining in the body for a long dormant period, up to years. The diseases that might be caused this way include a number of types of cancer. Even considering all these factors, however, he still wants to make the trial.

      A week later the parents of the sisters come in and ask, for the umpteenth time, whether anything can be done for their children.

      Do you tell them about the scientist's proposal? If so, do you recommend to them that they adopt it or not? If you think the experiment itself is ethical, how do you go about obtaining adequate, voluntary informed consent?

      (Adapted from case of the Hastings Center, printed in <u>Medical World News</u>, July 14, 1972.)

---

589       It is clear that this case fits the category of a therapeutic trial, so that from a legal view, the parents are competent to consent on behalf of the girls. If there is any chance that the treatment might help, would it be ethical for you to withhold information about the possibility of this from the parents? Recalling the doctor-patient "contract," we would like to say no immediately. But there might be another consideration here. In this case, the risks are of a fairly sophisticated nature and require a fair amount of biological knowledge to interpret. If the parents do not appear to be well educated, the physician might think twice about their ability to assimilate the information and weigh it properly to reach a rational decision.

As to how the risks and benefits are to be weighed—what is your opinion of the scientist's reference to the quality of life of the girls? Suppose in addition to the severe mental retardation the older sister also had a heart defect requiring major surgery, and the question arose of whether to do the surgery or allow the girl to die. How would you decide in that instance? Does your willingness or unwillingness to allow the girl to die in that instance suggest how much weight you might give to the risks of the experiment? (That is, if you are prepared to allow the girl to die due to her low quality of life, would it be inconsistent to reject this experiment because it carries an unknown risk of a fatal disease in the future?)

590 ↓

Case 37 illustrates fairly well the kind of risk-benefit ratio calculations that are required in instances of therapeutic experimentation, and the problems of informed consent by proxy. Incidentally, this case was based on a real one which was reported in Germany. The pediatrician did agree to the experiment; but, as of three years after the treatment was begun, it has apparently been unsuccessful.

591 ↓

CASE 38

In late March, 1973, a three-judge panel of the Wayne County Circuit Court began hearings on the case of "John Doe," who had spent the last 18 of his 35 years in Ionia state mental hospital after confessing to murder and rape. According to hospital authorities, he has been subject to uncontrollable rages and has not responded to any therapy.

John Doe was scheduled to undergo tests to see if he should have psychosurgery, under a research project financed by the state of Michigan and to be carried out by Wayne State University faculty at Lafayette Clinic in Detroit. However, a suit was filed charging that Doe and other Ionia prisoners were being held unconstitutionally without trials, and that no person so confined could consent voluntarily to become part of such an experiment.

The court is hearing conflicting testimony. The director of the experiment says the operation is to destroy a part of John Doe's brain responsible for his "uncontrollable aggression," and that no surgery would be done unless electrodes implanted into the brain reveal a localized abnormal brain wave pattern. A psychiatrist on the faculty defends the research protocol as fully adequate, and adds that the experiment is not psychosurgery since the abnormal waves would be indicative of local organic pathology.

A neurologist attacks the view that abnormal brain waves are diagnostic of abnormal behavior, and further notes that implantation of electrodes for such a test is itself a very risky procedure. A second psychiatrist attacks the research protocol as wholly inadequate and states, "If it produced any useful information, it would be almost by accident."

A third psychiatrist who spent five hours interviewing John Doe states that he found no evidence for any anger other than a normal and justified response to the poor conditions of the institution. He adds that it cannot be said that John Doe did not respond to conventional therapy, since no adequate therapy exists at Ionia.

John Doe's parents testify that they had signed the consent form for the experiment without reading it, without ever talking to any of the doctors, and without realizing that surgery was involved.

John Doe himself testifies that he gave his consent because he saw it as the only avenue to freedom; and that he has changed his mind after the court suit began, and the testimony indicated that the risk was much greater than he had first realized.


1)    Review the discussion on psychosurgery vs. neurosurgery in Chapter 9. Based on your understanding of the testimony, is this a therapeutic, societal, or manipulative application of behavior control?

2)    Is this a therapeutic or a non-therapeutic experimental situation?

3)    Which of the persons mentioned is John Doe's "doctor," if anyone?

4)    Was informed consent obtained? If not, what would you have required to assure that it was obtained, or is informed voluntary consent not obtainable at all under such circumstances?

5)    If you were a judge on the panel, what would you order done with John Doe, and what would be your ruling on the continuation of the experiment?


(Adapted from newspaper accounts in the Detroit Free Press, Detroit News, and New York Times, March 29—April 9, 1973)

Let's zero in on the question of voluntary informed consent, which is quite messed up in this case. On the one hand, John Doe is clearly being imprisoned against his will, and the idea of freedom is being held out to him as partial coercion to get him into the study. (Compare this case with the more futuristic Case 34 in Chapter 9.) These factors would lead us to be suspicious of the "voluntary" nature of the consent. On the other hand, there is at least some semblance of therapy about the case, so it is not like the prisoner experiments we have been discussing previously. If an experimental treatment is the only treatment for a disease, and a person thereby feels forced to enter the experiment because he wants to maximize his chances of being cured, we do not usually consider this "involuntary" consent, although the label could certainly be applied.

If we are confused about the true therapeutic intent of the experiment, our confusion probably arises out of the confusion of involuntary mental hospitalization itself. In the typical institution, the therapeutic, societal, and manipulative components are so mixed up together that an analysis of the situation is nearly impossible.

Incidentally, note that from the brief amount of information we are given in Case 38, we cannot say that John Doe is mentally incompetent to give informed consent, even if he is constrained by circumstances from giving truly voluntary consent. If anything, he seems more competent than his parents, who signed the form without reading it.

Also note that if the possibility of freedom might constitute coercion in the case of John Doe's consent, the same thing might equally act as coercion upon the parents, if they see the experiment as the only way to free their son. In such a case, is a proxy consent any better than the subject's own consent, as far as protecting the subject's best interests? How do you feel about requiring the court to appoint a disinterested party to serve as the one who consents or denies consent in such a case?

It is not possible, from the testimony cited, to reach any firm conclusions on the design of the experiment from the scientific viewpoint. However, based on the conflicts of testimony, and on the scientific credentials (not cited in the case report) of some experts who testified against the experiment, one has some evidence for concluding that there were significant defects in the experimental design. How does this factor influence your decision as to the ethics of the experiment?

As a point of fact, the court ordered John Doe freed, because he had originally been sent to Ionia without a trial, and the state law that had allowed this procedure had since been repealed. While the court could then have considered the question of the experiment itself to be a moot point, the judges went on to hear more testimony. They eventually concluded that no prisoners in state mental hospitals could be used as subjects in the experiment.

593

594

595

596

597     Now that we have looked over the primary aspects of the ethical decision on any particular experiment, we might ask what the responsibility of the medical profession and the entire society is regarding human experimentation in general. One question is how to enforce the provisions of ethical codes such as the Declaration of Helsinki. We already noted that some agencies will not grant funds unless the experimental protocol includes ethical safeguards; but in a case such as the Lafayette Clinic psychosurgery, the investigators may have escaped this critical review by getting their funds from the state. Another suggestion is that, since the entire career prestige of a scientist is dependent upon having his works published in a reputable journal, the editors of journals have a responsibility not to publish the results of unethical research.

598     Beecher advocated this view in his 1966 expose: "...It is not enough to ensure that all investigation is carried out in an ethical manner; it must be made unmistakably clear in the publications that the proprieties have been observed. This implies editorial responsibility in addition to the investigator's. The question arises then, about valuable data that have been improperly obtained. It is my view that such material should not be published. There is a practical aspect to the matter: failure to obtain publication would discourage unethical experimentation. How many would carry out such experiments if they knew its results would never be published? Even though suppression of such data...would constitute a loss to medicine, in a specific localized sense, this loss, it seems, would be less important than the far reaching moral loss to medicine if the data thus obtained were to be published. Admittedly, there is room for debate."*Another suggestion is to publish such results with a stern editorial condemnation of the methods; Beecher felt that this was likely to smell too much of hypocrisy.

599     A current suggestion among journal editors favors the publication-with-critical-editorial view. It is suggested that if the editors feel that a piece of scientifically valid research is unethical, they ought to print it with a critical editorial, and ought also to inform the investigator that they intend to do this. The investigator might then either withdraw the article, or make his own written reply if he feels he has been unjustly criticized. Beecher's view, on the other hand, has no provision for redress where a researcher genuinely feels that he has taken every necessary ethical precaution.

600     Another question is who is to be selected to be the subjects of medical research. That is, we do not only have to ask if the burden imposed is worth the benefits; we also have to ask if the burden is being distributed over society in an ethical manner. Traditionally this has not been the case, with the vast bulk of subjects for the higher-risk human experimentation coming from the prisons, the mental institutions, and the charity wards of hospitals.

*Reprinted, by permission. From the New England Journal of Medicine 274:1354, 1966.

Sullivan (in Barber, Research on Human Subjects) did a survey of experimental 601
subjects, noting the relationships between whether the patients were low-income
patients from clinics or high-income private patients; whether the potential
benefits outweighed the risks as far as the individual subject was concerned;
and whether the overall benefit to society was great or small as compared to
the risks of the subjects. He found that not only were clinic patients more likely
than private patients to end up in studies with an unfavorable risk-benefit ratio
for themselves, but also that the clinic patients were more likely to be in studies
where the overall societal benefits were low in relation to the risks. A traditional
justification has held that society has a need for medical knowledge which only
experiments on the poor can provide, and that low-cost or subsidized medical
care is society's repayment. Sullivan's data suggest rather that there are some
experiments of potentially low benefit which might never be done at all, except
for the ready availability of poor bodies to do them on.

A number of proposals have been made to change the social distribution 602
of the burden of being an experimental subject. One which is easily rejected is
to halt all human experimentation. This is easily rejected because if one feels
that this experimentation is unethical, in order to be ethically consistent he
ought to be willing to refuse for himself all medical treatment that has been
developed in the past through human experimentation; how many sick people
would be willing to do so?

Another proposal is that since the supposed benefits of these researches
fall upon society as a whole (or is it just upon those segments of society that
can afford ready access to medical care?), there ought to be some sort of
national draft or lottery to select subjects, similar to serving on a jury.

Another question: what happens if an experimental procedure turns out 603
to have severe long-term side effects which had not been anticipated, and the
subjects are left with the need for extensive medical or custodial care? This
problem is analogous to the problem of the children in Europe born with
malformed or absent limbs after their mother took the drug thalidomide. This
was not an experiment per se, but rather a case of a drug being approved for
therapeutic use without adequate testing. In England, after years of court
battles, the company which marketed the drug has finally agreed to pay the
medical bills and damages of these children (which by now has amounted to
many million dollars).

604    In a similar manner, it is also being proposed that a drug company or whoever else sponsors research should be responsible for paying damages if a similar tragedy should occur. This proposal holds that this is fitting even if it raises the cost of drugs. The suffering and risks undertaken by experimental subjects should be calculated as part of the real cost of the product, and the consumers who benefit from the product should pay the price. If some sort of national subject pool chosen by lottery were to be formed, presumably some sort of national experimentation insurance would be a feature of the plan, unless passage of a comprehensive national health insurance plan renders this unnecessary.

605    We have now seen how human experimentation creates problems in the area of the doctor-patient relationship and in informed consent, and we have touched upon some of the societal implications of research in human subjects. To conclude this chapter, we present a case which is complicated by elements of the issues of experimentation, quality of life, and control of reproduction. We offer this for discussion and will attempt no answers, since at the time of this writing the issue is a new one.

---

## CASE 39

606    A certain government's Committee on Research Review is meeting to examine the ethical ramifications of a proposal submitted by the prestigious Institute of Embryology at Y University. The Institute has long been concerned with the plight of women who are prone to spontaneous abortions. While new techniques for care of premature newborns allows medicine to save infants born with birth weights as low as 1200 grams, many women cannot carry a baby even that long and thus are deprived of the opportunity to have children. The Institute is therefore interested in the development of an artificial placenta, which might sustain infants as low as 300 grams birth weight. To perfect this technique, it is necessary to use human fetuses; all possible work in animals has already been done.

The Institute proposes to obtain the fetuses voluntarily aborted by hysterotomy (surgical removal of the fetus from the uterus) under the country's abortion laws which allow abortion up to the 24th week of gestation. At first, the research team feels that they would be able to maintain vital signs in such fetuses for only a few minutes or hours. As the techniques are gradually perfected, survival time will gradually increase.

Because it cannot be known what types of long-range damage the fetus may suffer as a result of these techniques (e.g., brain damage), the Institute wishes to keep fetuses alive for no longer than a two-week period at this point. The institute cannot venture to say what it will do as the techniques are perfected to allow maintaining the fetus to a full-term stage of development, since it has no data at present.

(Adapted from: Case No. 138, Hastings Center Report, April, 1973)

**Questions on Case 39:**

1) Who are the experimental subjects? Are the mothers who abort the fetuses party to the experiment or not?

2) Is it possible to obtain informed consent for these subjects? If so, from whom is the consent to be obtained? In what form?

3) Suppose one feels that a woman may abort a fetus because of her right to control of her own body. Does this right extend also to the right to allow the fetus to be used as a research subject—or is this an unwarranted additional presumption? How about the right to deny permission to use the fetus for research?

4) If the fetus is maintained for a week or more beyond the time when, by law, it has become viable, would "disposal" of it constitute the killing of a human being? Of a "person"?

5) Disposal is justified because of possible unforseen damage, which would not have occurred, however, had the fetus not been used in research to start with. Does this disposal then constitute an attempt to rectify one moral wrong by committing another?

6) Suppose you are now at the point where evidence indicates that the fetus can safely be brought to term without deleterious side effects. Is there now any justification for "disposal"? On the other hand, are you justified in bringing to term an infant which has already been rejected by its mother?

7) The NIH proposed guidelines state that it is wrong to maintain heart beat and respiration in an originally non-viable fetus for research purposes, or to do a research procedure which itself will terminate respiration or he heart beat. It also states that, for purposes of in vitro fertilization, the safety of the technique ought to be demonstrated on non-human primates before a fetus raised that way can be allowed to be brought to term. Do you agree with these policy statements?

8) The NIH also proposes (interestingly, in light of the Supreme Court decision on abortion) that for research purposes, a fetus is a child and consent must be obtained from both parents. For an aborted fetus, only the mother's consent must be obtained. Do you agree? Ch. 12 ↓ 608

# 12. Allocation of Scarce Resources

Up to this point we have been looking at medical-ethical issues from the viewpoint of the individual patient, and have gone on from there to consider longer-range implications at the levels of the family, society, and the human species. If we were to do this with the problem of resource allocation, we would run a serious risk of looking at the issue through the wrong end of the telescope. We will have to anticipate our discussion of "Bioethics" in Chapter 18 and deal with the whole spectrum of resource-allocation decisions.

608

This spectrum of decisions is nicely outlined by Leon Kass: "Personnel and facilities for medical research and treatment are scarce resources. Is the development of a new technology the best use of the limited resources, given current circumstances? How should we balance efforts aimed at prevention against those aimed at cure, or either of these against efforts to redesign the species? How should we balance the delivery of available levels of care against further basic research? More fundamentally, how should we balance efforts in biology and medicine against efforts to eliminate poverty, pollution, urban decay, discrimination, and poor education? This last question about distribution is perhaps the most profound."*

609

A reasonable strategy for approaching a question of resource allocation would be to first define just how much of the resource is available to begin with, or, if partially man-made, how much of the resource is to be made available; and second, determine how that amount of the resource is to be divided among those who stand in need of it. This last problem is the ethical question of "distributive justice." Therefore, let's start off by considering the availability of resources as a global issue, first looking at resources in general and then focusing on medical resources.

610

At the outset we have to get some basic things clear in our minds. The first of these is the concept of the "spaceship earth" that is rather belatedly making itself known in the public awareness—the idea that our resources are finite, and all human beings are part of the same community as far as the use of them goes. For one segment of the human community to use up resources without regard for the needs of the other segments is the same as a person in a rowboat in the middle of the ocean saying, "I don't have to worry about that leak; after all, it's in the other end of the boat."

611

Next, we have to remember that no resource is scarce or plentiful by any isolated objective standards. Rather, it is scarce or plentiful in relation to certain human needs. It is often said that there is a population problem in the world, but this is a misnomer. There would be no population problem if all resources were infinitely extensible. The real problem is a mutual balance between population, food supply, land, and other needed resources.

612

*From L.R. Kass, "The New Biology: What Price Relieving Man's Estate?" Science 174:779, 1971. Copyright 1971 by the American Association for the Advancement of Science.

613    Further, we have to be more specific about what we mean by human needs; we might want to establish at least three categories. First we would have the needs that must be met to maintain survival at a minimal biological level—food, water, etc. Next would be the needs that must be met to provide the environment suitable for what we have been calling a minimal "quality of life." Things such as public educational facilities might fit into this category. In the last category would be the "needs" which go beyond this, such as the needs created by advertising in this country for items such as deodorant sprays, canned dog food, snowmobiles for recreational use, and a host of others. If we are forced by scarcity of resources to eliminate some of these needs, it is not hard to see which category will go first. The problem is that placing an item in the second or the third category is to a large extent a value judgment rather than a decision based on firm biological data. For instance, it is clear that advocates of gun-control laws place handguns in the third category, while most sportsmen place them in the second.

614    The philosopher John Rawls, in his A Theory of Justice, makes use of the idea of "self-respect," which he defines as having a "rational plan of life" which is respected by one's associates, and having confidence in one's general abilities to carry out one's intentions. In his scheme for social justice, Rawls gives highest rank to those "primary goods," as he calls them, which are most closely tied to individual self-respect. A more detailed working out of "self-respect" might very likely aid us in sorting out human needs among the three categories.

615    Where does medical care fit into these categories? The talk of the "right to health care" would seem to suggest that this is a basic survival need. However, we can't deny that the human species has survived throughout most of its history, and continues to do so today in many parts of the world, with only a mere fraction of what we consider to be minimal medical care in this country. Therefore, the bulk of medicine would seem to fit into the quality-of-life category ("second-class needs"). Certain aspects of medicine, such as cosmetic surgery, might be placed in the third category as a relative luxury item. Much of the new medical technology predicted for the future fits into the third-class-need category. For instance, the idea of dying at age 70 or 80 is consistent with our present notion of quality of life; therefore it could be argued that medical advances which would extend the life span greatly beyond this would constitute a response to third-class "needs."

616    Now to interject the question of distributive justice. We might say that ideally the resources needed to meet all first-class needs should be distributed equally among all the peoples of the world. While we might call medical care a second-class need, nevertheless it seems to occupy a particular place in our value structure, and so we might want to include it in the universal distribution scheme also.

Suppose that a benevolent director came to power as ruler of the world tomorrow and set about to implement universal justice; what would be the result? As to food, it is a calculable fact that if the total food supply were to be distributed among the entire world population, everyone would be hungry, though many would be less hungry than before. There is simply not enough food being produced right now to supply every man, woman and child with the number of calories, let alone the nutritional balance, that the experts have set as minimal nutritional requirements.

The situation with medical facilities would be even more acute. In the U.S., with an average of one doctor for every 700 or so persons, we are talking about a physician shortage and attempting to increase the number of new doctors graduating from medical schools. Under the benevolent dictatorship, all these new graduates, as well as many of the doctors in practice, would be shipped overseas to countries such as Kenya which now has one physician for every 11,000 inhabitants.

This picture of worldwide redistribution points out some of the political aspects of the resource problem. Simply put, it seems to be a tendency for humans who have enjoyed second-class or third-class needs being met effortlessly for a period of time, to unconsciously redefine these as first-class and second-class needs. If someone then tries to take away those resources, all hell is likely to break loose. In 1973, the U.S. public was faced with the prospects of relative shortages of food and fuel. Public demands included stepped-up food production and cuts in foreign exports of food; and the immediate construction of the Alaska pipeline with stepped-up offshore drilling. If anyone recommended a lowering in the level of expectations in order to get along with less resources, his voice was lost in the general din. And even the worst shortages envisioned still would have left the American public with far more supplies than would be the case under our hypothetical benevolent dictator.

These illustrations are not included to show that the American people, who have always fancied themselves the unselfish friends of mankind, would be the first and strongest opponents of any true attempt at global resource distribution. Rather, the main point is that the scarcity of resources issue as pertains to medicine is a very real one; as in the case of the food problem, anyone who says that the whole difficulty can be solved by better distribution or transportation techniques is dreaming. Therefore, as we go on to deal with problems of distributing resources within the U.S. health care system (such as whether Social Security should pay for kidney machines), we have to remember that we are describing a highly artificial and potentially unstable system. At some time in the future, the other three billion passengers on the spaceship may knock at our doors and demand their rightful share, and the whole house of cards will collapse.

617

618

619

620     It is, nevertheless, within that artificial and unstable system that we will have to practice medicine for the foreseeable future. And even within the confines of American society, the prospects are disturbing. Not only has the cost of basic medical care and hospitalization increased several-fold in the past decade, but very expensive technologies for treating illnesses which used to be untreatable are increasing in use. One patient on an artificial kidney machine for one year may run up a bill of $20,000 to $40,000, and right now only a fraction of the people who could use such machines have access to them. This was changed by the Social Security bill of 1973 which would, in principle, provide Federal funds to anyone in need of dialysis who cannot afford it. Based on such trends and the likelihood of even more expensive treatments in the future, such as artificial hearts, it has been estimated that within a few decades, the U.S. could find itself devoting over half of its gross national product to health care.

621     It would seem that we have a clear conflict between these economic considerations and the sanctity-of-life demand that the physician do everything possible to preserve life. If we presume that if the physician has an individual ethical obligation to do something, then the medical establishment has a social responsibility to provide the resources to allow him to do it; then it would appear that the obligation to preserve life at all costs would definitely lead us down the road of total resource allocation, regardless of how much the society's quality of life in other areas may suffer as a result. (Of course we get to a critical point where the allocation of economic resources to medicine begins to threaten other first-class needs and thus produce more illness by malnutrition, inadequate sanitation, etc.)
        REVIEW
        SANCTITY ¦ 218

622     If the sanctity-of-life approach leads to this dilemma, can the quality-of-life view do better? We have been making reference to some kind of quality of life of a society. Does this mean merely the best possible quality of life for the greatest number of people, or is there more to it than that?
        We have seen in Chapter 6 how the quality-of-life approach can help us determine whether a certain patient should receive a certain treatment, given the assumption that the treatment is available. We could envision an ethical system which restricted the use of expensive life-prolonging technologies such as kidney dialysis, by means of establishing very stringent quality-of-life criteria for the use of the treatment so that only a few would qualify. Since we have seen that all quality-of-life criteria so far proposed tend to have a hint of prejudice or elitism about them, the political ramifications of such a course might very well doom it, regardless of the ethical difficulties involved.
        REVIEW
        BIAS    ¦ 233

We are led to the conclusion that if treatment of a certain type is not available to all who have the strictly medical indications for it, it might be socially and politically most acceptable to have it available to none. Implementation of this would entail careful monitoring of research funds presently being spent, in order to emphasize research that promises new low-cost therapies, or better ways to utilize existing therapies. This may be partially self-defeating in that it is often necessary to develop an expensive and inefficient prototype first before a cheaper modification suitable for large-scale use can be designed. (In the case of dialysis, note that the scarce resource is not the dialysis machine but the teams of trained personnel needed to work a dialysis program. While the machine itself could be modified to some degree, the idea of a year's course of dialysis therapy costing as much as weekly allergy shots seems highly unlikely at any time in the future.)

623

The problem of possibly removing some therapies already available to a small number is much more sticky. As the case of the Social Security legislation has shown, once a treatment becomes available at all, the political pressures to make it much more widely available become close to insurmountable. It should also be remembered that the medical establishment is accountable to the public to some degree, even if medical leaders refuse to recognize this at the time. The medical profession has been brought down from the pristine pedestal it previously occupied in public opinion by the present controversies about unequal distribution of health care and about questionable human experimentation. If it also became known that the medical profession was going into the business of withholding treatment from sick patients, the political pressure would be very great for a total regulation of medicine by government. While greater political regulation of medicine is not necessarily a bad thing, under these circumstances it is very likely that ethical considerations, or even rational ones, would be thrust into the background.

624

While political control spurred by such emotions might have more bad consequences than good ones, nevertheless we have to face the conclusion that society as a whole has a right of participation in any decision involving the allocation of medical resources on a large scale. This implies that if the removal of some existing treatment options is necessary in order to avoid unavailability of resources to meet other needs, the public must be made aware of this and educated as to the consequences of ignoring the issue. Needless to say, this is going to require a level of public awareness and far-sightedness that has not been often seen in the past; the question of how this awareness is to be accomplished before the damage has been done can best be postponed until Chapter 18.

625

**626**    The question of resource allocation between medicine and other social needs is a question that the physician can neither answer nor duck. He cannot answer it because such a question demands a type of sociological and economic expertise not possessed by most physicians. He cannot (ethically) duck it because the answer to the question will have a profound impact on the way he practices medicine. The medical establishment ought to have a say when such matters are debated, but it must share the arena with other professionals; and medicine must give way to these other expert opinions when the other experts are looking at the matter from a broader perspective.

**627**    After this very brief overview of the resource problem on the global and societal levels, we have to focus in on the doctor and the patient. We shall consider this in two parts: first, the effect resource allocation problems have on our model of the doctor-patient relationship; and second, how the doctor ought to handle problems of distributive justice when he must choose among patients.

**628**    We have noted that one element of the doctor-patient "contract" is the expectation that the doctor will inform the patient about all the alternatives that might be open from a medical point of view, and offer them as options among which the patient may choose. It is taken for granted that the physician is limited in his range of alternatives by forces outside of his control, and that he is not obligated to describe options that are not his to dispense. For example, if society decided that kidney machines were a waste of resources and should be gotten rid of, the physician would not be obligated to inform his patients in renal failure about dialysis treatment. (We argue also that in some cases the physician might be ethically obligated to describe an option he was not prepared to give, if it was his own moral compunctions and not medical or societal restrictions that prevented him from offering the treatment—as with sterilization and contraception.)

**629**    What happens if, as we recommended, the medical profession takes an active role, along with other segments of society, in restricting certain treatment options by the resource-allocation restrictions that are agreed to? We could envision several ways in which this might or might not affect the doctor-patient relationship. Most simply, the doctor might decide that while organized medicine is making resource allocation decisions, he is taking no part in it, and is content simply to live with the results. If the doctor plays Pontius Pilate in this way, we might question his degree of social responsibility, but he seems to have preserved the old doctor-patient contract intact.

In another case the physician might take an active role in making resource decisions, while keeping this activity separate from his patient contacts—very much as a doctor who is running for political office might compartmentalize his activities. For instance, the doctor might be arguing in a committee that kidney machines are an unaffordable waste of resources; but so long as the committee has not taken final action on his proposal, he could continue to offer dialysis as a treatment option to his patients who might benefit from it. 630

We might imagine this same doctor saying to himself that his activities were really not consistent if he argues against wasting resources on kidney machines while recommending the machines to his patients. Therefore he decides to avoid giving the treatment that he is opposed to. This constitutes a moral judgment on his part. He might then still notice an obligation to the patient to at least mention the existence of this treatment and note that the patient could go to another doctor if he wished to receive it. This is essentially what we recommended in Chapter 10 where the doctor's own moral values prohibited him from giving out a certain treatment, but where the patient's right to adequate and comprehensive health care would be violated if an alternative were not provided. 631

Recall, however, the argument of the hypothetical pious physician in Chapter 10 who objected that if he told the patient about another doctor who would give the treatment, he would be leading the patient into sin, and that would be sinful for himself. Similarly, a doctor who feels strongly that a treatment constitutes a misuse of resources might argue that if he gives the treatment himself, or if he allows the patient to go to another doctor for it, the end result is still the misuse of those resources, so either action would be prohibited. 632

This argument sounds more plausible than the religious one because something is involved here beyond an insoluble disagreement about sin. In the other case, the doctor insists that if the patient gets the abortion or what-ever, the patient will burn in hell, while the patient insists she won't; and only after we are all dead will we know who was right.

REVIEW ↑
"SIN"   ¦ 491

The resource argument sounds more plausible because what is at stake are the interests of the whole society, and the patient, as a member of society, will be damaged if these interests are disregarded. 633

Of course, this plausibility is only superficial because of the point we raised earlier, that the physician as a physician has no special expertise in deciding what are wise and unwise use of resources. If the patient is a member of society, then he has as much right to participate in societal decisions as the physician, up until the time when the properly situated societal institutions agree on a final solution to which both patient and physician must submit.

## CASE 40

634
As a prominent physician, you have been called upon by a joint House-Senate committee which is discussing legislation on research into the development of a workable artificial heart. Since you know that your prestige will cause the committee to put great weight on your testimony, you are preparing your position with care.

In your readings on the subject, you are most impressed by two articles. One summarizes succinctly all the arguments against the development of this new technology: the problems inherent in the task; the great cost of the research alone; the considerable cost of each artificial heart after it is perfected, which would mean either that it will be available only to the rich or that the government would have to subsidize its use; the possibility that the living would keep having one heart put in after another in order to keep on living, without regard for the needs of generations of humans yet unborn; all the pressing social needs which the several million dollars needed just to begin the research could better be spent on.

The other article is much briefer and confines itself to one argument. It states the obvious, that an artificial heart would constitute a treatment option not now available to physicians. And, it argues, we have an obligation not only to our own good sense but also to society and to posterity to increase the number of options open wherever possible. Only by "keeping our options open" can mankind maintain adaptability in the face of a changing environment, and thereby hope to survive as a species.

What is your testimony before the committee going to be—in favor of or opposed to the allocation of the research money?

---

635
While you can argue the merits of this case, we will focus on one argument—the business of "keeping your options open," which is often thrown about loosely in ethical discussions of this type. As we did in Chapter 6 with "playing God" and "primum non nocere," we might ask whether this phrase is a meaningful one, or whether it is used as a smoke screen to dodge the really hard ethical questions.

Back in Chapter 2 when we described the steps of the decision-making process, we observed that a common error was to assume that for any decision there must be two and only two alternatives. We saw that the world is not a binary computer, where at each decision point there are only two choices, "yes" or "no" or "0" or "1". Our experience indicates that there are some actions we can take which genuinely increase the net number of options open to us, and other actions which decrease the number. An example of the former might be going to college, so far as job opportunities are concerned. An example of the latter, so far as alternative life styles are concerned, might be joining a monastery or convent.

REVIEW
ALTERNATIVES 32

In science, certain discoveries also seem to open up a whole range of new options; these usually fall into the category of pure research. The artificial-heart project is applied research, with its research goal sharply focused. How does that fit into this picture?

Also recall the point we raised about the resource-allocation element that is present in all ethical decisions—that a decision to do one thing is at the same time a decision not to do all the other things that we might have done at the same time. Any decision we make automatically entails closing off options, whether we like it or not. Therefore, we have to come up with some sort of "net" number of options that are left after the decision is made, in order to compare two alternative courses of action. In the case of college, suppose that going to college increased your job opportunities greatly over those of the high-school graduate. However, if you go to college you cannot join the Army, and it happens at this time that there are more job openings for Army veterans than for college graduates. Under those circumstances, to decide to go to college because it "opens up options" would be a decision based only on one fragment of the total picture.

Thus, while "keeping your options open" is a good thing to do in the abstract, the idea that it logically follows that therefore one should manufacture an artificial heart is full of flaws. The options opened by having the heart have to be weighed against all the options that will be closed when the several million dollars is used up for research purposes.

Besides, notice that once we have chosen a goal, many options may lead to consequences that are incompatible with that goal. For example, suppose we have firm evidence that the continuation of the present rate of population growth will lead to the extinction of the human species, by starvation or pollution or both, within two hundred years. The phrase "keeping your options open" would seem, in its unqualified state, to demand that we keep open the option of everyone having as many children as they wish. Do we truly want to "keep all our options open" in that instance?

Let's now turn to the problem of distributive justice, or allocation of resources on the patient-by-patient level. This problem is no stranger to busy practitioners, who apply it every day when they decide how many appointments to schedule or whether they can accept any new patients.

636

637

638

639    Any such problem is usually handled in two stages. First, one selects a pool of possible recipients of treatment by excluding all those who do not meet certain objective and medical criteria. Then one selects out of this pool the appropriate number of people who will actually get the treatment.

In the example cited with the practicing physician, the pool is formed by taking all those who call for appointments and eliminating those whose medical problems do not coincide with the doctor's specialty. From this pool, those to receive appointments are selected on a simple first-come-first-served basis, with exceptions being made for those referred by other physicians, personal friends, etc.

640    Since the problems of kidney dialysis and kidney transplantation have received a great deal of attention in the literature, we might use these as examples for this discussion.

When dialysis programs first began, the pool was selected by medical criteria designed to select those who were most likely to benefit from dialysis in terms of their lengthening of biological survival time. These included such things as age between puberty and 55, absence of complications such as diabetes, etc. Since machines have become more common and since the teams have become more experienced, these limits have been loosened up to a certain extent.

641    Next, one has to choose from that pool the patients to get the machines, assuming that there are not enough to go around and that those patients turned down will, if a machine does not become available in the near future, die of end-stage uremic poisoning. Here the groups have tended to go in one of two directions. One was the phenomenon referred to in Chapter 7 as the "Let's form a committee syndrome." In this case it was assumed that if the committee was given the right composition from the start, with the proper mix of clergy, laymen, physicians, and what have you, that "ethical" decisions would magically arise from the subsequent deliberations. Hence, the attention was directed to the criteria to select members of the committee instead of the criteria that the committee was to use to actually select patients for the kidney machines.

642    Once these committees were formed (and immediately dubbed "God Committees" by the cynics), the members belatedly came to the problem that those dialysis groups who took the second direction came to in the first place— by what kind of criteria do you select the patients who will live and who will die? The way in which the committees handled this problem provided a field day for medical sociologists, but the results represented less than a bumper crop of ethical insights.

(For instance, one conclusion the sociologists reached was that physicians tended to make poor members of the committee as far as the actual decision-making went. It seemed that their prior training made it nearly impossible for a physician to say "no" to putting anyone on a life-saving machine. Eventually the lay members had to step in to take the burden of the final decision off the doctor's shoulders.)

The most basic way of approaching the problem of criteria is to decide to have none at all. Everyone will be chosen by purely random procedures, so that there can be no question of favoritism or unfairness. This sounds attractive in its simplicity. How does it measure up when one is faced with a specific case?

643

## CASE 41

You are a one-man God Committee (all the others called in sick today) who has two kidney machines and five patients who are ready to die of renal failure if they do not get a machine. The information you have been given on them is as follows:

644

| Patient | Sex | Marital Status | Age | No. Children | Occupation |
|---------|--------|----------------|-----|--------------|------------|
| A | male | married | 35 | 2 | ? |
| B | female | single | 28 | 0 | ? |
| C | male | married | 38 | 3 | ? |
| D | female | married | 32 | 1 | ? |
| E | male | married | 30 | 0 | ? |

Are you going to select your two lucky winners at random? If not, what criteria are you going to use? What further information would you need to apply those criteria? How can you obtain that information in a way that will not bias your results?

One interesting feature that the medical sociologists have observed is that given the amount of information presented in Case 41, the majority opinion tends to favor a random selection. However, as more information is added, people want to start to apply specific criteria. For example:

645

## CASE 42

646        At your next meeting you are still alone, and again five patients are vying for two machines. This time, however, you have an additional item of information for each.

| Patient | Sex | Marital Status | Age | No. Children | Occupation |
|---------|-----|----------------|-----|--------------|------------|
| A | male | married | 35 | 2 | Mafia hit man |
| B | female | single | 28 | 0 | Concert violinist |
| C | male | married | 38 | 3 | Accountant (currently unemployed while on trial for embezzlement) |
| D | female | married | 32 | 1 | Manager of house of prostitution |
| E | male | married | 30 | 0 | Researcher on kidney physiology; last year became youngest man to win Nobel Prize for his role in developing the kidney machine |

Are you going to select the two at random? If not, by what criteria? Are these criteria different from those you adopted in Case 41?

647        Unlike most of the other cases we have presented, we cannot claim that Case 42 is a true situation. However, it illustrates the way that emotional components are bound to enter into the decisions of such a committee. If the committee operates on an <u>ad hoc</u> basis the emotionalism will influence the decisions directly. If the committee operates by criteria the emotionalism will influence the choice of the criteria.

One observer, noting the tendency of the committees to emphasize middle-class church-going virtues in their criteria for selection, commented that Henry David Thoreau with bad kidneys would never stand a chance.

648        A model committee made up of medical students chose as its criteria the number of years of biological survival that the patient could expect. It might have been only a coincidence that since medical students are uniformly young, they would have been at the top of the list according to their own criteria.

On the other hand, when dialysis machines were first introduced into use in Sweden—a culture with a longer heritage of respecting older persons as valuable members of society—preference was uniformly given to older patients over young ones.

Possibly the most bizarre while still entirely rational criteria are recounted in this anecdote. One committee had continually given preference to men who were happily married and who had children dependent upon them. The crunch came when the committee had to choose between two men about the same age, both married, and with identical numbers of young children. After deliberation, the committee decided to proceed by figuring out which of the two wives, by virtue of good looks, bank account, or whatever, would have the easiest time getting another husband and remarrying. The decision was then to give the access to the dialysis machine to the husband of the other wife.

649

These illustrations may help to explain why, in those situations in which it is still necessary to select patients for life-or-death matters, the idea of forming "God Committees" to do the job is losing popularity. But is anything gained by this? An individual still has to choose, either at random or by some set of criteria similar to the ones discussed. The only gain is that these decisions are more private than committee meetings, so that if a complete lack of ethical consistency and a mockery of distributive justice is what is actually taking place, at least one is not making a public spectacle of it.

650

However, as we said at the beginning of Chapter 7, it is important not to let the "committee syndrome" distract attention from the actual features of decision-making. If committees use social-worth criteria, what are the implications of this choice?

651

---

## CASE 43

At long last another member of the committee has shown up for work. In the last case, you elected to employ a set of social worth criteria (since the five candidates had already been chosen by virtue of the fact that medical criteria had been met). As a result, patients C and E are receiving renal dialysis, and you have sent flowers for A, B, and D. However, at this meeting, two new candidates have applied. Both are reasonably upstanding individuals. One meets the medical criteria better than either C or E, in that she has fewer medical complications outside of the primary renal problem. The other is a highly placed politician whose particular interest has been to get additional government funds for research and development of dialysis programs. Since you can always train more physiologists, while enlightened politicians are hard to come by, you conclude that this candidate meets the social worth criteria better than either C or E.

652

You state that it is indeed a pity that no opening in the program exists for either of these two individuals; but your fellow committee member says that this is no problem; you will simply put C and E off the machines to allow these new candidates to have them. When you object that it is improper to stop treatment on people once they have been accepted, he replies that if one takes the medical and social worth criteria seriously——i.e., that certain individuals are more worthy of being saved——his proposal is the logical conclusion. If not, really you are simply allocating resources on a first-come, first-served basis; and this is random allocation and not medical and social worth criteria.

Do you accept this argument? What do you do with the new patients?

653    Considerations such as those in Case 43 led Childress to reject social-worth criteria in favor of some sort of random selection, which he felt would better serve the notion of the dignity of the indivdual and trust in the physician.

Westerveldt has noted that there are problems with the first-come, first-served means of selection. Dialysis is only the last stage of medical treatment for renal failure. How do you motivate a patient to stick to his treatment regimen to prevent or postpone the need for dialysis, if his compliance might result in someone getting the kidney machine ahead of him when he finally does need it? But presumably such problems could be worked out in a practical scheme.

654    Up to now we have been touting the idea of quality of life as a means of approaching many difficult ethical issues. Can we select recipients of scarce medical resources on the basis of quality-of-life criteria instead of social worth or at random? Westerveldt, a renal specialist, insists that "God Committees" have tried to do just that——by looking into the patient's psychological and social environment, they have tried to select those who will lead the nearest-to-normal life and will make the best adjustment to dialysis. We must conclude that either the critics of the committees failed to see this; or else that in practice the committees strayed from this ideal and went instead to social worth criteria.

655    By social worth criteria, the committees approached their task as one of dispensing a limited number of gifts. Without dialysis, everyone, not just some, would have died; so the natural approach is: "Society is doing this for you. Now what are you doing for society?" Within this framework, the idea of judging the candidate on the basis of his own interests would not occur to anyone. (Not only have patients been denied dialysis because of their lifestyles; in a few cases, patients obviously unable to make the psychological adjustment to the machine-dependent existence have literally been forced to continue therapy.)

656    This approach stands out as a glaring inconsistency with the now-popular notion of medical care as a right, not a privilege. Which is it? If medical care is a right, and dialysis is medical care, committees have no more right to inquire into the social worth of the recipient than a public health nurse would have asking a person if they are Democrat or Republican before she will give them a polio booster. On the other hand, we might decide that some medical care, such as polio vaccine, is "normal" and is a right, while other care, such as dialysis or transplant, is "extraordinary" and is a privilege. This dichotomy between "ordinary" and "extraordinary" care has already cropped up in the Catholic Church's position that one must give one, but not necessarily the other, to a dying patient. But we already observed that in practice the distinction is often hard to make.

Now we have to go back to the problem of resource allocation on the societal level, since problems that crop up in questions of patient-by-patient allocation might be indications that our societal-level priorities are out of whack.

Let's assume that we have adopted the two-level view of medical care, with some of it being a "right" and some being a privilege. Now we must compare this with our scheme of the three classes of human needs. Wouldn't it seem that privilege-care must be a third-class need (a relative luxury item that society can dispense with) while right-care must be a second-class need (one which would result in a lowering of quality of life below a minimum level if not met)? And can we not therefore conclude that if there is any scarcity of resources, the privilege-care ought to be the first to go? This might not have been the intention at all of those who labeled that kind of care a "privilege" to begin with.

REVIEW ↑
NEEDS ┊ 613

The people who want to have kidney machines to fall back on if their kidneys give out are thus in a bind. If they want to define that kind of care as a right, they have to expend the resources to build enough machines and train enough personnel so that they can share their machines with the natives of Kenya, among others. If they want to define that kind of care as a privilege, they are setting it up as a sitting duck to be the first to go under any sort of truly just system of distribution. The reason that these people are not in this bind, of course, is that such a system of resource allocation does not now exist. As we conclude this discussion of scarce resources, the most fitting question might be for how long the natives of Kenya, among others, are going to stand for this.

657

658

Ch. 13 ↓ 659

# 13. Euthanasia and Allowing to Die

In Chapter 6, "Determination of the Quality of Life," we stated what the ideal of ethical consistency would require that decisions made about the beginning of life and about the end of life should both be related to some clear and easily applicable unifying principle. We argued that some kind of quality-of-life approach was the most useful way to set up such a principle. However, we also said that as of now, the medical profession has not come close to this ideal state, and tends to deal with these issues in a more fragmented fashion. Therefore, in Chapter 10, we gave some additional discussion about abortion; and in this chapter we will have some additional things to say about allowing a patient to die and about euthanasia or "mercy killing."

REVIEW
CONSISTENCY    237

We'll begin with a quick summary of what was already said on this subject. We have already outlined the features of a quality-of-life approach, given an example of a set of quality-of-life criteria upon which life and death decisions could be based (Appendix III), and pointed out the strengths and weaknesses of such a method.

From a medical-sociological standpoint, we listed eight "stages of involvement" ranging from vigorous treatment to active involuntary euthanasia, and made some observations about the current attitudes of physicians to these stages and about how far many physicians will go along this spectrum.

REVIEW
STAGES    243

We then considered the argument that allowing a patient to die at his request (and, therefore, euthanasia as well) was wrong because it was the same as suicide. Several arguments against this view were offered. The basic point of these was the presumed right of a person to control his own body, although we saw in some court decisions that the state was not ready to relinquish all its rights in the matter.

We did, however, see other court decisions which seem to establish some precedent for the right of a competent individual to refuse life-prolonging treatment. (Since it was also argued that once one accepts the position that it is right to allow a person to die, it is hard to make a firm ethical distinction between that and actively bringing about the death, these court decisions might, at some time in the future, provide the basis for judicial approval of euthanasia by consent of the patient.)

It is obvious why the issue of euthanasia has become more prominent lately—the recent advances in medical technology which allow an almost indefinite preservation of existence on a merely biological level. (These same life-prolonging technologies have provided the impetus for the "brain death" redefinition described in Chapter 6.) Interestingly, while modern technology has increased the support for the idea of euthanasia, it has almost completely eliminated one of the indications that has traditionally been considered as the primary case in which euthanasia might be applied—intractable pain. With narcotics and other drugs, or surgery on nerve roots where drugs fail, it is generally possible today to bring any pain to within bearable levels. With drugs, however, the price paid for this might well be the total loss of any higher-level mental function; and we might well ask what we have gained in such a case by not killing the individual outright instead of doping him into oblivion.

659

660

661

662

663    Even if intractable pain has been virtually eliminated, we can assume that there are other kinds of "suffering" which might also lead a rational person to desire death; therefore, we shall use "suffering" as a general term to describe the kinds of reasons one might have for desiring euthanasia.

On the political and educational fronts, a number of organizations have taken up the cause, and in some cases have had bills introduced into state legislatures, under the rallying cry of "the right to death with dignity." Since this seems on the surface to be another one of those self-proclaimed rights which do not specify whose responsibility it is to deliver the goods, we might be suspicious of this "right" until it is examined more critically.

REVIEW
"RIGHTS" 157—165

664    First of all, just exactly what do people mean by death with "dignity"? At the vaguest level, there might be some reference to "lying in bed stuck full of tubes." Since in modern hospital practice it is more rare than otherwise to come across a patient who does not have at least one tube in him somewhere, this could easily degenerate into the ridiculous question of how many tubes a person must have before he is undignified.

A better approach, one which is more in keeping with some of the quality-of-life criteria, would say that the essential feature is some degree of conscious self-awareness and a sense of having control over one's fate. Death is undignified, in this view, when the person becomes a "vegetable" and cannot communicate.

665    One writer stated on this subject, "My father and mother both died on the farm at about sixty. Until their last illnesses, they were active and vigorous, and life seemed good to them in spite of the lack of modern sanitation or lighting in the house. All of their brothers and sisters went to the city, lived in modern houses and openly pitied my mother's lot of farmer's wife. In their protected environments, they have gone on living, until their average age is eighty. One is blind, one has been terribly crippled with rheumatism, the keen mind of another is entirely faded, and the oldest...is cared for by a paid attendant. With all his contemporaries scattered, I hardly wonder that he longs to die."*

This seems to represent a view of dignity depending on the overall functioning of an individual, or what others might call having a "meaning" in one's continued existence, and thus gives a particularly holistic view of what might be meant by quality of life.

666    On the other hand, it has been argued that death with dignity is a poor term because death is inherently undignified; and thus, in a perverse sort of way, those who go around promoting "death with dignity" are making death even more undignified than it would be otherwise. This line of thinking also draws upon the argument which often follows "death with dignity," that is, that death is a normal part of life (we shall have more to say about this at the end of the chapter). The retort is that if death is a part of life because it is inevitable, then suffering is a part of life also, but there is no lobbying effort going on for "suffering with dignity." This whole line of argument derives its best support from a religious framework of beliefs, although many clergymen are active supporters of the euthanasia movement; clearly different theologians are reading the revealed signals of religion differently.

*Reprinted from Lucy G. Morgan, in the <u>Hastings Center Report</u>, Vol. 1, Dec. 1971, with permission of the Institute of Society, Ethics and the Life Sciences, Hastings-on-Hudson, N.Y. 10706.

The only conclusion possible out of all this, from an ethical viewpoint, is that in a pluralistic society, any reference to what is dignified and what is not has to be more a matter of taste than a matter of morals. *Therefore, granted that one wishes to maximize "dignity," whatever it is, about the only way to accomplish it is to let the patient decide for himself how he wishes to make his exit, within the reality constraints that are imposed by circumstances outside his control. It might follow from this that the doctor ought to favor laws that would allow him to take positive action to end life, since that is one of the options that a minority of patients may request, so long as the law has enough safeguards to prevent abuses.*

667

The argument against this is that it would be impossible to write a law with enough safeguards to prevent all abuse, and so any such law is too dangerous to allow, even if the goal is a laudable one. Recall that this was the same objection raised by the sanctity-of-life proponents against any set of quality-of-life criteria, and that it was related to what we called the "domino theory" in ethics. The only answer to both objections is to actually design a law, or a set of criteria, that seems comprehensive enough to satisfy all but the extreme die-hards, and then try it and see empirically what the results are.

668

REVIEW
DOMINO THEORY | 227

While we cannot make any list of do's and don't's about how to achieve dignity, one simple and practical suggestion is worth noting. If the outcry against undignified death and "tubes" and all is a recent development, the implication is that death was more dignified twenty years or so ago than it is now. This might be seen as mere sentimental nostalgia with no basis in fact; or it could be seen as the reflection of the fact that several decades ago many or most people died at home while today the vast majority die in hospitals or nursing homes. And, whatever your dignity criteria might be, it is almost certain to turn out that one's home is a more dignified setting than a hospital. Therefore, if medicine were to re-orient its practices toward more home care for terminal patients, "death with dignity" would automatically increase. (Medicine is just now finding that home care pays dividends for the non-terminally ill as well.)

669

Since we have been using the term of euthanasia in its more modern (and etymologically incorrect) sense of "mercy killing," we ought to stop a bit and look at the implications of this. *While we are doing this, it is important to remember that mercy killing, even though practiced by a small number of physicians on infrequent occasions, is still murder in the eyes of the law everywhere in the U.S.* Since, however, there is a possibility this may change in the future, we are justified in divorcing the ethical from the legal issue, and discuss in what situations we might advocate euthanasia if it were legal to do so. At present, a physician who wishes to kill a patient must make the ethical decision on civil disobedience as well as the ethical decision on euthanasia.

670

REVIEW
LAW | 261–262

671    We made it clear in Chapter 2 that the ultimate test, when compared against our values, was the <u>consequences</u> of an action, thereby implying that in ethical justification the <u>motives</u> of an action took second place. We have had further occasion to bring up the motives of actions in a number of places in this unit, but these were mentioned in order to clarify the basic assumptions upon which the argument was proceeding. At no time has it been stated that an act was to be judged ethically valid or invalid on the basis of the motives <u>alone</u>.

With euthanasia, therefore, we come across a peculiar word compared to our previous discussions. If euthanasia is defined as "mercy killing," the inclusion of "mercy" means that the motive of the action, or its presumed motive, is included in the definition of the action. Therefore, a question, "Is euthanasia right or wrong?" is an invitation to judge an act on its motives, which we have denied as proper ethical method.

672    The philosophical messiness of having the action and motive mixed up in one word might suggest that euthanasia is a bad word, as so defined, and we need a better one. However, there does not seem to be a better word that compresses the essential idea in so short a space.

Therefore, we have to conclude that "mercy killing," like "killing," is an ethically neutral term, and cannot be judged right or wrong independent of the circumstances (i.e., the consequences). Instead of asking if euthanasia is right or wrong, we can clarify the matter by asking what kinds of acts fit the definition of euthanasia.

673    One instance might be that of allowing a patient to die, or ending his life, because of the resources that would be used up and "wasted" if he were allowed to live as long as he might otherwise have done. The motive is the benefit to society of conserving scarce medical resources. This is not euthanasia if we make the reasonable assumption that "mercy" implies a concern for the best interests and the wishes of the individual patient himself. As to whether this kind of allowing to die or killing is allowable, our discussion of resource allocation in Chapter 12 has suggested a good way to escape this decision— resource allocation is a societal matter and should be decided on the basis of societal policy, not on <u>ad hoc</u> individual decisions by individual doctors.

674    The next typical instance is a sticky one—the desire to allow a patient to die, or to kill him, because his continued biological existence at a continued low quality of life is an emotional and financial drain on his family and upon those who are required to care for him. This instance will come up more frequently if home care again becomes the norm for terminal patients—what about the mother with several young children, whose nerves are worn and whose attention is distracted by having to care for an aged parent at the same time? Is this fair to the children?

This is a sticky case because most writers on euthanasia slip easily back and forth between this case and a genuine euthanasia case, in which the person is either demonstrably suffering or else has voluntarily requested an end to his life. We often hear talk of "Euthanasia should be allowed if the patient is suffering and if the family is under financial or emotional stress" as if these were just two variations of the same theme.

In approaching this borderline situation, it is important to avoid two extreme positions which are tempting in their simplicity, but are equally erroneous. One is that the genuine interest of the individual is indistinguishable from the interests of society; therefore if one is a burden upon family or community, one's true self-interest lies in ending one's life quickly. The dangers here are easy to spot.

The other extreme position is that the interest of the individual has to be judged in isolation from the interests of others. But this position contradicts the obvious truth that a conscious, aware patient will notice the financial hardships and emotional trials that his illness causes to those close to him, and that awareness of these may be a source of genuine suffering.

675

One problem in seeking a reasonable middle ground between these two extremes is that as the patient's quality of life worsens with progressive illness, his awareness of his surroundings is likely to deteriorate as well. At a time when a strict quality-of-life approach might be expected to declare the patient deserving of a quick death, the patient is least likely to be undergoing any active suffering because of hardships to family and friends.

676

This consideration might lead to a conservative argument that the killing of a patient because of hardship to others cannot, per se, be called "euthanasia." This is not to say it might not be justifiable on other grounds, such as weighing the patient's low quality of life against the cost in terms of decreased quality of life of the family. We might even want to invent another term to label this particular motive.

If it seems like nit-picking to be so concerned over definitions, remember that vagueness in use of words can lead in practice to intolerable ethical confusion and abuses. The obligation to be as precise as possible is increased when human lives will hang in the balance. Any euthanasia advocate who is not as clear as possible in his definitions is laying himself open to serious criticism from opponents of euthanasia.

677

However, a reply is possible to the more conservative argument just cited. Suppose you are given information that next week you will fall ill in such a way that your chance for any sort of useful recovery is nonexistent, but that you will linger on for months in a semicomatose state at great cost and emotional trauma to your loved ones. Now someone brings you a paper which calls upon the physicians to end your life early in that illness. Would you sign? If you could be sure that the circumstances were as described, it is likely that you would, barring specific religious objections. It could then be argued that such a death would be a "mercy" to you, and that it ought not to be withheld from you simply because you did not actually sign such a paper prior to the illness.

678

679    We might conclude from this more liberal argument that to bring about the death of a person in an irreversible state of low quality of life, in order to prevent hardship to the immediate family, could indeed be classified as euthanasia without evidence to the contrary. Relevant contrary evidence might be strong religious sanctity-of-life views in the individual, or possibly evidence that the family, in communicating with the patient, are in fact exaggerating their hardships out of self-pity or other motives.

680    But even in this view we must be careful to distinguish personal cost to the individual's loved ones from a general cost to society as a whole. While resource allocation and social justice questions must be taken into account, realization of societal cost cannot be said to cause "suffering" in the sense that personal costs and hardships do. As we concluded above, "euthanasia" does not apply in this case.

681    Now let's suppose that a physician has accepted the quality-of-life approach and has decided that in some cases it is morally justifiable either to allow a patient to die or to kill him by injecting an overdose of morphine or by some other painless means; and let's suppose that the legal problems have been dispensed with. *In attempting to implement his beliefs in practice, the physician might run across serious problems in two categories—first, the problem of making accurate predictions as to the patient's future prognosis; and second, the problem of determining the real will of the patient.*

682    The dilemma of prognosis is not peculiar to the euthanasia instance, but is a general feature of the art of prognosis itself—that is, that medicine has achieved a good deal of certainty as to what will happen to so many patients in a large group, while doing relatively little to dispel the uncertainty as to what will happen to a particular patient. Euthanasia or allowing to die is a highly individual decision, all the more so for being irrevocable and untestable (since after the patient is dead we can never know if he would have recovered); and knowing that the five-year survival rate for the disease is 35% seems to be of precious little help in deciding what to do in the individual case. Where statistics are nearly 100% or nearly 0% the answer seems clearer, but just how near does it have to be?

# CASE 44

Your state's liberalized euthanasia statute had been in effect for one year when 11-year-old Timmy R. was first brought to you by his parents. He had been bitten in a field by a strangely acting skunk, but no one had captured the animal and, for various reasons, there had been a considerable delay before seeking medical care. With considerable misgivings you began the series of rabies vaccinations. Your worst fears were confirmed when, despite the shots, Timmy began one week ago to show some neurological symptoms. You are now convinced that he has clinical rabies.

Given the prolonged and painful course of rabies prior to death, you feel that this definitely is a case in which death would be more merciful. You are also aware that rabies is one of the few diseases which is invariably fatal once clinical symptoms appear—or was until 1972. In that year there was a report of one case in which a child who had the clinical signs of rabies was aggressively treated and survived. As far as you have been able to learn, there is only this one well-documented case on record of successful treatment.

Timmy's parents are completely crushed emotionally and are of no help to you in reaching a decision based on Timmy's best interests.

Is Timmy a candidate for euthanasia or for aggressive therapy?

---

We stated before that a valid rule was when in doubt, treat. Does one case constitute sufficient doubt to subject Timmy to weeks of possibly useless therapy? If not, would two cases? Ten cases?

Dr. Alfred Jaretzki III summarized the problem of statistics: "If we had ten patients and put them through an ordeal and eight of them were to come through successfully, there would be no great problem. True, we should be thinking of individuals, but if it is that great a yield, I think nobody would argue. If we, on the other hand, are thinking of ten patients who were put through a great ordeal and only one or two or at most three benefit from it, then this becomes a major moral issue and a very difficult decision."

As Dr. Jaretzki said, true, we should be thinking of individuals. So why don't we? Mainly because we were all trained in science and math and nurtured on the unspoken fiction that medicine is, or ought to be, an exact science. Given that background, whenever we are faced with a dilemma and at the same time are offered some mathematical data, we are apt to grab hold of those data and cling for dear life, whether the data get us out of the real dilemma or only seem to do so. The problem is that we have a mathematics of the aggregate, but no one has developed a mathematics of the individual.

At least with statistical data, there is something that can be laid out on the table and debated in some semblance of a rational fashion. In many cases even the statistics are not available, and one has to argue from even more vague concepts, thus making any chance of agreement less likely. This often arises when the patient for whom death is being considered is not terminally ill, and is considered a candidate for euthanasia because of a prediction of a very low quality of life for an indefinite period of time in the future.

## CASE 45

687    A child has been born with meningomyelocele, a congenital defect of the lower spine and spinal cord coverings which allows the spinal cord to be exposed. If untreated, 60 to 80 percent of such children die within the first year of life, due to meningitis, hydrocephalus (accumulation of fluid around the brain), or kidney disease. There are new surgical techniques with which such infants can be aggressively treated soon after birth, However, this child has a large area of defect with some hydrocephalus already present, and in such cases the benefits from surgery have been minimal.

A pediatrician on the staff argues that this is a case in which it would be appropriate to intervene to end the life of the infant quickly. He points out that if it had been possible to diagnose this defect at early gestation, as one can with Down's syndrome, few would object to aborting the fetus, which would have amounted to the same thing. He adds, "Having seen children with unoperated meningomyeloceles lie around the ward for weeks or months untreated, waiting to die, I can't help feeling that the highest form of medical ethic would have been to end the pain and suffering, rather than wishing that the patient would go away."

To this view the chief of pediatrics retorts that it makes no sense to talk about the infants "waiting to die" and suffering in that light, since they do not, at that age, have the capacity for self-and-future-awareness that such suffering would require. He goes on, "The word 'suffering' is often appropriate to the parents. Yet how many of us in pediatrics have seen love and devotion, not misery, come at least occasionally to the parents of the handicapped? Surely all of us know of many cases in which a severely handicapped child has brought great joy to a family." He concludes that therapy even where cure is not possible is still a major goal of medicine, and that one can't get off the hook by doing away with the patient.

Assuming that in either case the parents agreed with the pediatrician, which of these views would you find most acceptable?

Positive euthanasia ↓ 689

Treat surgically ↓ 693

---

688    While the patient in Case 45 is fictitious, the arguments used are quoted almost verbatim from an editorial debate printed in the Journal of Pediatrics, May, 1972. The opponents were, in fact, two pediatricians from the same hospital.

You will be able to compare the two views from a number of angles, but we will focus on one here. In the arguments cited, both pediatricians were arguing from experience; one, that of seeing the children lying alone in the wards, unwanted and presumably enduring suffering; the other, that of seeing the child as the center of a loving family relationship. It seems likely that so long as one doctor is saying "let it die" with the one picture in mind, and the other doctor is saying, "let it live" with the other in mind, no agreement is
690 ↓    possible.

If you advocate active euthanasia in this case, you have some support. Rachels, whose arguments on the absence of any moral distinction between active and passive euthanasia were summarized in Chapter 6, cites just this type of case, in which causing suffering by refraining from action negates any "humane" impulses that might have been present to start with. But the argument for the quickest and least painful end still presupposes that the end, and not continued life, is best for the child. How firm do you want the statistics on the prognosis of meningomyelocele to be before you decide this?

689

688

---

Similarly, when it comes to a particular case, the one doctor's view of the child's likely future will be shaped by his past experience, while the other will reach a different conclusion about the child's expected quality of life; so again the disagreement will be total.

690

Of course, as we saw in Chapter 2, these are very inadequate grounds on which to proceed with an ethical discussion. Each doctor could go on indefinitely recounting specific anecdotes which tend to support his own mental picture.

Another example of this occurred in a public forum in the fall of 1973. A Detroit newspaper carried a story about parents of a Down's syndrome child with multiple congenital defects, whom they wished to allow to die by withholding feedings—given the equation of euthanasia with murder under present law, this apparently barbarous practice is as far as most hospitals will allow toward the same goal. A number of persons wrote letters defending the parents' right to make such a decision; one cited memories of seeing such babies lingering on in the dingy wards of state institutions, incapable of any sort of mental development. Another parent taking the opposing view sent in a snapshot of his own happy, smiling Down's child who is going to school in special education classes and watches Sesame Street on TV. Since the category of Down's syndrome embraces this whole range of possible prognoses, it is impossible to argue a general proposition such as, "Babies with Down's syndrome should be put to death in a merciful way." But clearly many of the letter writers equated "Down's syndrome" with the mental picture of their own experience, and did not consider the wide range of variation.

691

Now, assuming that one has reached a satisfactory conclusion about the actual prognosis of the individual patient, one is faced with the other major problem—determining accurately the patient's true desires. In the case of the unconscious or incompetent patient, the question of who ought to be allowed to speak for the patient would be answered along the lines of the rights-of-participation decisions described in Chapter 7. However, this area presents some special problems, because our entire society is infected with an almost unbelievable degree of irrationality pertaining to anything connected with death and dying. While an attempt to answer the question, "What would I want done to me if I were in that state?" might provide reasonably good ethical guidelines in other instances (within the restrictions noted in Chapter 2), in the case of allowing to die or performing euthanasia, such an approach might be so overlaid with emotionality as to be useless.

692

694

REVIEW
PARTICIPATION   340

**693** If you are unwilling to kill the infant by direct action, surgical treatment does seem more humane than allowing the baby to die a drawn-out death. But the surgery, plus the hospital (and most likely later institutional) care of the child represents a considerable outlay of resources. By arguing for the joy that a severely handicapped child can bring to the family, the second pediatrician seems already to have ruled out the idea that the treatment is that much help for the child. Is bringing joy or meaning to the life of the family worth that outlay of societal resources, where the child is not helped? And are all families likely to find benefit in the care of such a child, or only certain families with **688** certain values?

---

**694** One approach to an accurate statement of one's values on this subject is the "Living Will" distributed by the Euthanasia Educational Council (Appendix V), which the patient may sign at a time of presumably sober reflection and which may then speak for him at a time when he is incapacitated in the future. For now, of course, the will asks only that extraordinary therapy not be employed; in the future it might be modified to include a request for active euthanasia without any major changes in format. While the will has no legal force, its authors point out that by giving a copy to the physician and to a relative, the person is putting a considerable moral obligation on those parties to carry out the agreement.

**695** There are, of course, some important problems with such a document. First, how can one come up with foolproof wording? The document as it now stands mentions "physical disability" as grounds for withholding life-prolonging treatment. Does this mean, for example, that if a blind person has a cardiac arrest, the physician ought not to attempt resuscitation?

You might want to try writing your own will of this sort to see if you can improve upon the present version in this regard.

**696** Because of these considerations, a document personally prepared and tailored to the individual's own values may be preferable to any standardized form. One such individualized will was reprinted by Modell in the New England Journal of Medicine (see references), and could serve as a useful model. You might try writing your own will; it would point out some of the difficulties as well as providing a useful clarification of your own values.

**697** A bigger problem with any document, however well worded, is that it provides no inherent mechanism for recognizing a change of mind. A person could easily sign such a will in the comfort of his living room, and then change his mind when he is actually staring death in the face. Which of these two opinions represents his "true, rational" will? Arguments could be raised plausibly to defend the rationality of either; and when in doubt, our procedure is usually to give greater weight to the most recent. But here the patient may be incapable of communicating his most recent opinion, while the outdated one is enshrined on an official-looking document, signed and witnessed.

# CASE 46

Mr. L.J., an elderly pharmacist, has a constricting cancer of the esophagus which makes it very difficult for him to swallow. This cannot be cured and major surgery would be required even to give some temporary relief.

When he was brought in by the family, Mr. L.J.'s children told you, "He doesn't know he has cancer; he couldn't take it if you were to tell him." As usual in such cases, however, when you ask Mr. L.J. what you can do for him, he responds, "I know I am dying, and I want you to know I am not afraid of dying. I am afraid of suffering." He tells you of a friend of his with cancer of the pancreas, who was made to suffer through several operations, and he extracts a promise from you that when events reach a terminal state you will merely try to keep him comfortable. When you tell the family, they are uncomfortable about it but agree that this is the right course.

After six months and one palliative surgery which is pretty much a failure, you feel that it is time to fulfill your part of the bargain. However, when you engage him in conversation about his wishes, you find that he no longer wants what he originally asked for; in fact, he seems to have retreated from his acceptance of reality.

All of Mr. L.J.'s questions to you now are along the lines of: When am I going to get well? When can I go back to work? What are you going to do to relieve this and that symptom? You realize that while his reality sense has deteriorated, the patient is still alert; and his knowledge would tell him if you were giving him a drug simply for comfort instead of trying for aggressive treatment.

You discuss this new turn of events with the children. One son, a physician, is upset at this new evidence of his father's flight from reality, and says that you should fulfill the wishes of Mr. L.J.'s "better self" as told to you six months ago. Another son and daughter dispute this and say that you should respect his wishes as of now.

What do you do in planning Mr. L.J.'s future treatment—do you choose a palliative, non-surgical course or an aggressive course of therapy?

(Adapted from a case recounted by Dr. Alfred Jaretzki, III)

---

Judging from the discussion immediately preceding, one would have some obligation to treat the disease more aggressively than you would otherwise, because of the patient's apparent change of heart. The patient's new outlook might represent a flight from reality, in your mind; but if he has chosen this psychological mechanism to deal with his inner problems, it does not follow that you ought to insist that he face reality squarely at this moment.

This case is offered as further illustration of a point made earlier—that the hypothetical person named "A" or "B" who makes up his mind once and for all is found on the pages of ethics textbooks but has few counterparts in real life. It is quite likely that Mr. L.J.'s denial of his actual prognosis is only one phase of his process of dealing with death, and that he will change his mind again at least once in the remaining course of his treatment.

## CASE 47

700
Your patient is a 78-year-old man with a terminal carcinoma and severe arteriosclerotic disease in his brain. He is too senile to communicate his desires effectively or to decide matters on information that you give. He might linger on for six months or more if you treat aggressively, or else he could go quickly if you allowed it.

The patient's children are adamant that everything possible should be done to prolong the patient's life. However, you are somewhat surprised to get a visit from another party, who is also elderly and an old college classmate of the patient. It seems that in the state of New York where you are practicing, there is a rather innovative law—Section 100-A of the 1966 Mental Hygiene Law—which allows a court-appointed "Committee of the Person" who can act in a person's capacity if he later becomes mentally incompetent. The "Committee" need be only one individual, and the method of selecting him is identical to the way a will is filed and an executor chosen. However, this "Committee" has no say over a person's property, but only over how the individual is to be treated as a person. If there is any dispute over how the "Committee" should fulfill his duties, the Court must take up the matter.

Your patient's "Committee" tells you that the patient asked him especially to act to prevent any useless prolongation of life beyond the time of functional capacity, since the patient did not wish to be a financial burden on his family or on society when he no longer had use of his mental faculties. The "Committee" also notes that the patient chose him, instead of a family member, because there had been some disagreements, within the family, and the patient distrusted his children with the responsibility of carrying out his instructions in this matter; he felt more comfortable in the hands of a person the same age who could see matters his way.

When you acquaint the patient's children with the instructions you have received from the "Committee," they are absolutely horrified. They want to know how you could even think of accepting the word of an outsider over the instructions of the patient's "own flesh and blood."

Do you treat the patient vigorously or allow him to die?

---

701
In Chapter 7, we referred to a fictional character as the ideal person to decide matters were the patient to become incompetent to decide—a momentary reincarnation of the patient, with all his values, but having momentarily regained his mental capacity and the ability to communicate. This New York law has provided the doctor in Case 47 with about as close an approximation to this fictional character as possible. The doctor then has to weigh the opinion of this person against the wishes of the family.

Recall also in Chapter 7 the observation that the impending death of a relative often gives rise to guilt in the survivors about various things not done in the past, and this guilt may find expression as "do everything you can, doctor." How could you determine in Case 46 if this was what was happening? If the children are carrying a burden in Case 47, and you decide to follow the instructions of the "Committee," do you have any responsibility toward the children to help them work out their guilt feelings in another way? (Note that if their attempt to work out guilt by keeping the parent alive is frustrated, an alternative means of working it out is to direct it in the form of anger toward the doctor who would not listen to them.)

One other twist to the problem of determining a patient's true wishes arises from the fact that a patient's request to be allowed to die, or to be killed by euthanasia, can be considered a form of suicide. We already saw that this does not make it ethically wrong. However, if this is a form of suicide, then psychological insights into the act of attempted suicide may be applicable to this situation also.

702

In particular, we are interested in a case different from those we have been considering. In those, the patient was in a weakened state and confined to bed, so a request to the doctor to put an end to his sufferings could be seen as a request to an agent to do what the person himself would do if he were capable. But what about the case where a terminally ill, but still active and not bedridden patient comes to your office requesting a prescription of a potent drug so that he can take an overdose at the appropriate time? (This is stage No. 6 in the stages of involvement listed in Chapter 6.)

703

There are two possibilities in this case, and it is hard to choose between them. One is that the person may be completely rational and is simply expressing a reasonable request for your assistance in controlling his own destiny. The other is that this person is indulging in a behavior common to those who express suicidal wishes or attempt suicide ineffectually—they do not really want to die but consciously or subconsciously see their acts as ways of "getting attention" which they need to work out their real emotional problems. In this case, the request cannot be taken at face value. What the patient really wants to say is that he is scared about facing death and needs moral support. If you fail to read his real message, he will conclude that you do not care, and will then go home and possibly use the prescription that he originally did not really want.

704

One could rationally argue from these considerations that a person who requests a drug under those circumstances should <u>never</u> be given it: if he truly wanted to die, he would do as most successful suicides do, and find his own effective means of ending his life. The very fact that he has gone out of his way to announce his intentions to you means that his request is in the call-for-help rather than the real-intention category; so you would be doing him a disservice to fulfill his request.

This argument has a certain psychological appeal. Besides, it is hard to go wrong by giving emotional support to the patient. However, this argument seems as rigid in its own way as the opposite injunction (in line with the "Engineering Model") simply to give the patient what he asks for.

705

**REVIEW**
**"ENGINEERING MODEL"** | 106

706    Right now, presented with such a patient, most doctors not only would not prescribe the drug; they would do everything possible to dissuade the person from a suicidal course, up to and including psychiatric commitment. (Note that by so doing it is just as easy to avoid giving the patient the true emotional support he needs as it would be by writing the prescription.) The suicidal patient fills most doctors with extreme anxiety. On the other hand, we might well wish to guard against a pendulum swing too far in the opposite direction, with doctors never trying to dissuade a suicidal patient, as a few of the more radical psychiatrists would recommend.

You might also want to consider whether the decision presented by the patient who requests a suicidal drug is one that ought to be made with the assistance of psychiatric consultation.

707    Now that we have discussed the two major dilemmas present in cases of euthanasia and allowing to die—determining an accurate prognosis and determining the patient's true desires—we can end this chapter with a couple of speculative matters. First, it has occurred to some that much of the debate over euthanasia and allowing to die can be reduced to a basic philosophical difference, in much the same way that the difference over the "humanhood" of the fetus seems to be at the root of the abortion controversy. We noted that the "right to death with dignity" group seems to be treating death as a normal and expected part of life, and to be viewing it with an attitude of inevitability. On the other side, the "heroic treatment" physicians seem, by their efforts to stave off death and by their exasperation and dejection when death triumphs, to be viewing death in much the same light as disease, which in some sense is preventable and treatable.

708    In this way, the philosophical basis of one's attitude toward death hinges on the answer to the question: is death a physiological phenomenon or a pathological one—is death a normal part of the human condition or is it a disease? (Of course, in most cases, one or the other of these two attitudes may be operating depending on the circumstances. Thus, a doctor might see death in the abstract as inevitable but death at any specific moment in time as preventable.)

709    Is there any definitive answer to the question? Either view seems open to attack. It seems a strange use of terms (though not logically inconsistent) to call something a "disease" which happens to all of us sooner or later. By the same token, it seems strange to argue that something is "normal" just because everyone is subject to it. If everyone in the world became infected with measles simultaneously, would measles thereby cease being a disease?

On the face of it, the question looks like an empirical one; and it is interesting to decide what evidence would prove or disprove either of the two answers. For instance, suppose someone found a "cure" for death. This would tend to make us think of death as a pathological process, but it would not be conclusive, since we can intervene to change a number of normal physiological processes also, and we could arbitrarily call such interventions "cures" if we chose.

On the other hand, the failure to find such a "cure" would not be evidence  710
that death is physiological for the same reason, and also because there are
many entities which we call "diseases" for which we have no cure.

As one scans the problem in this way, it might occur to one that maybe
this is not really an empirical question at all, but rather a value judgment.
As we showed in Chapter 2, an ethical question or a value question is not
solved simply by the accumulation of data. This discussion here anticipates
the topic of Chapter 17, in which we shall argue that all definitions of "health"
and "disease" are basically value judgments rather than empirical decisions,
even through empirical data play an important role in them.

Finally, we might consider a practical point regarding active euthanasia.  711
As we saw back in Chapter 6 when we listed the "stages of involvement" of
physicians in death questions, the doctor tends to approach these questions
from the point of view of what he has to do, even though we would ideally
prefer that he approach them from the overview of maximizing quality of
life. We also saw that even though a strict ethical distinction between allowing
to die and killing might not be justifiable, doctors in fact do make a very
strong emotional distinction. It seems that so long as doctors are trained to
save lives, most of them will have a very hard time accepting the proposition
of ending lives by direct means.

Indeed, Kass, who has no absolute prohibition against euthanasia, is willing  712
to consider the relatives of the patient giving him an overdose of a painless
drug, presumably after the doctor has supplied it. But he states firmly that in
his view of medical practice, it would be absolutely wrong for the doctor
himself to perform this function: doctors must not kill.

Therefore, if we get to the point where there seems to be no ethical  713
barrier in the way of active euthanasia in certain carefully selected cases, and
yet this emotional barrier persists, could the problem not be solved by assigning
the role of carrying out the death decision to another person besides the
doctor? Could not hospitals have "executioners" who could be called in to
do the dirty work upon the decision of the health care team, thereby leaving
the doctors, nurses, and other health workers free to devote all their emotional
energies to saving lives?

714    While a number of rather gory points could be made about such a proposal, we shall find fault with it on other grounds. First, we could argue in general that it is ethically a poor practice to do the Pontius Pilate routine, and approve of a thing while leaving the undesirable implementation to others. Also, we could object on the grounds of continuity of health care. If among the legitimate goals of medical practice we want to include 1) relieving suffering and 2) helping where possible to implement the patient's own decisions about the control of his life, then it would seem that active euthanasia, as we have envisioned it, is squarely within the realm of good medical practice; and to hand it off to an outsider would be to deny this status. Finally, we noted that even when the doctor has bad news for the patient, the promise of ongoing emotional support to the end may be the crucial ingredient that prevents truth-telling from being cold and unfeeling. If, at the final moment, it is the "executioner" and not the physician who is at the bedside, this would seem to be a serious gap in the promise of support.

715    If these objections to the "executioner" idea are indeed as conclusive as they seem to be, then we are led to a conclusion: if we base our medical ethics in this regard on the quality-of-life approach, there is no a priori reason to oppose active euthanasia, in addition to passive euthanasia or allowing to die. But when it comes to commission of an act, it is the doctor, or the health care team, which is going to have the personal responsibility; it will not be possible to hand the job to someone else and still say that one is delivering good medical care.

716    Thus far, the debate over euthanasia has tended to be a polemical one, with people more interested in scoring points than in making important distinctions. What needs to be done now is precisely what is suggested: to place euthanasia within the context of "good medical care," at least on a conceptual level until the legal problem is settled one way or the other. All other forms of medical treatment are discussed in terms of indications and contraindications. What are the indications and contraindications for euthanasia? And we can be sure that if we do move from the stage of polemics to practical applications, more unforseen and perplexing ethical issues will present themselves. Ch. 14 ↓ 717

# 14. Mass Screening Programs

Most medical people are happy that the science of preventive medicine, often neglected in past decades, is receiving new emphasis. Even though our present medical care delivery system is geared toward treating the sick, it is acknowledged that it would be better to prevent the sickness from occurring. And, once the public is sufficiently educated on this score and the required medical manpower is made available, then patients will come to see doctors (and to enter into the doctor-patient "Contract") in order to prevent future illness. This sort of preventive medicine is purely in keeping with the nature of the doctor-patient relationship as we have been describing it, and so presents no new ethical problems on that score.

717

However, at present, the technology available to detect potential disease has gone beyond the public's general level of education on its availability. Therefore, in order to put these new techniques to good use, the medical establishment has found itself going out into the community as part of mass screening programs, instead of waiting for patients to come to them. While it has always been held contrary to professional etiquette for an individual physician to sing his praises and recruit patients by advertising, the profession itself now sees nothing wrong with pushing sickle cell screening in the black community through newspaper ads, church campaigns, and various subtle forms of coercion. These facts suggest that the mass screening concept represents a fundamental departure from the doctor-patient relationship, and that ethical problems may arise as a result of this.

718

As we saw in Chapter 4, the transmission of knowledge from doctor to patient is an important part of the relationship. However, in the model we have been using, the knowledge of something "wrong" is intimately tied in with the treatment to set it "right"; the doctor who provides the one is standing by to provide the other. Mass screening programs, on the other hand, tend more to deal with knowledge alone. If treatment is offered, it is often by another agency or by another wing of the program. If the screening is for the carriers of genetic defects, no treatment as such is offered or is possbile; the "treatment" given is a set of risks for the defect appearing in the children of the couple screened, and the couple has to decide what to do with this new knowledge. This knowledge, gained in this manner, is much more likely to be resented or even rejected than knowledge gained within the continuity of the doctor-patient relationship.

719

720    Also in Chapter 4, we saw that one of the most time-honored "clauses" in the "contract" was the expectation that the physician would respect the patient's desire for privacy and for confidentiality of communication. In Case 8, it was shown how the goals of a community screening program might well conflict with this desire on the part of the patient. Where the doctor is serving as an agent of a social program, he would seem to be more easily persuaded of a need to divulge information that the individual might wish to conceal, especially for purposes of compiling statistics or of directing the attention of public health agencies to people needing treatment.

REVIEW
CASE 8     141

721    And even where a screening program is designed to maintain confidentiality, it may be very hard to convince the screened population that this is the case, especially when socio-cultural factors intervene. A perfect example is provided by screening programs for sickle cell carriers in the black community. The inner city has for decades been exposed to adequate medical care only when it served the purposes of the white community to do so—such as when patients were needed as "teaching material" for medical schools, or for research projects. So now, when the people in the white coats march in and explain that the screening program is strictly for the greater good of the black population, the people are bound to be suspicious. This suspicion is bound to be fueled by the provisions of some of the hastily enacted laws for mandatory sickle cell screening, such as compulsory screening of grade school children. It is interesting to ask if, when a cheap and reliable means is developed to detect the carriers of a genetic disease present only in whites, whether legislators would be willing to enact laws with some of these same provisions.

722    The concern over confidentiality is bound to be exacerbated by the general level of public ignorance where genetic disease is concerned. Although in most cases of recessive traits, a carrier with one gene for the trait is completely normal from a medical viewpoint, there is often a social stigma attached to a known carrier; as Case 8 showed, this may be seen as a threat to masculinity or femininity or as an insidious "disease in the cells." Worse, in sickle cell, the practice of calling the carrier state "sickle cell trait" has blurred the distinction between this and sickle cell disease, even though persons with the trait are completely healthy except for very particular circumstances (such as very high altitudes). Following in the wake of some screening programs, blacks found to have sickle cell trait were fired from their jobs or refused military service, despite the total lack of medical justification for this.

These problems again bring up the question of conflicts between the interests of the individual and of society. In several places previously, we have argued that it is wrong to draw a sharp line between these two types of interests, since to ignore the needs of society would eventually lead to damage to individual interests, and vice versa. However, we have also argued that it is possible to have a conflict of these interests in a specific instance, even where the interests are in agreement overall; and we stated that for the purposes of ethical justification, it aids clarity to distinguish societal motives from individual motives.

723

We can see how it might be in the interests of an individual to know that he has, or carries genes for, a certain disease. How does it aid the interests of society for individuals to have this knowledge? If we are talking about a communicable disease, it would appear to be in the interests of the whole society, as well as of the as yet unaffected members, that affected individuals are found out and given treatment. That is the ethical justification for requiring vaccinations before children can enter school. However, genetic defects are not "communicable diseases" in any meaningful sense of the term (although one legislature committed the absurdity of arbitrarily defining sickle cell disease as communicable in order to establish a mandatory screening program).

724

The victims of genetic disease do put a measurable burden on the rest of society through the finances required for their care and for the loss of economically productive members, etc. Therefore, a potential societal benefit from mass screening, as perceived by those who set up such programs, is the possible reduction in the number of affected individuals. But in order for this to occur, it is not enough merely to give the knowledge to the parents—the parents must take action by not having children or by aborting fetuses at risk or whatever. Furthermore, the idea that having children is both a natural activity and a "right" is so ingrained in society that many parents will elect to have children even when faced with very high odds that the children will be genetically diseased to a serious extent.

725

Given the societal desire to decrease the number of individuals with genetic defects, coupled with the observation that as things now stand, the mere knowledge of risk is often insufficient to deter childbearing, the stage is set to include along with genetic screening an implied or explicit coercion to avoid having children if one is found to be at risk. Furthermore, since it is necessary to identify those whom you intend to coerce, this is often accompanied in turn by subtle coercions to take part in the screening program. Besides the obvious means of legislating mandatory requirements, this coercion can take more subtle forms, such as exploiting the bandwagon sense of "everybody else is doing it," or by tying the screening program with some sort of economic pressure.

726

CASE 48

As director of the county health department, you are approached by an official from the U.S. government food stamp distribution program. The food stamp people are concerned about the high incidence of iron deficiency anemia among children in lower socio-economic groups in this country, as revealed by national surveys. It has also been feared that due to cultural patterns and to poor nutrition knowledge, the foods purchased by food stamp users might not be the most nutritious and therefore the children might be exposed to dietary deficiencies.

The program proposes to have public health nurses at the distribution center to take finger-prick blood samples from the children of food stamp recipients to test for anemia by hematocrit, the same procedure that you routinely carry out in the well-baby clinic. To assure compliance, the blood test would be made a requirement for the mother's obtaining food stamps. Since your department already has provisions for treating anemia with free iron supplements, immediate therapy would be made available whenever a case of anemia is found.

You are in agreement with the objectives of the idea, and you acknowledge that since many mothers do not bring their children in, your existing facilities are not detecting all the iron deficiency in the community. However, you are concerned about the compulsory nature of this screening proposal.

The official replies that since the amount of blood drawn is miniscule, the deficiency disease may have few outward symptoms, the disease is perfectly treatable by oral supplementation, and free therapy will be provided, that therefore no reasonable mother could refuse to have her child tested anyway. Even if the mother were unreasonable, the child has a right to good health care regardless. Anyway, just to make it all officially proper, each mother will be asked to sign a consent form for the testing.

The food stamp program has no trained personnel to do the blood tests and thus is dependant on your providing nurses for the proposal. Do you agree to the proposal as it now stands?

---

The proposal in Case 48 meets one of the requirements for screening programs that was just hinted at—that of providing treatment along with the knowledge. The hangup, obviously, is the question of compulsion. First, it ought to be clear that making the test a condition for obtaining food stamps represents coercion, regardless of how many forms may be signed. The question is then: on what grounds might such coercion be justified?

Is a child's "right to good health care" adequate justification? In addition to the problems we mentioned before when there is no specification as to who is obligated to fulfill a right, we have a problem in that we usually assume that a right will be asserted by the party whose interest is actually involved, and that that party may choose to waive the right. We assume, therefore, that a "right to health care," if it exists, can be met by providing opportunities for care. We do not think of this "right" as requiring us to sally forth into the streets to recruit patients actively.

However, an exception might have to be made here, as in the case of the presumed "right to life of the unborn," where the party to whom we attribute the right is unable to claim it himself; under such circumstances it does not seem so odd to appoint ourselves as stand-ins.

We can suppose, also, that if the program were established at the food stamp distribution center on a voluntary rather than a compulsory basis, some children with anemia would be missed in the screening. (Just how many would be missed might be information that would be of value in making this ethical decision. Therefore, an alternative proposal might be setting up a voluntary testing program to see how high compliance is, with the option of altering the program later if expectations are not met.)

729

↓

Presumably we know the consequences of a compulsory program—ill feelings on the part of the "patients," increased distrust of governmental agencies with a possible carryover against the health professions because of their participation in the program, etc. We put a minus weight on these consequences in our ethical calculations. Now, we have to decide: how many anemic children put on the other side of the balance would outweigh these consequences? There could be wide disagreement here. Some who are particularly sensitive to the social discontent of the underprivileged citizens might say that no matter how many anemic children are missed, the social ills would not be outweighed. (Note that while moderate anemia in children may slightly retard physical and intellectual development, and may help predispose toward infection—the results of research are unclear—it is hardly a life-threatening illness.) On the other side, someone who is gung-ho for the "right to adequate health care" may insist that these social consequences are of minor impact if even a single anemic child is missed in screening.

730

↓

There is one flaw in this latter view, however, that might indicate that the ill feelings generated by such a program have to be taken more seriously. The idea that it would be bad to miss some anemic children supposes that identification will automatically lead to treatment and cure. But treatment does not take place when you give the mother the bottle of iron syrup, but rather when the mother actually gives it to the child. A mother who is upset by the element of coercion in the program and who therefore cannot identify with the program's goals seems much more likely to forget or neglect to give the child his medicine. A voluntary program, on the other hand, if it is combined with a genuine attempt at education, might miss some children but increase the long-range benefits of those that are identified.

731

↓

When weighing the consequences of any social program that involves coercion, it is well to remember that people's behavior in a state free of compulsion is not necessarily a good indicator of how they would act if compelled to do these same things. This is shown by some of the public outcry concerning mandatory auto seatbelt legislation; from some of the angry letters to editors, it would seem that a few would refuse to wear seatbelts just because the government wanted to tell them to do it, regardless of their own safety considerations.

732

↓

733    Now that Congress has just passed a comprehensive and compulsory national health insurance act, you have been appointed to the panel of experts who are determining just what the provisions of national insurance coverage shall be. You have come to the question of screening for genetic disease, and it has been generally agreed that if the physician feels that a patient is at risk to have a child with a diagnosable and untreatable genetic defect, the insurance ought to pay for amniocentesis or other diagnostic procedures as well as for an abortion carried out because of the findings.

The panel has not turned to the question of paying for the institutional care of mentally retarded individuals with genetic defects; this is a controversial issue because of the large sums involved. One panel member (named M.) states that a provision should be added to the program that would deny reimbursement to parents who received prenatal diagnosis of the defect or of the strong likelihood of a defect, and failed to abort the fetus. He argues that if one has the means to prevent the birth of such an individual and chooses not to, one should pay for the consequences and not expect society to pick up the tab. To have society pay for such children, argues M., is simply an encouragement of what he calls "irresponsible parenthood."

The debate continues:

R.:   What if the parents' religious beliefs forbid an abortion?

M.:   If your religious beliefs say your kids should go to a parochial school, you pay for it yourself. Either you give up your religious beliefs or you pay for them. You are free to have the beliefs but not to charge taxpayers who do not share them

L.:   What if the person had normal diagnostic results but an error was made, and a deformed child was born anyway?

M.:   We ought to pay for that. It wasn't the parents' fault; they took every reasonable precaution.

T.:   It seems that then you ought not to pay for amniocentesis unless the parents sign a form or something to say that they will abort if the child is abnormal.

M.:   I agree, that sounds logical.

R.:   It seems that if you are going to be consistent, you have to provide for the killing of these "mistaken diagnoses" that L. was talking about, since you were prepared to abort them had the diagnosis been correct rather than have the taxpayers foot the bill.

M.:   You're twisting what I said. Once they are born they are citizens and you're stuck. All I'm saying is that we should provide for reasonable precautions and preventive action, before you get to that stage.

B.:   I don't see how your proposal would work. If parents thought they might not want to have an abortion, they would avoid having any prenatal diagnosis in order to protect their insurance payments.

M.:   I would propose that the failure to have prenatal testing, when the doctor had recommended it and it was available, would also constitute grounds for nonpayment of costs of institutionalization, just as would be the case if they had the tests but ignored the results.

Do you accept M.'s proposal or not?

Like the previous case, Case 49 presents the prospect of utilizing economic compulsion to get individuals to submit to testing; and in addition to get individuals to have abortions if the test comes out positive. We found fault with the iron deficiency testing on the basis of coercion. Do we therefore reject this insurance provision on the same basis? Or is this insurance provision more or less justifiable than the compulsory anemia screening?

This case goes back to the topics raised in Chapter 7 and asks under what circumstances society as a whole, or specific social institutions, have rights of participation in the decision. In the iron deficiency screen, to reject mandatory testing would be to say that the cost of not detecting the disease will be borne by the individual (even if the individual who will have the problem did not have any say in whether to be tested or not), so society has no business interfering. Of course, society pays some price whenever any of its members are in less than optimal health, but it could be argued that this effect is negligible in the iron deficiency case.

On the other hand, in the case of genetic retardation, if non-detection of the disease leads to the birth and survival of an individual who must be cared for in an institution, society would have to bear the costs, and in monetary terms these are considerable. Therefore, the argument goes, society has a right to participate in the decision of whether or not to do the test, and whether or not to do the abortion if indicated. No one is being forced to have the abortion; they just have to pay for the results of not having one. If the result of this was that the rich were able to keep deformed babies in institutions while the poor were denied this privilege, this would merely be placing such a privilege in the same category as owning three Cadillacs or some similar luxury; no one is arguing that the poor ought to be able to do anything the rich do.

This argument based on social costs would be rebutted if one could show that the institutionalized individuals do in fact contribute something of value to society that "reimburses" the cost of their upkeep. It is generally assumed that no such compensating value exists, but our failure to find one could be related to putting the argument in dollars-and-cents terms. (How many of us could calculate in monetary measure what we are worth to society, if anything?)

Some could argue that each individual, whatever his mental capacity, has an infinite worth as an individual human being, so that any social costs would be outweighed. However, this is not a true argument from the consequences, but rather an appeal to sanctity-of-life dressed up in consequentialist terms, and we would deal with it as we would any other sanctity-of-life, a priori principle.

REVIEW SANCTITY ⬆ 218

738    Through all this we have been ignoring the individual. We could assume that at serious stages of retardation, whether a person lives or dies is a matter of indifference to that person; so then we are justified in weighing the social consequences to decide what to do.

A greater problem (similar to the problem of abortion in general) occurs when we ask if it is a matter of indifference to a fetus (of which even normal ones are "mentally retarded") whether it is allowed to be born or not. As a person, I might feel an objection to the idea that I ought not to have been born; but I could not feel that objection had someone actually implemented that idea at the appropriate time. To attribute indifference or concern to a fetus seems to be talking nonsense. On the other hand, one could argue that if I abort a fetus, I am responsible for the fact that it never develops consciousness and therefore never has any objections to my act; so therefore I cannot use the lack of objections to justify the original act.

739    Depending on the quality-of-life criteria we have adopted, we could argue that it is a positive kindness for such individuals not to be born, and so we are merely using financial coercion to force parents to be kind to these children in that way. An objection might be that to apply this consistently, we should be prepared to pass a law forcing parents to abort such children regardless of financial ability to pay. However, we could argue back that this would entail a significant increase in the degree of coercion. The kindness to the aborted individual may be enough to justify the lesser degree of coercion but not the greater.

740    If the discussion of this case has appeared even more disjointed than usual, it is because of the ethical imponderables involved in assigning precise weights to the various consequences. Early on, we saw pretty clearly what had to be weighed on both sides, but that still left us with the problem of assigning the weights in a consistent and rational manner. (For this reason, this case is a good one for small group discussion.)

741    The last two cases have dealt with coercion in a screening program resulting from factors independent of the screening itself. However, is screening intrinsically a coercive activity, in a more subtle sense? From the point of view of the individual tested, the major or the only "product" of a screening program is knowledge. And knowledge may not only be extremely burdensome, but may also profoundly affect the life of the person afterwards. A person going to a program to be tested may come out with reassuring good news or with crushing bad news, and the odds of the two depend on the type of disorder being tested for. If no outside coercion is present, it is very likely a weighing between the reassurance and the crush that leads an individual to decide whether or not to be tested. What would people do if the chances are exactly 50—50?

## CASE 50

Huntington's chorea is an inherited disease of the nervous system whose symptoms usually develop in an affected individual at age 35-45. The disease leads to progressive mental and physical deterioration with death occurring 10-15 years after first onset; the final stage of the disease has been described as, "The patient presents the pitiful picture of the complete ruin of a human being." The inheritance is autosomal dominant with complete penetrance—therefore, one-half the offspring of an affected individual will carry the gene, and all who carry the gene will develop the disease ultimately. There is no treatment. Because of the late age of onset, most patients have had several children before they become aware that they have the gene.

One of the patients in your practice is a 42-year-old man who has shown Huntington's symptoms for a little over a year; he has two sons, aged 19 and 17. The fact that each has a 50% chance of carrying the gene weighs heavily on their minds, since each hopes to start a family and have children soon. Each would have serious reservations about having children if they knew they carried the gene.

You are aware that a new experimental test is available in which a patient at risk may be given a drug, levodopa, for a period of time. Apparently, if he carries the gene he will develop symptoms—facial grimaces, tics, or other involuntary movements—typical of the early stages of the disease itself, and these will disappear with withdrawal of the drug. If the person is not a carrier, no symptoms will appear.

Do you inform the sons of your affected patient about the existence of this test? If you do, and they seem uncertain about what to do, do you encourage them to have the test, or not?

---

In an article on this subject, Hemphill assumed that the test had been fully developed experimentally, and then listed what he felt to be the major "pro" consequences of adopting the ethical proposition, "All people with a known family incidence of the disease should be tested before childbearing if possible":

1) If all those with positive tests refrained from having children by natural means, the level of the gene in the population would be significantly reduced.

2) Those with positive tests would know the approximate span of their active years and could plan their lives accordingly, without engaging in false hopes.

3) The knowledge of the disease per se could be considered good in that it increases the humanity of the knower—it allows him to make a wider range of informed choices.

As a supplement to No. 1, we would add:

4) By not having children, the person would avoid the bad consequences of knowing that he had passed the gene on to his children, with the feelings of guilt, resentment, etc., that would be bound to develop within the family in that case.

**744**   Hemphill also considers the following "con" consequences:

1)   Early diagnosis of Huntington's can make no difference in the terminal course of the disease, since there is no treatment.

2)   By doing the test, one gives the patient a "sneak preview" of the actual symptoms that inevitable fate has in store for him. Thus, his feelings of anguish and dread, that he is bound to carry with him for 10 or 20 years, will be heightened.

3)   While the option is supposedly "free," the psychological factors determining acceding to the test or not must be powerful. A patient may take the test in an unrealistic hope of being reassured by a negative result, and then be totally crushed when a positive result occurs.

4)   Given social demands, there is no reason to believe that a test which starts out free of coercion will remain so. Life insurance companies may demand that individuals at risk take the test before a policy will be sold; employers may follow suit.

On the basis of these consequences, Hemphill concludes that the negative consequences are weighty enough to force "careful scrutiny" before giving the test. Do you agree?

**745**   We could argue plausibly that the good consequences of making the test available outweigh the bad. Either an individual has the gene or he doesn't. If he or she does not have the gene, he will have some very significant emotional reassurance as well as useful information on which to plan his family life. (Keep in mind that the test today is still experimental and has not been shown to have the degree of accuracy we are assuming. We assume, for example, that there are no false-negative results.) If the individual has the gene, he gets an emotional wallop in the stomach, but he also gets useful information which he may (or may not) use in his future planning. One use he can make of this information is to avoid passing the gene on to his children and thus decrease the potential misery that otherwise would be repeated generation after generation. The emotional anguish which Hemphill emphasizes should not be minimized. But it is treatable, even if the disease is not. And many patients conjure up such dismal pictures of their prognoses that hearing the true picture from the doctor may actually reassure them—as we noted in the section on truth-telling in Chapter 4.

**746**   How do you weigh Hemphill's social consequence, that coercion may be applied by insurance companies, employers, etc.? It seems this cannot be dismissed lightly. If medicine provides a test knowing that other societal institutions may react in a certain way, and they subsequently do, medicine can hardly wash its hands of the affair and deny any share in the responsibility. Therefore these social consequences must be weighed in the equation, but it is not at all clear that they outweigh, all by themselves, the good consequences of providing the knowledge to the individual.

## CASE 51

You are a counselor for the New York City Sickle Cell Counseling Service. Before you is a black couple in their early 20's who plan to be married in three months. The wedding plans were already underway when the man came in to be tested. When his test came out showing him to be a sickle cell carrier, his fiancee—a volunteer worker in your program—realized that she had never been tested, and she was shocked when her test came out positive as well. From having worked in the program, she knows that therefore each of their children will have a 25% chance of getting two sickle-cell genes and having sickle cell disease, while each will have a 50% chance of being a carrier like the parents. As is usual with recessive traits, none of the relatives on either side has sickle cell disease, so the couple has no firsthand experience with the disease; they will consider trying to adopt children or having a childless marriage depending on what you tell them.

You tell them about the effects of the disease. You also know that experiments are under way with the use of urea and cyanate ion as a possible treatment for people with sickle cell disease in crisis; if these are successful (they have not been to date except in the test tube) a person with the disease might be able to lead much more of a normal life, possibly with a normal life expectancy.

You also know that work is being done on diagnosing sickle cell disease by amniocentesis, which would allow selective abortion of affected children while carrying normal babies through to term. This has been done so far only on aborted fetuses, and if the experiments are successful it will still be several years before such a test will be available to the general public. As with the treatment of the disease, you are afraid to give the parents any ground for false hopes if these experimental possibilities are not realized.

What do you tell the couple?

(Adapted from Case 137, Columbia University Program in Medical Ethics, courtesy Dr. Robert Veatch)

---

As far as the experimental treatments and prenatal diagnoses go, Case 51 is a "condition of doubt" case similar to one noted in Chapter 7. We mentioned then that if you don't know, there is no a priori reason not to tell the people that you don't know, and then do your best to put what you do know into perspective. What we want to emphasize here is that the "knowledge" that is the product of a screening test, however problematic when it is precise knowledge, is even more difficult to handle in the more common case when a considerable level of uncertainty is involved.

With this in mind, go back to one of the points raised in favor of doing the test on the person at risk for Huntington's chorea—the idea that knowledge per se is a good and that its possession makes one more human. It is an observable fact that people do tend to place a great deal of weight on knowledge for its own sake, and that the idea of knowledge as good in itself is hardly ever challenged within the scientific or medical communities. However, from an ethical viewpoint we cannot take any such assertion of a priori good at face value until we have examined the consequences. If we had to find fault with a sanctity-of-life view for this reason, we can't let a "sanctity of knowledge" view slip by unexamined.

750      According to our ethical method, knowledge is good mainly for one thing—as a guide to action which is most likely to be consistent with our values (and to determine in this way whether our values themselves are consistent with each other). This would lead us, perhaps not to reject that argument as a reason for doing a diagnostic test, but anyway to assign it a much lower weight than the other arguments which point out how the information gained will be useful for taking concrete action. Surely if the only gain is knowledge itself, and the test either was very expensive or else involved a risk of physical harm to the patient, we would hardly approve of doing it.

751      Similarly, a high degree of uncertainty will render the knowledge less useful as a guide to action than it would be otherwise. Therefore, in these "condition of doubt" cases, we might have to weigh the knowledge to be gained on a sliding scale, and there would come a point where the uncertainty was so great that the value of the knowledge was nil. (Don't forget that where that point comes will vary from patient to patient, with their ability to assimilate increasingly sophisticated information to make a rational decision.)

752      We in the scientific world have been led possibly to over-emphasize the utility of knowledge. Since knowledge can be a grave burden, it is natural that there is a view at the other extreme, and this view has favored us with yet another candidate for "righthood"—the "right not to know." This phrase (thankfully, in quotation marks) was used in a journal article on sickle cell screening, in defense of those who did not want to take the opportunity to be tested. One physician wrote to object that "surely, this must represent the nadir of human rights. One might well ask if this right to ignorance should be cherished; indeed, should it be encouraged and pursued by all right-thinking men of good will?"

753      The original author replied as follows: "It seems to me that the answers to the question of whether the 'right not to know' should be implemented must be based on the consequences of not knowing. With sickle cell screening, if an unmarried black person elected not to find out...and married another black person without becoming aware of the spouse's sickle cell status, there would be a 1:100 chance (approximately) that the prospective parents would both have the trait.

     "I suspect that some persons will prefer to take this chance rather than burden themselves with knowledge of their own sickle cell status, deliberate over the point in the relationship at which they should attempt to ascertain their partner's sickle cell status and agonize over the role that this information should have in deciding whom they date or court."*

     Do you agree with this reply?

754      So long as the general rule is followed by attempting to keep coercion to a minimum in mass genetic screening, it would appear that the "right not to know" will be protected. It remains to be seen what is gained on a rhetorical level by enshrining this as a "right." It might be more useful, when people do indicate a desire not to know, to inquire why, and whether this might be indicative of some more important problem. If people do not want to know what genes they carry, this may arise in part from the general level of ignorance and superstition on genetic matters, and point out the need for a serious improvement in public education.

*Reprinted, by permission. From the New England Journal of Medicine 288:972, 1973.

Now consider a different type of uncertainty—not what the results of the screening test mean, but what the results of the screening test are. No lab test is 100% perfect. Many people in public health regret the day when the legislatures rushed to enact statures requiring mandatory testing of all newborn infants for phenylketonuria (PKU) in order to institute the special diet that would prevent subsequent mental retardation; it was later found that the test had many false positives, and that many of these normal babies may have been harmed developmentally by being placed on the PKU diet. And in some cases the rate of "false positives" can be quite high as a result of the design of the procedure itself—as Case 52 shows.

---

## CASE 52

You are having lunch with two of your obstetrical colleagues and mention one of your patients who is now about 8 weeks pregnant. She has one son with classic hemophilia who has had a number of serious medical problems due to his bleeding disorder. Your statements about the many hemophiliacs who lead almost normal lives have been to no avail—she does not want to have another child with hemophilia, and she came to you because she read in a woman's magazine about amniocentesis to detect some disorders in utero. She is likewise adamant in wanting more children if she can possibly have them. She has an appointment at 3 this afternoon at which you are to give her your answer and advice.

One colleague points out what you already know—since hemophilia is sex-linked, and the mother is now proven to be a carrier, 50% of her male children will be expected to have it, and 0% of the female children (though 50% of them will be carriers). There is no prenatal diagnosis for hemophilia per se. However, Dr. M. goes on, some centers have adopted the strategy of doing amniocentesis to determine the sex of the baby by karyotype, and then aborting all male fetuses. While the mother can have only female children, she is assured of having children free of the disease.

At this point Dr. D. chokes on his sandwich and begins to object strenuously. An opponent of "abortion on demand," Dr. D. can accept abortion when the baby is known to have a genetic defect. But here, he says, you are 50% of the time aborting a perfectly normal fetus. "Since when in medicine do we treat an individual for a disease we think his brother has?" demands Dr. D. "Especially when the treatment is death." He feels that it would be immoral even to mention this possibility to the patient.

You disagree with Dr. D., since you have read the section above about withholding information from patients due to one's own moral values. But, if the patient has amniocentesis done, you, as her obstetrician, will be the one to do the abortion. Are you prepared to abort a male fetus if she requests it?

757    Duck, because here comes another "right." The physicians who do abortions of this type often prefer not to say that they are aborting fetuses—rather they are protecting the mother's "right to bear a normal child." One stated, "[These families] are incredibly desirous of having a normal child" (does incredible desire constitute moral justification?). If this "right" were elevated to sacred proportions, the consequences might be truly staggering. Right now, obviously, this right is being neglected, since about 1 out of 65 births results in a child with some sort of clinical genetic defect, ranging from mild to lethal. We can now test for several dozen genetic defects by amniocentesis; this is done only where the mother is known to be at risk because of previous births or family history, because the amniocentesis itself is not without risk and in addition costs a minimum of several hundred dollars to test for just one trait. Does the "right to have a normal child" mean that every pregnant woman should have amniocentesis to test for every trait which we can detect (at a cost of possibly $5000 per mother)?

758    Opposing this rather extreme idea of a "right" is Dr. D., whose arguments sound like those of ethicist Paul Ramsey. Ramsey opposes all ethics based on consequentialist theories of the "greatest net good," calling this statistical morality: "To screen by means of sex determination and to catch a normal male fetus in a statistical net is in no instance to deliver medical care in his case. Such mistaken identification is rather like operating on the wrong patient—which no one would excuse by saying that the condition to be remedied was graver than the operation."

759    Ramsey does not restrict his objections to the case where there are 50% false positives. He quotes another author, a physician, as saying,"'the rare normal pregnancy that would be lost' (through routine laboratory error) would be 'an undefendable catastrophe.'"

760    As we saw in the discussion of abortion, Ramsey takes an ethical position which is practically indistinguishable from a sanctity-of-life view, so his position is logical. As a practical matter, if you are anti-abortion, the "treatment" here will be indefensible; if you are willing to perform abortions upon the request of the mother for emotional or financial reasons, then you are not likely to get squeamish about the 50% of normal male fetuses who will be lost through this procedure.

There is, however, another dimension to this case which cannot be lost    761
sight of, and which has to do with just what one means by "statistical morality."
Genetic counselors have great difficulties trying to explain to lay people that
to say that "each child will have a 50% chance of having the defect" does
NOT mean the same as "50% of your children will have the defect." It is
completely possible, although improbable, that the family might have 10 children
and all would have the defect.

It is true that one consequence of aborting male fetuses in hemophilia
carriers will be that about 50% of those aborted, in a large enough sample,
will have been normal. But which is which is known only in retrospect if at
all. All that is known at the time is that there is a 50% chance that the fetus
has the disease, and if abortion is allowable in principle, this may or may not
be grounds for abortion depending on the seriousness of the disease. If we have
only statistical knowledge to go on, either we practice "statistical morality"
(in that sense) or we do not act at all.

We have now touched upon the major issues involved in mass screening    762
programs, with an emphasis on genetic screening, which, along with the so-
called "right to bear a normal child," blends nicely into the topic of genetic
engineering in the next chapter. We have seen that the implications of screening
run the gamut from the highly individual to the broadly social contexts. In
conclusion, we might cite another long-range consequence of genetic screening
which is alluded to by Ramsey in his discussion of the issue.

Ramsey starts from the point that we will develop in Chapter 17, that    763
"normal" and "abnormal" are concepts based on value judgments and thus
are subject to change. In particular, we include many things as "normal" or
"borderline" simply because we have no way of preventing them. Ramsey
states, "As screening becomes a part of standard medical practice, the concept
of 'normality' sufficient to make life worth living is bound to be 'upgraded,'
and the acceptance of 'abnormality' and care for abnormals is bound to be
degraded in our society." Thus, even the best screening will allow some mistakes
to slip through, and as the "mistakes" decrease in numbers, society will presumably be less and less willing to care for them in an adequate and humane
manner.

Ethicists who are prone to "domino theory" type arguments are also prone    764
to stating possible consequences as if they were certainties. Ramsey may well
be right in fearing such an attitude, given the human tendency to sweep anything, or anyone, who reminds us of an unpleasantness underneath the nearest
rug. It is quite possible to prevent this from forming a basis of future policies,
however, if we take Ramsey's warning seriously.                Ch. 15    765

223

# 15. Genetic Engineering

We have referred before to the general level of irrationality in our society pertaining to death, and how this complicates decision-making on a number of ethical issues. If our society is irrational about death, it is at least as irrational, if not more so, about parenthood and having children. Furthermore, our society is far from being alone in this regard. These societal attitudes can throw a monkey wrench into any attempt to rationally approach issues such as genetic engineering, as well as control of reproduction and population control policies.

765

Back in Chapter 10, it was noted that there is overlap between what we are calling genetic engineering and what we have called control of reproduction. While we made the distinction then between deciding whether an individual will be born and deciding what genetic makeup the individual will have, this can only be a rough distinction. For example, the decision of a couple, both of whom are known to carry a deleterious recessive gene, not to have children is a decision that certain individuals will not be born, and also that certain genetic combinations will not be allowed to occur.

766

To be clear what we intend to talk about under genetic engineering, see Table 4, which lists both broad categories and specific techniques for controlling the genotypes of individuals.

Some people might be tempted to dismiss discussion of genetic engineering on the grounds that these are "science fiction" types of future technologies, and that we should restrict our attention to the real issues of today. As you can see from Table 4, however, it is impossible to generalize in this way. Under "selective mating" we have to include the avoidance of inbreeding, which is a social practice dating back to prehistoric times. Among those techniques which are purely medical, the first recorded pregnancy resulting from artificial insemination in humans was in the 1780's. The first experiments in which fertilized eggs were removed from one animal and transplanted into another animal was performed in 1893.

767

Of those techniques listed in Table 4 that are not now in common practice, in most cases it is not because of any theoretical obstacle to their accomplishment. All that is lacking in these techniques is the purely technical detail of putting a theoretically well defined idea into actual practice. If society were to decide that these techniques ought to be developed, and supported a crash program of research and development, some of them could be in general use within two or three years.

768

We saw in discussing resource allocation that it is much easier not to develop a technology than to restrict its use after large segments of the public had come to accept it and to expect it. Thus, in genetic engineering, we have the luxury, as of now, of discussing the consequences of these technologies without that kind of social pressure. Medical ethics would be lax in its duties if it did not take advantage of this opportunity.

769

Table 4

Some Possible Technologies for Human Genetic Engineering

A. Selective Mating
1) By phenotype of parents
   a) Sterilization of "unfit"
   b) Encouraging mating of selected pairs
   c) Artificial insemination with selected sperm donor
2) By genotype of parents—as in 1) but with specific knowledge of parental genotype
3) By relationship of parents—avoidance of inbreeding, incest, etc.
4) By age of parents—encouraging earlier pregnancy when incidence of chromosomal defects is less
5) By genotype of gametes
   a) Differentiation of sperm carrying "normal" gene from those carrying defective genes, followed by artificial insemination with "good" sperm
   b) "Vaccination" of mother so that defective sperm will be rejected by immune mechanisms

B. Technologies Involving Developing Zygote
1) Parthenogenesis—development of unfertilized egg (genotypically identical to mother)
2) Cloning—development of multiple individuals, all with same genotype, by separating cells at early embryo stage
3) Extracorporeal gestation or "test tube baby"
   a) Egg fertilized outside body, implanted in mother's uterus as treatment for infertility
   b) Egg or embryo already fertilized removed and developed to term in artificial placenta, as treatment for tendency to abort spontaneously
   c) Development of individual completely outside of body from conception to birth

C. Technologies Involving Somatic Cell Genotype
1) Directed alterations of genes
   a) Using viruses as DNA transmitters—naturally occurring viruses, or viruses modified specifically to replace missing genes
   b) Specifically induced mutations—no good approach now known
2) Random mutation with selection of cells with altered properties, followed by re-fusion of selected cells to host

Before going any further, we ought to make note of some terms used in this context. An individual's <u>genotype</u> is the complete set of genes that he carries, as determined (normally) at the time of conception; while his <u>phenotype</u> is the observable set of traits of the individual, as determined by the constant interaction between his genes and his environment. <u>Eugenics</u> is the practice of genetic engineering by selecting which genes are to be allowed to combine to form the genotype; one might distinguish <u>positive</u> eugenics as selective breeding in hopes of producing superior individuals, while <u>negative</u> eugenics is the avoidance of the production of inferior individuals. <u>Euphenics</u> does not change the genotype; rather it alters the inner environment of the somatic cells so that either bad genes are not expressed in the phenotype, or good genes are expressed more fully. <u>Euthenics</u> also leaves the genotype alone, but instead alters the outer environment, so that what might have been a bad trait in the old environment is turned into a neutral one. The meanings of these terms can best be clarified by applying the terms to specific examples, as we shall do in the course of this chapter.

769

Table 4 presents a formidable list—are we going to have to go down item by item and evaluate the ethics of each technique? Or can some useful generalizations be made? To start off, we might take note that traditionally, applications of these techniques toward the end of negative eugenics has been tolerated much better than any attempt at positive eugenics. Obviously this is because most people can agree that a severely retarded individual represents a lamentable situation which ought to be avoided if possible, while few of us trust someone else to decide what human traits are "ideal" or "better" and therefore ought to be selected.

770

Therefore, for now, let's restrict the discussion to what we could call negative or neutral eugenics applications—in one case, the prevention of the development of, or the return to normal of, individuals who would otherwise have what the textbooks class as genetic diseases; and in the other case, the application to allow parents who cannot have children through natural means to have them in some other way, with the assumption that the resulting children will be neither genetically superior nor inferior to the children they would have had by natural conception and birth.

771

On this issue, it might help to come through the back door, by first seeing why we might reject some kinds of ethical arguments as inadequate. Two we can dismiss without much discussion: first, the idea that genetic engineering is necessarily wrong because we are "playing God", second, the argument that it is positively required because technology will allow it, and we always ought to do what is in keeping with "progress."

772

REVIEW
"PLAYING GOD"     281

773    A somewhat more substantial argument is that the experimentation that would be necessary to perfect these techniques (such as means of in vitro or "test tube" fertilization and gestation) would almost invariably produce "mistakes," or fetuses who have had defects introduced as a result of the experimental technique's unforseen consequences. Presumably these fetuses would not be allowed to develop beyond that point (if indeed the damage could be detected at the time it occurred). Therefore, it could be objected that this experimentation is immoral because you will have to kill your "mistakes." (For an example of this problem, review Case 39 in Chapter 11 on using aborted fetuses for such an experiment.)

774    One could reply to this by saying that there are plenty of risks to a naturally developing fetus, which may fail to implant in the uterus, spontaneously abort, or develop a congenital defect; and the risk to a fetus in a "test tube" is not significantly greater. The rejoinder is that this is an illegitimate justification, even if your statement about the relative risks is true, because the fetus would not have been exposed to any risks at all had you not meddled in the first place; the fetus would simply not existed to begin with. A rough way of paraphrasing this argument is that if you run over a person with your car and break his back, you cannot justify your action by pointing out that people run over by automobiles quite frequently get broken backs.

775    However, this argument cannot be begun unless we attribute some degree of "personhood" to the fetus being experimented on, and so one's view of this ought to depend on what one feels are acceptable quality-of-life criteria. At any rate, it does not seem to make any sense to say that such an experiment, terminated with the death of the fetus if it was found to be deformed, would cause the fetus any "suffering." And while the fetus is dead at the end, the consequences of our not doing the experiment would have been that either the fetus was not conceived or that it would have died earlier; so these have to be weighed in as well.

776    But what if the fetus has been deformed and we are unable to detect it, and allow the fetus to come to term? This leads to Paul Ramsey's major ethical objection. He insists that we can never be certain until the child is actually born, if then, that damage has not been done as a result of the experiment. For example, we could hypothesize a very subtle effect of the artificial placenta so that the children it produces end up with an I.Q. 5 to 10 points below what they would have had otherwise; this would be almost impossible to detect. Therefore, since we cannot exclude the possibility of such damage, the experiment constitutes unethical experimentation on the child-to-be without his or her consent.
    REALISTIC? *780

This argument has greater plausibility than the former, because we are not hypothesizing "suffering" to an unconscious fetus; we are suggesting the possibility of real damage to the individual who is to be born and who will have to live his life with the results of that damage (unless we also approve infanticide or euthanasia to cover our "mistakes"!). However, Ramsey seems to lose our sympathies by the strictness of his criteria. He demands absolute certainty that damage will not occur before he will pronounce the results ethical. In Chapter 5, we noted that one ethical "error" is to set impossibly high criteria and then reject your opponent's view because it does not meet them. It would seem that if Ramsey is going to demand absolute certainty before we can "meddle" in this way, he would also demand certainty for any of the other types of "meddling" that make up medical practice.

777

Possibly an even deeper problem with Ramsey's position has to do with the idea of the lack of consent of the child-to-be. Did any of us give our consent to be born? The world is full of risks, both in utero and outside it; nobody asked our opinion before exposing us to them. If the experiment  1) gives existence to a child who otherwise never would have been born, and  2) as a side effect produces some defect or handicap, to say that the experiment is unethical implies that even a slight harm is worse than not existing at all. If this were the case, Ramsey might be expected to be in favor of abortion, but we already saw how he stood on that. These implications of Ramsey's deontological approach to ethics may suggest why we have favored a con-sequentialist mode instead.

778

Note that the problem with this argument of Ramsey's is the all-or-none form with which it is stated. It could be stated in a weaker form: the ends to be served by such techniques, such as the desire of parents to have their own children, are less important than other ends served by medicine such as preservation of life and relief of suffering of individuals who have already been born. Therefore, while X degree of uncertainty would be tolerable in another medical situation, because of the important ends at stake, this same degree of uncertainty is not tolerable in genetic engineering. When stated this way the argument is plausible. But, since anything done by human beings is bound to include some uncertainty, a demand for certainty is the same as saying the genetic engineering is not appropriate as a human endeavor.

779

781

We should note in passing that the problem of subtle influences on the developing fetus seems a very real one. For instance, the normal fetus is ex-posed, in the uterus, to the levels of hormones circulating in the mother's blood; and these hormone levels often change in the form of episodic bursts of activity, rather than remaining at a steady state or following well-regulated cycles. It is at least conceivable that the exposure to these episodic bursts of hormones is a necessary condition for the normal development of a fetus; and that a fetus raised in an artificial placenta in which levels of these hormones followed a pre-determined, cyclic pattern would be defective in some subtle way. If it indeed turns out that the subtle effects of a normal placenta are as important in this regard as the gross effects, the creation of a workable artificial placenta might be much farther off in the future than is now imagined.

780

777

**781**     And that, in fact, is precisely Ramsey's next argument against "test-tube-baby" technologies. He decries the abandonment of human procreation of babies to be replaced by the inhuman manufacture of babies. But is this not rather an assertion of rational control over gestation, and is not rationality the highest human property? Ramsey quotes Leon Kass: "Human procreation is human partly because it is not simply an activity of our rational wills....Human procreation is begetting. It is a more complete human activity precisely because it engages us bodily and spiritually, as well as rationally."

**782**     Few would argue with this value judgment so long as it concerns the procreative act and the participants in it. Just as most would hold sexual intercourse in an atmosphere of love and trust to be superior to the same act in a less conducive atmosphere, most of us would rather "procreate" our babies, when possible, rather than have them "manufactured." This alone is a good reason why the practices Ramsey fears are unlikely to become any more widespread than would be necessary to correct for infertility problems, or to prevent severe genetic defects.

**783**     However, some people of this persuasion (as the accompanying editorial to Ramsey's articles in JAMA shows clearly) do not confine their value judgments to the procreative act, but attribute a loss of humanity to the child that results. That is, the child who is "manufactured" by genetic engineering—even by something as apparently innocuous as artificial insemination—is held to be less of a human being than one "called into being" through a "natural" sex act. Presumably the criteria are those of Kass—that a procreative act ought to engage the participants emotionally and spiritually as well as rationally. By these criteria, a child conceived as a result of rape is, for that reason alone, less of a human being than another child. This is not only a weird position for someone who opposes abortion and euthanasia because they deny the "humanness" of the victim; it is a particularly cruel throwback to Medieval thinking which ought to have no place in a contemporary ethical debate. (To be fair, Ramsey makes no explicit statement to this effect, but some of his comments could be construed in this way.)

**784**     The final argument against genetic engineering we shall consider here is also mentioned by Ramsey, when he speaks of "turning the profession of medical care into a technological function." Elsewhere he states that in vitro fertilization in the case of an infertile woman is not medical treatment, because it does not correct the underlying defect; the woman is just as infertile after the genetic engineering as before. (Would we then say that a patient given exogenous insulin for diabetes is not receiving medical treatment, because his own pancreatic islet cells remain incapable of insulin secretion?)

What is the point of saying that something is not medical treatment? 785
Does that mean it is unethical for doctors to do something in their professional
roles which is not medical treatment—that "not medical" equals "unethical"?
From an opposing point of view we could argue that anything that doctors
do in their professional roles is medical treatment simply for that reason.

Therefore, there are two questions here: 1) what we are going to label
as "medical treatment," and 2) what ethical significance we are going to
attach to the label. As far as the label goes, we might want to have some non-
arbitrary criteria. If our criterion is correction of an underlying defect, we
already saw that genetic engineering has as much right to the label as many
other things which are routinely accepted parts of medical practice.

We might well ask whether there is, in fact, any non-arbitrary way of 786
distinguishing what is medical treatment from what isn't; this whole problem
ties in closely to the question of what is a disease, which we shall come to
in Chapter 17. If the label is indeed somewhat arbitrary, that makes it harder
to pin any ethical judgment on it. At any rate, to argue against something
because it is not medical treatment is to make an ethical judgment by definition—which, as we saw with the suicide argument under euthanasia, cannot
stand alone without supporting reasons.

We are now obligated to turn to the "good" arguments for and against 787
genetic engineering. The arguments opposed, especially when they come from
within the scientific community, tend to center on one issue: uncertainty.
In raising this issue, a distinction is usually made between further basic research
into genetic mechanisms and the applied technology. A good example of this
is the following statement by two physicians, Friedmann and Roblin, at the
conclusion of a review article on therapy by gene manipulation:

"In our view, gene therapy may ameliorate some human genetic diseases 788
in the future. For this reason, we believe that research directed at the development of techniques for gene therapy should continue. For the forseeable future,
however, we oppose any further attempts at gene therapy in human patients
because (i) our understanding of such basic processes as gene regulation and
genetic recombination in human cells is inadequate; (ii) our understanding of
the details of the relation between molecular defect and the disease state is
rudimentary for essentially all genetic diseases; and (iii) we have no information
on the short-range and long-term side effects of gene therapy. We therefore
propose that a sustained effort be made to formulate a complete set of ethico-
scientific criteria to guide the development and clinical application of gene
therapy techniques."*

*From T. Friedmann and R. Roblin, "Gene Therapy for Human Genetic Disease?"
Science 175:949, 1972. Copyright 1972 by the American Association for the Advancement
of Science.

789    Note how this argument differs from the one of Ramsey—there is no statement to the effect that no uncertainty is permissible. Rather there is the assertion of too much uncertainty at present, while leaving open the possibility that the uncertainty will be reduced to tolerable levels in the future.

Note, however, that there is a danger in this approach. Because the argument is so scientific and objective, we might tend to place decisive weight on it and to neglect other "non-scientific" arguments which may be every bit as valid. Then, one day in the future when we wake up to find that the uncertainties have been reduced, we may well see the therapies going into widespread use before we have time to formulate these other objections. The opportunity referred to earlier, of having a thorough ethical debate on the merits before the technology is actually breathing down our necks, will have been lost. Hence the importance of the Friedmann-Roblin call for a "sustained effort" to formulate "ethico-scientific criteria."

790    Scientists as a rule tend to call for continued basic research even where they oppose implementation. But even here ethical considerations are being taken into account. Berg, as chairman of a committee of the National Research Council, has called for a halt to certain types of research in which DNA from different bacteria, viruses, or other species is artificially linked together. The group sees a danger that the products of such research might provide a route for the spread of dangerous genes to naturally occurring organisms——for instance, genes for resistance to antibiotics may be spread among bacteria that infect humans. (Such DNA research is needed in order to carry out genetic engineering of type C-1-a in Table 4, but this was not the reason the researchers oppose it.) It remains to be seen whether such a voluntary research moratorium, the first attempt of its kind, will be effective.

791    At this point it might be wise to focus the discussion more on specific features of certain types of technologies listed in Table 4. While we can postpone the complicated question of long-range consequences until later in the chapter, we might at least want to think about the short-term side effects. A good place to start might be to examine the goals of some of the technologies and to weigh them according to a scale of societal values. This might then lead us to an idea of what level of side effects is permissible. Going back to Chapter 12 and our levels of needs, we might decide that we can tolerate significant side effects in a technology which meets a very basic need, but that much smaller side effects will be prohibitive if the technology is in the superficial-need category.

Indeed, this point may explain the position of the more enthusiastic advocates of genetic engineering such as Joseph Fletcher; they are often led by their position to deny or to minimize the importance of the various side effects, or else to overestimate the degree of certainty of a desirable outcome. Another mistake they might make is to forget about the resource-allocation consideration, as Fletcher does when he suggests that women ought to have babies by in vitro techniques in preference to natural childbirth.

792

Looking at Table 4, we see that the procedures under "Selective Mating" and the "Technologies Involving Somatic Cell Genotype" (gene therapy) are both aimed at changing the genetic endowment of the individual—the former before, the latter after conception. Since for now we are considering only negative or neutral eugenics, this means for practical purposes the use of genetic engineering to prevent the occurrence of genetic disease. On the other hand, the technologies involving the developing zygote, particularly the test-tube-baby processes, have their practical aim more toward allowing women who are now infertile or who tend to spontaneously abort to have their own children. These fit under the category of genetic engineering because they can also be used in conjunction with the other techniques to change genotype.

793

As far as the techniques to prevent genetic disease go, one has pretty much already made the relevant value judgment if, in the preceding chapters, one had determined that the prenatal diagnosis of such a condition was grounds for abortion, or that euthanasia might be considered in the case of an individual with such a disease. It would seem quite inconsistent to say that a condition was so bad that death of the individual was desirable, and yet not be willing to apply therapy for that disease if it were available. (Unless, of course, one's real motive was population control and not medicine in its more traditional sense.) This would suggest (remembering that we are temporarily postponing discussion of long-range consequences) that the allowable side effects from the therapy can be weighed against the bad consequences of the disease. In the case of a genetic disease such as cleft palate, which responds to postnatal surgical treatment, we might decide that even with minor side effects, gene therapy or selective mating procedures are not warranted.

794

The problem of weighing benefits against side effects is much easier when there is only one individual or one conception under consideration. As Ramsey showed with his condemnations of "statistical morality," the answer is less clean when individuals-to-be are involved.

795

In the year 1987, you find yourself counseling a couple who have been married three years and who wish to start a family. In the genetic screening test that is required by the government to get a license to have children, it was found that both Mr. and Mrs. L. carry one recessive gene for a disease which leads to severe mental retardation with a life expectancy of 11 years average. This means that each child conceived by the L.'s is at a 25% risk to develop the disease.

You see two options open to the L.'s, who wish to avoid the birth of an affected baby. One is artificial insemination of Mrs. L. by sperm from a donor who has been screened and found free of the gene. This gives a 0% chance of a child being born with the disease, but the L.'s seem initially opposed to the artificial insemination idea using the sperm of another, unknown male.

The other option is a technique which has been in use for 9 years, in which sperm are collected from Mr. L. and a fluorescent-tagged antigen added. This can be made specific for the recessive gene in question, so that those sperm which carry the gene will be labeled and, by a complicated process, separated from the others. Mrs. L. can then be artifically impregnated with the "clean" sperm from her husband.

The hitch is that since the technique of sperm immunoselection has been used, epidemiologists have noted an increased incidence of leukemias and lymphomas in children conceived by these treated sperm. While in the late 1970's great strides were made in the treatment of these cancers, the particular strains involved in these children have proved relatively resistant to therapy. The latest figures available to you is that such children have a four-fold increase in risk of developing cancer, which is still a small chance since the normal risk is less than 1%. Of those children who do develop these cancers, only 32% survive for five years.

You are aware that the L.'s are not too sophisticated in biological knowledge, and therefore how you present these data will very likely sway their decision. If you say that with the sperm immunoselection, each child conceived will have a 2—3% risk of cancer as opposed to a 25% risk of mental retardation in normal mating, and a 0% risk in artificial insemination, the couple will very likely opt for the immunoselection.

If, on the other hand, you say that in normal mating 75% of the children would be free of defect, but under immunoselection some of these otherwise normal children will be exposed to an increased risk of cancer, the L.'s might decide that that is wrong and decide reluctantly to have artificial insemination by donor. But this is not necessarily a good thing; you suspect that their reluctance stems from Mr. L.'s masculinity hangups if another man's sperm impregnates his wife. You have seen such cases in which the husband later got so emotionally disturbed that he rejected both wife and child.

What do you tell Mr. and Mrs. L. about their choices?

Which of the two possible presentations of the facts do you deem most accurate—or are they both equally accurate? The first is the statistical morality approach: we don't know which child will have the defect and/or which will get cancer, so we have to regard each child as having such-and-such risk of each. Since we then have to weigh the risks, these figures are the best thing we can use. The second approach is the Ramsey formulation: even if we don't know which, some of the children who later got cancer would have been normal as far as the genetic disease goes, but they were exposed to the same "treatment" as the affected sperm, so the result is unethical. Ramsey is not concerned about the inability of this method to weigh risks; he has no intention of weighing risks, since he believes that ethical reasoning should proceed from established rules and principles and not from the consequences (see Appendix I).

797

As we indicated before, the so-called statistical morality seems a more valid approach in this sort of case. To apply the other, we get into a string of what-if's and otherwise-would-have-been's which have the nagging quality of a child's question: "Where would I be if I hadn't been born?" Our difficulty in getting a handle on such questions severely limits their usefulness as guides to ethical reasoning. From a strictly practical viewpoint, weighing risks seems to be superior. (Another application of "statistical morality" would be to decide that it is all right if a small percentage of the population suffer if the overall happiness will be increased as a result. In this case we might well object, since we are here talking about individuals who are alive and who will suffer real, not hypothetical, consequences.)

798

Now, let's turn to the test-tube-baby propositions—those which are mainly being advertised as means for mothers to have children of their own. This relates to our discussion of last chapter about the "right to bear normal children," which we saw was a highly suspect right which led to absurdities if any attempt were to be made to implement it across the board. Here we run across the point mentioned at the beginning of this chapter, about the irrationality of our society in matters regarding parenthood. Since, despite the fact that there is manifestly a lot of incompetent parenthood going on, the institution is hardly ever attacked, it is worth while to spend a little time on an argument against genetic engineering which is seldom stated.

799

In trying to evaluate just where we are to rank the need to have one's own children—and surely this has traditionally been placed as a very basic need—we might do well to ask just why it is people have children. Psychologists have concluded that there are several motives for parenthood, which occur in varying mixtures in each parent. There are several kinds of what we might call selfish motives—the frontier need to have children to work the farm; the equation of children with immortality and perpetuating one's name; viewing children as surrogates who will achieve the success in the world that was denied to the parents. There are also altruistic motives, which emphasize the child's identity as a unique individual and the parent's job of cultivating that individual to allow him or her to reach the fullest potential.

800

801     It is known that when the parents' needs are given much more emphasis than the child's needs as an individual, trouble may result in the child's development. It seems fair to say that the woman with marital problems who decides to get pregnant so that her husband will "start loving her again" is committing an injustice to the child-to-be (as well as actually increasing the chance of a marital breakup). It is not clearly known what dangers may accompany the more subtly selfish motives, although surely factors such as parental disapproval of the child's career plans, when the plans do not coincide with the parents' expectations, is a source of significant family friction. We might thus hazard a generalization that a relative increase in altruistic motives and a corresponding decrease in selfish ones would tend to increase the quality of life of children. And the overall social benefits of raising children with better quality of life after they are born might surpass anything that could be gained by tampering with them before birth.

802     At present, there is little attempt being made to further altruistic parenthood or to expose selfish parenthood for critical discussion. As one noted economist said, one of the prime causes of deteriorating social institutions is the fact that child-raising in our society is done by almost completely unskilled labor. Among the extreme answers that have been proposed is the one mentioned in Case 53, of licensing parents and forcing conditions on them before allowing them to have children. We might well shy away from such a solution. But, as an alternative, we might at the very least want to look very critically upon any new developments which seem to give further impetus to the selfish parenthood motives.

803     So what does all this have to do with genetic engineering? Well, it could be argued plausibly that by offering guaranteed parenthood as a "right" of all individuals, society will be reinforcing the selfish aspects of parenthood—the desire to have a baby because it will make me feel good, and a corresponding decrease in awareness of the obligation that I am undertaking toward that baby. We would hesitate to make this any sort of absolute judgment. After all, infertility is not distributed only to those who are emotionally unfit to be parents. However, the problem becomes even more serious when we add the possibility of altering the child's genes or prenatal environment to achieve certain positive goals.

# CASE 54

1987 again, and you are on a committee of the FDA to screen new drugs and approve them for use. Fortunately, by a recent Congressional action, the FDA has been charged with looking at new drugs from a resource-allocation viewpoint as well as the safety angle, so that you can reject a safe drug if you judge that society could better devote its resources in other areas.

The two pills now up for discussion have curious properties. They started out as pills for nausea of pregnancy and were tested and approved for use in pregnant women. Subsequently a strange feature was noticed by chance. Of mothers who had taken pill A, 98.3% of the offspring showed up with blue eyes, while in the case of pill B, 97.9% of the children had brown eyes—all with no apparent alteration of the genotype.

While the mechanism is unknown, the specific chemicals responsible for the eye color control have been isolated, and the drug company has applied for permission to release the pills for the express purpose of altering eye color in unborn children. The chemicals have been tested further and again no significant side effects have been noted.

The company acknowledges that certain chemicals, such as diethylstilbestrol, have been found to produce deleterious effects in the offspring when ingested during pregnancy, and to show the effects when the child reaches adolescence or later. Since this set of pills has not been tested long enough to observe this, these long-range side effects cannot be completely ruled out.

In its resource-impact statement, the company contends that the cost of the pills will be quite cheap, and the resource allocation for this purpose will be negligible from the viewpoint of the entire industry. Therefore, even though choosing the eye color of one's baby is not a pressing social need, releasing the pills for general use seems justified.

Are you going to vote for or against the licensing of these pills?

---

Consider for the moment just one aspect of the proposal in Case 54—the consequences for shaping social attitudes. What concept of parenthood is conjured up by the vision of parents going to the drug store to buy the eye-color pills, possibly with the husband and wife getting into an argument over what color to choose? If anything, it would seem that the idea of the child as a unique identity has taken second place to the child as a sort of plaything which the parents go shopping for. This would in turn have grave implication for the "humanness" of the child—not by the parents' attitudes during prenatal development, but rather due to the fact that the way the parents raise the child is likely to reflect these attitudes. Are you condoning and encouraging these attitudes by putting the pills on the market?

What we are suggesting is a rather tenuous and abstract connection between a particular action and societal attitudes. We know that societal attitudes do have a profound effect on behavior, and vice versa. But how can we measure the effect, and how do we measure the likelihood that action X will produce attitude Y? Present attempts at these psychological measurements, such as the question of whether TV violence encourages violent behavior, are full of problems of interpretation. While such considerations are certainly ethically relevant, we also have to be careful not to use them to justify paternalistic control in the absence of good data.

807      Thus, as Case 54 shows, the problem of weighing possible attitudinal consequences is great enough when the selfish and the altruistic motives for parenthood are clearly distinguished. But Case 54 was written so as to be strongly biased toward what we would tend to consider a frivolous use of genetic engineering. Now go back and look at Case 31 in Chapter 9, which proposed an I.Q.-boosting pill which could be given to school kids. Suppose it was this pill instead of the eye-color pill that was being proposed for prenatal use.

REVIEW
I.Q. PILL    440

808      Parents often say that they want their children to have good opportunities in life—we would have to call this an altruistic motive, though the definition of a good opportunity might be clouded by self-centered ambitions rather than the child's own potentials. As a general rule, we would also have to admit that in our society, a person with higher intellectual capacity has a better chance at success, although there is no positive correlation between I.Q. and the actual attainment of success. What are your views on releasing this kind of pill for use by pregnant mothers in order to alter their children-to-be? If you had one answer for the eye-color pill and another for the I.Q. pill, where do you draw the line in between them?

809      In conclusion, we have seen that where genetic engineering is intended to prevent or correct genetic disease, it is possible to weigh the risks against the benefits for the child, even though we might have to rely on statistical data. In the case of genetic engineering to fulfill the desires of the parents, side effects to be suffered by the child have to be weighed against the benefits to the parents. Is it ethically permissible to put individual A at risk in order to make individual B happy, when (as Ramsey said) A has no choice in the matter? (Some might say A has no gripe, because if it were not for the desire to make B happy, A would never have been born. But since this leads us back into the thicket of what-if questions, we are forced, in self-defense, to consider the question of whether or not one is born as an ethically neutral issue.)

810      As a general rule in society, we are very suspicious of such an action relating to A and B; we tend to demand that the benefit to B be large and that the risk to A be small before we will permit this. But where A is an unborn child and B is the parent, these usual relationships are obscured, because we have grown used to thinking of the parent as the primary spokesman for the child. *Therefore, when genetic engineering is put to use to allow parents to satisfy their procreative desires, the ethical guidelines drawn ought to place strong emphasis upon the interests of the child, to make sure that these considerations do not get left out.*

811      It is now time, before proceeding to the long-range consequences of genetic engineering, to say a few words about positive eugenics. In negative eugenics, we assumed that it was agreed that certain things constituted genetic diseases, and that diseases are bad; having decided on the ends to be served, we only had to discuss the means. In positive eugenics (which Case 54 would have been if the pills had altered the genes for eye color), we not only have to decide upon the means to breed superior individuals; we also have to reach some sort of agreement about the end results that are to be considered desirable.

To start on the practical side, can we breed humans for positive traits, such as good looks or high intelligence? You can do this with animals, and human beings are animals. There is, however, a problem in that most of the complex traits we might like to breed for are determined by the mutual interaction between heredity and environment, with the role played by each component unclear. Where environmental factors are important, manipulating the heredity alone may produce no change or in fact a worse specimen. Even when we can produce the direction of change desired by manipulating heredity, it is impossible, where there is an interaction of a number of genes, to predict the rate of change; the improvement may be too slow to be practical.

812

Assuming you can get over these practical difficulties, what are the ends toward which the positive eugenicist should aim? Since negative eugenics aims at the elimination of genetic disease, it seems logical and laudable that his positive-minded counterpart should aim for genetic health. While we promised to talk about definitions of health and disease in Chapter 17, this creature called "genetic health" has enough peculiar features to justify considering it separately.

813

It is revealing to watch how one geneticist, Lappe, tries to elucidate the concept of genetic health. He points out a number of problems along the way. First of all, there is the problem that as far as recessive genes are concerned, the phenotype does not reflect the genotype. A person can be normal in a phenotypic and medical sense and yet carry a gene which, if matched up with another like it, would produce a lethal disease. Since this gene can be passed along to children, and can be expressed in the phenotype if the wrong mating occurs and two genes come together, it might make sense to say that anyone who carries such a gene is genetically unhealthy.

814

The only problem with that is that we are all genetically unhealthy. According to calculation, we all carry up to 10 recessive genes which, if matched up with another to form the homozygous condition, would produce a lethal disease. Does it make sense to have a definition of health which fits no one?

815

A further problem exists with the differences between the homozygous (two identical genes) and the heterozygous (one each of two varieties of gene for the same trait) states for certain traits. A good example is sickle cell anemia, which appears with the homozygous state or ss. The ss individual will, without treatment, have a shortened life span, so this seems definitely to be an evolutionary disadvantage—so much so that it was a mystery as to why the gene was relatively common in the African population, since natural selection should have been working to eliminate it. It was then found that the heterozygous individuals (Ss) were more resistant to malaria than the normal or SS individuals. If you were Ss and married an Ss, out in the jungle, 25% of your children would be ss and would be expected to die early, but 50% would be Ss, would have no anemia, and would be more resistant to malaria. Therefore, the net effect of the s gene was beneficial. (Nature practices statistical morality even if we don't.)

816

817    In conclusion, the s gene is genetically unhealthy, in terms of fitness to the environment, only in the ss state; given a malarial environment, it is very healthy in the Ss state. How do you arrange your concept of genetic health to account for this? (It has been suggested more recently that the Tay-Sachs gene, in its heterozygous form, tends to protect against tuberculosis, which would certainly have been of benefit to Jews in Eastern Europe.)

Also suppose you call the Ss person genetically healthy because he is resistant to malaria. Now he comes to the U.S. where there is no malaria, but he can still have children with sickle cell anemia. Did he change from healthy to unhealthy in the middle of the Atlantic?

818    As a thorough geneticist, Lappe lists all of these problems, but he fails to draw what might be a logical conclusion—namely, that there is no such thing as genetic health. This actually makes more sense. Health should be a property of a biological system (we won't say organism, because we might want to talk about, say, a healthy cell or healthy tissue). Any biological system is the result of a complex mutual interaction between its genetic program and its environmental inputs. If one of those elements, by itself, is messed up, the system will suffer, so we can have genetic disease. But one of those elements, by itself, cannot insure the overall balance and harmony of the system, so we cannot have genetic health, or environmental health either.

This approach to health, if it is unclear here, may make more sense when we discuss concepts of health and disease, and the nature of man as a biological system, in Chapter 17.

819    If we have no concept of genetic health, what else is there for the positive eugenicist to aim at? He is left with little more than his own view of the future, or his own Utopian view of what human beings ought to be and can become. As we had occasion to note earlier, people in general are (with good reason) reluctant to entrust someone else to design a Utopia for them, if there is any hint of a variation in fundamental values. Therefore, it seems unlikely that any sort of consensus on the ends of eugenics could be reached for purposes of formulating a policy of positive change.

Recall the argument of uncertainty as it related to negative eugenics. If negative eugenics was hampered by uncertainty, it seems that positive eugenics has gotten a double dose of it.

820    What sort of uncertainty are we referring to when talking about positive eugenics? Essentially, the problem is one of understanding multiple interactions, as opposed to strictly one-way cause and effect chains of events. Even if we neglect the outer environment, it is clear that most traits result from the actions of sets of genes. Each gene produces its own biochemical product, and the products do not only interact with each other, but also interact with the other genes. Unless genes are turned "on" and "off" through these biochemical interactions, the genes are simply inert pieces of a DNA molecule, incapable of having any effect on the traits of the individual. Thus, until we understand those interactions pretty well, we are on shaky ground if we try to create new traits by changing genes.

We argued back in Chapter 9 that many techniques of psychosurgery may be based on fallacious views of the brain, by attributing behavior to specific brain locations instead of to a complex interaction of many nervous elements. In a similar way, we would have to avoid any eugenic gene-manipulation which focused on one gene instead of upon the whole complex network; else the unwanted and unforeseen side effects might totally overshadow the hoped-for result.

As in the case of psychosurgery, these side effects could be devastating to the individual upon whom the gene therapy or gene selection was performed. However, in psychosurgery, the major bad effects are limited to the individual, while in genetics, the change is inheritable and so all future generations could be affected as well. This is important when we realize that the result of much animal and plant breeding has been the reduction in the total number of genes in the species "gene pool." The result seems to be a limitation upon the ability of the species to adapt to changes in the environment. This is especially clear regarding infectious disease—if you selectively breed a plant or animal that is resistant to a microorganism, you are putting selection pressure on the microorganism to form new mutant strains which can overcome that resistance. And since the length of the reproductive cycle is much shorter for the micro-organism than for the plant or animal, you may well be fighting a losing battle, with a new disease appearing as soon as you breed resistance to the old disease.

In plants such as wheat and corn, where the gene pool has been narrowed very drastically, the result has been an increase in new plant diseases. Plant geneticists are now going back to the older, less productive varieties that have been in danger of extinction in order to preserve samples of them; that way, if a new disease comes along which threatens to devastate present strains, these older types will still be available for attempts to breed newer resistant species. Thus, while the previous breeding practice has been to diminish the number of different genes in the gene pool as a result of selecting out the superior traits, geneticists are now trying to increase the number of genes in order to restore the species' adaptability.

Population genetics seems to be one area where the injunction to "keep your options open" is very good advice. If we close out important options by seeking to eliminate genes which we think are harmful (and which may, like sickle cell gene, actually be beneficial in a heterozygous state), and by increasing the incidence of a few genes which we think are beneficial, the options are closed not only to us but also to all of posterity (if we ignore the chance of re-emergence of these genes through spontaneous mutations). Genetic engineering is tampering with posterity when we have no information about the changes in environment that posterity might face. Ramsey would surely want to point out that we have gotten no informed consent from posterity for these manip-ulations.

825    These considerations ought to give pause to the more enthusiastic advocates of genetic engineering, such as Fletcher, who states, "Not to control when we can is immoral." This follows from Fletcher's claim that rationality and concern are the most important "human" attributes. But sometimes, where we are dealing with complex and interrelated systems, "rational concern" can best be expressed by including an element of chance. We can all think of situations in which social justice might best be served by choosing people by lot; and all but the most extreme economists would admit to certain circumstances in which it is most efficient to let the vagaries of the marketplace determine prices instead of rationally trying to set prices beforehand.

826    Basically, the argument so far holds that genetic engineering may do damage to the future of the human species by reducing the variation in the gene pool. Another argument holds that we are already doing damage to the species by thwarting the processes of natural selection—and that maybe genetic engineering will be required to repair the damage. This other argument is that of the so-called "genetic deterioration" of the species that results when individuals with hereditary diseases, who would normally die before reaching the age of reproduction, are allowed to live by medical treatment and thus can pass on their defective genes to offspring. Diabetes is often cited as an example, since it was usually fatal at an early age before the advent of insulin. Since diabetes is at least partly genetic, the contribution of several genes, it is argued that by allowing diabetics to live normal lives, the incidence of diabetic genes will increase in the species until eventually all humans will need insulin to survive.

827    The scientific evidence for and against the idea of genetic deterioration requires some sophisticated genetics knowledge to evaluate, so we cannot do justice to the issue here. One geneticist, Crow, estimates that relaxation of natural selection by allowing individuals with bad genes to survive will, as a net result, produce very little change in average gene frequency. In the case of a sickle cell gene, where the selection pressures are different for the heterozygous and the homozygous states, the frequency of the gene might go up or down depending on which selection pressure predominates. A similar process occurs where selection works on groups of genes instead of on a single gene, as with diabetes. Even in the case of a single recessive gene, Crow estimates that if the original frequency of the gene in the population is 0.5%, and the gene did cause total sterility but with new medical treatment has no effect on the individual, with random mating it would still take 70 generations for the incidence of the gene to double to 1%.

828    Because of all these factors, Crow estimates that the rate of new mutations to form harmful genes might be much more important in determining genetic deterioration than the problem of relaxed selection. Since we know of a number of environmental hazards, notably radiation and certain chemicals, which can increase the mutation rate, our efforts to prevent genetic deterioration ought to be directed against those hazards instead of trying to manipulate the genes directly.

It is also important, with regard to the question of relaxed selection, that humans do not randomly mate and have children; and social factors can have more influence on the gene pool than strictly medical ones. These social factors are reflected in the "Selective Mating" types of genetic engineering listed in Table 4, which, as we have seen, have been in use for long periods and thus are known to be relatively free of "side effects." Lappe notes that when Japan passed a law which did no more than introduce legal abortion and encourage earlier marriages, the number of births of Down's syndrome children was reduced by 1/3, and the births of children with all other congenital defects dropped by 1/10. Therefore, these kinds of social factors may be keeping up with or even surpassing medical advances in their effects on the gene pool.

829

Another ethical issue sometimes raised in genetic engineering is cloning. Table 4 lists cloning in regard to manipulation of the developing zygote; but it is also theoretically possible to take one cell from an adult person and cause it to develop into a new individual with the identical genotype. (In this way one could have a "spare" in case one needed a kidney transplant.)

830

You can see immediately a number of ethical issues. We will not discuss them in any depth, mostly because, while the technology of cloning is not so far-fetched, the motives that could lead society to undertake it on any scale do not seem very prominent.

831

Fletcher, who sees no a priori ethical objection to cloning, makes one point that helps clarify the debate. Recall our point with regard to "genetic health" that a person is the product of the interaction between his genotype and the environment, and in no sense is "determined" by his genes. Thus, even though the person cloned from one of your cells has your genotype, his environment is certainly different and he is thus a unique individual, not a "Xerox copy" of you. And so presumably you would have no more right to demand that he give up one of his kidneys to treat your disease, than you would to demand it of anyone born in the normal way.

832

Moreover, as scientists learn more about somatic cell mutations and mutation-inducing environmental factors, we come to the conclusion that mutations in our body cells occurring since fertilization (which are not inheritable unless they chance to occur in our germ cells) may be much more widespread than we had thought. Thus there may be no guarantee that a cell taken at random from our skin, say, represents our own original genotype; and cloning "Xerox copies" may thus be even more unlikely.

833

834   For our final case discussion in this chapter, we return to the problem of genetic deterioration. We have discussed it from the larger context of social policy. But what are the individual responsibilities?

CASE 55

835   Mrs. T.H. is a somewhat special patient of yours. Twenty years ago, she was among the first babies with phenylketonuria (PKU) to be saved from developing progressive mental retardation by being fed a phenylalanine-free diet. Having been taken off the diet at age 9, she now has a high serum phenylalanine level; but since the amino acid is toxic only to the developing nervous system it does not affect her health in any way.

Now Mrs. T.H. comes to you to ask about having children. Assuming her husband is free of the PKU gene, half their children will be carriers but none will have the disease. But of more concern is the fact that any infant, in utero, will be exposed to the high phenylalanine concentration. While of course no data from previous patients are available, your best guess is that this is a severe risk to the developing fetal brain.

Mrs. T.H. is aware of the situation and asks what can be done to manage a pregnancy to give her some chance of having a healthy child. You reply that while some experimental procedures might be of some benefit, there is simply no therapy. "But if I should happen to get pregnant and come to you, you would pretty much have to do what you could, experimental or otherwise, wouldn't you?" she says.

Rather disconcerted by this prospect, you tell her that not only does she have a responsibility toward her potential child; she also should be grateful that the PKU therapy was able to save her 20 years ago and should feel a debt not to further tax medical resources. "I didn't agree to anything back then," says Mrs. T.H. "The goal of medicine is to help people lead normal lives, and for me that means having children of my own."

What do you tell Mrs. T.H. concerning pregnancy?

836   It is sometimes asked whether diabetics, who would have died in childhood had not medical science developed the treatment for their condition, should feel an obligation not to have children so as not to pass on the genes for their condition. While the problem with Mrs. T.H.'s prospective baby is not its own genes but rather the environment in utero, the case is analogous.

If you feel indeed that Mrs. T.H. ought not to have children, you might hope to persuade her by further explanation of the risks to the fetus—it may be that the success of a new therapy in her own case has made her unrealistically optimistic about the possibilities of medicine. Or you might try to counsel husband and wife together. Unfortunately in a case such as this artificial insemination would be no help; and with liberalized abortion there may well be a shortage of adoptable babies. But what do you do if Mrs. T.H. says that she wants a baby so much that she will take the risk of raising a retarded child?

837

If you oppose a pregnancy here, it might be strictly on the basis of the quality of life of the infant. What do you think of the argument of social obligation? Recall our criticism of the kidney transplant selection criteria utilized by "God Committees" in Chapter 12. In that case the criticism was that they treated a transplant as a social gift and then demanded that the recipients be socially and morally worthy of it. The argument here is not dissimilar, except that Mrs. T.H. already received her "gift" 20 years ago and now society wants to collect on her account. What is your opinion of this argument? If you accept the social gift view in Mrs. T.H.'s case but not in the transplant case (or vice versa), what are the relevant differences?

838

In summation, we can state that the question of possible long-range consequences of genetic engineering is a controversial one, and that with the present state of biological knowledge, we may not have enough data to reach any firm conclusions. While it is important to begin making ethical decisions now, it is also important to keep the decision-making process open and flexible, so that the new information can be fed into our ethical thinking as it arises in the future.

839

We can predict that there will be major problems with the interpretation of this new information. A good part of this will be due to the fact that judgments about genotypes must be made in terms of the individual's fitness to the environment. While modern science has become very adept at measuring the quantity of something with great precision, it is still in a rudimentary state when it comes to getting some kind of mathematical concept of fitness. Because of these problems in interpreting data, it will be especially important in these issues to have close cooperation between the ethical decision-makers and the research community.

We have had to skim rather lightly over the details of the specific technologies involved in genetic engineering. Further information on these topics can be found in several readings listed in the references. You might also want to look back on several cases which relate to topics discussed in this chapter: Case 28 in Chapter 7, Case 37 and Case 39 in Chapter 11, and Case 49 in Chapter 14.

840

Ch. 16

841

# 16. Organized Medicine and Medical Economics

## CASE 56

You are a third-year medical student doing your clerkship in a community hospital in Michigan. Your patient is a 68-year-old lady who is suffering from multiple problems; your careful history leads you to the conclusion that several years of inadequate nutrition forms a major component of her problem. She lives alone in a rather run-down house, tends to be depressed, and has no appetite or incentive to eat adequate meals. You are ready to discharge her and feel that she can remain in pretty good shape for several more years at least if she could improve her diet. However, if she goes back to her old habits, you can expect to see her back in the hospital within six months.

You are aware that in the community there is a hospital-run program called "Meals on Wheels" which delivers one nutritious, hot meal per day to invalids, or convalescents; you feel that this program is exactly what your patient needs.

In discussing this with the hospital social worker, you discover that while the lady has both Blue Cross and Medicare coverage, neither will pay the nominal $1 per day fee for the meals program. Instead, your patient would have to pay out-of-pocket, and you know that her personal finances are very tight and that she would probably not agree to pay this extra expense. "Why pay them when I am perfectly capable of fixing my own meals?" you imagine her saying, even though you know that left to her own devices she will go home and eat toast and coffee day in and day out.

The social worker makes a cynical comment that apparently Medicare and Blue Cross would rather have the patient admitted to the hospital again to run up another $6000 hospital bill rather than pay $7 a week to keep her well. This is part of the whole problem of medical care insurance being slanted toward crisis, in-hospital care instead of prevention, she adds.

What do you do now?

---

Most of the cases so far discussed have had, as the alternatives in answer to "What do you do now," a series of things that you could do within the context of the daily practice of medicine. The only alternatives open to you in Case 56, except for shrugging your shoulders and doing nothing, all fall outside of the strict realm of medical practice. You could pay the weekly $7 out of your own pocket without telling the patient, but that would be in a capacity of private charity rather than of medical care. You could also write an angry letter to your Congressman, make an appointment to object to the president of the local Blue Cross, or bring the matter up at the next meeting of the county medical society. But all these are political rather than medical acts, although your status as a medical professional may be of significant benefit in accomplishing what you want.

843    Because all these things except doing nothing are outside of the strictly medical role, many doctors will choose to do nothing and justify it on those grounds. They may contend that that has nothing to do with ethics; it is merely a matter of how they choose to spend their time. Or they may argue that if one did those things it would be unethical, because it would take time away from seeing patients which is the doctor's ethical obligation.

844    We will argue that this sort of decision does have ethical significance. *It seems safe to say that, within reason, you are ethically obligated to provide the best medical care you can. It is possible and indeed likely that certain social, political, or economic circumstances prevent you from giving good care. If these circumstances are to some extent within your power to change, then to that extent you would seem to be obligated to work to change them—else your ethical commitment to the best possible care is questionable.*

    Let's re-emphasize that the obligation is weighted according to your power to cause change. If the offending circumstances arise from policies of the Federal government, then your powers to change are the same as those of an ordinary citizen; your obligation is to elect Congressmen who support a change in policy, etc. If the circumstances arise out of a policy of the county medical society, of which you are a member, then your ethical obligation calls for a more active role in seeking change.

845    If you accept this ethical obligation, you have to go through a complex process. First, you have to be aware of the instances when the medical care being given falls short of optimal—a hard task because while we quickly perceive new problems, defects of long standing are usually accepted as inevitable or else are not perceived at all. Next we must decide what factors are responsible— also hard because in complex socio-politico-economic networks, many factors impinge upon any one event, and none of those factors can be changed without influencing many other parts of the system also. Finally, when we have isolated which factors we think are responsible, we have to decide upon the most effective way of changing them, while keeping the "side effects" to a minimum.

846    Thus is it clear that while (as we saw in Chapter 2) knowledge is an important ingredient in any ethical decision, it is particularly crucial in these matters. If we identify five social factors that influence the problem but miss a sixth; or if we choose to attempt change through a hospital board of directors without having realized that a more effective route would be through the state health department, we can waste all our effort for nothing—or worse yet, we can end up making the problem worse than it started out to be. A further problem is that data about social and economic relationships may often be more imprecise, or more open to debate, than some of the other data we are used to dealing with.

However, before trying to grapple with any data, let's go back to the first step—identifying the problem. The real problem with this comes when you as an individual practitioner, or the medical profession as a whole, is part of the problem. We are always reluctant to accept this because, on an emotional level, we tend to treat motives and consequences on a direct, cause-and-effect basis: good motives lead to good consequences and bad motives lead to bad consequences. Since each of us knows that he or she has excellent motives, none of us is prepared to accept the idea that these motives might have bad results. In fact, as our ethical decision-making scheme showed, there are a number of intervening factors between motives and consequences, so this sort of simplistic thinking cannot hold up.

847

One result of always thinking of our own motives as benevolent is to fail to perceive conflicts of interest that may arise—and these conflicts of interest may be the prime ingredients in the problem situation. To deal with a specific example, we will note an article by Robert M. Sade, M.D., in which he offers refutation of the idea of a "right to health care." Sade takes pretty much the same approach we used earlier—he argues that if health care is a right, then the doctors have an obligation to provide health care, and the only way to enforce that obligation would be to use government force against doctors; and that would be clearly immoral and undesirable.

848

However, Sade takes a stronger line. He notes that saying that the patient has a right to the doctor's services is the same as saying (for example) that anyone has a right to a loaf of bread, whether or not he can pay the baker or if the baker wants to sell it. The result would be to deprive the baker of the bread which he himself produced, and of his own right to sustain his life in the long run. While Sade correctly points out that the doctor is a member of a service profession, not a production trade as the baker is, nevertheless the analogy of the baker catches the essential features of his argument.

849

Thus, all the way through Sade treats the doctor as simply an individual with goods to sell until the very end—when he says, "Nonparticipation [in coercive government programs] is the only way in which personal values can be maintained. And it is only with the attainment of the highest of those values—integrity, honesty, and self-esteem—that the physician can achieve his most important professional value, the absolute priority of the welfare of his patients."*

850

*Reprinted by permission. From the New England Journal of Medicine 285:1288, 1971.

851    Now, Sade here is pulling off a pretty neat trick. He has created this baker-doctor who is nothing more than a vendor with absolute right to his own self-interest—and who, we might assume, is not above selling us a stale loaf if he thinks he can get away with it. And suddenly this caterpillar has metamorphosed itself into a grand butterfly with all those good personal values and an absolute priority in the welfare of the patient.

We will resist the temptation to debate with Dr. Sade's politics in order to make this one point. It is accepted as a given, without analysis, that the doctor's first interest is in the welfare of his patients. From there the doctor can do all sorts of things, even if they are self-centered and selfish, and neither he nor his professional colleagues perceive any conflict between these actions and the so-called "absolute priority."

852    In this unit we have avoided this outlook from the beginning, although it might not have been clear at the time that that was what we were doing. The move we made was that of adopting the "Contractual Model" of the doctor-patient relationship, and then going on to refer to various "clauses" in the "contract." Now, in what sort of human relationships are contracts appropriate? *Two ingredients are required: 1) the awareness that the cooperation of the two parties is necessary to achieve a certain goal, and 2) the awareness that conflicts between the interests of the two parties may interfere with the accomplishment of the goal unless guidelines are drawn up to arbitrate those conflicts. Therefore by calling the doctor-patient relationship a contractual one, we have given implicit recognition to the fact that conflicts of interest between doctor and patient are likely to arise.*

853    While individual doctors and patients can have conflicts of interest, completely different types of conflicts can arise when either band themselves together to form organized groups. (The American Medical Association "Principles of Medical Ethics" states that "For the advancement of his profession, a physician should affiliate with medical societies...") And the same kind of motive-consequence confusion can exist at the organizational level—since each individual doctor is assumed to give first priority to the welfare of patients, the medical association as a whole must have this same priority. When the association goes into the policy-making field, this assumption has an important corollary—anyone opposed to the policy recommended by the association must be opposed to the welfare of patients.

The only problem with this assumption is that it is not true. Case 57 gives what may be an extreme example.

## CASE 57

In 1962, the provincial government of Saskatchewan adopted a system of publicly financed medical care. The physicians of the province, both individually and through their organization, opposed implementation of this form of "socialized medicine" on the basis that under such a system, they would be unable to deliver quality care, and that the best interests of their patients called for maintaining the old fee-for-service system.

Accordingly, when the plan was enacted, the physicians went on strike and refused to render care except in emergencies. They denied that any selfish interests of their own were involved and justified the strike in terms of their concern over their patients' care.

The government responded by filling vacancies in the government-run clinics and hospitals with physicians coming over from Europe. The local physicians attacked these new arrivals as "scabs" and challenged their ethics for failing to support their fellow professionals.

If you were a physician in Saskatchewan, would you join the strike? On what grounds?

854

---

This case, incidentally, is not irrelevant to the present U.S. situation. Several years later the entire Canadian medical care system was converted to government financing, leaving the U.S. as the only developed Western nation without a publicly financed medical care system. A survey of a sampling of U.S. physicians in 1972, conducted by the journal Medical Opinion, showed that a majority of them would go on strike given the appropriate provocation. Since many U.S. doctors are very much opposed to increased government control of medical care delivery, we seem to have all of the Saskatchewan ingredients boiling in our own pot right now.

855

The reason we stated that Case 57 was a rather extreme situation is because it presents the picture of doctors claiming that they are serving the best interests of the patients by not delivering care, and that other doctors who were delivering care were being unethical for doing so. This inversion of values shows how drastically the divergence between the interests of doctors and patients can be with the doctors still refusing to recognize it.

If you were debating with a striking physician who claimed to be motivated solely by patient considerations, and you felt that he was motivated at least in part by financial self-interest, is there any way you could convince him through argument of the correctness of your view? You can see why consequences and not motives ought to be the final focus of argument in ethical decision-making.

856

857    However, our view that the position of the Saskatchewan physicians represents a perversion of real interest in the welfare of patients is partly based on our knowledge that after the strike ended (as described by Badgley and Wolfe), the physicians went back to work, and that the quality of medical care in Canada since socialization has not suffered appreciably by any objective criteria of measurement (more on this later). Therefore, we know that the dire consequences predicted by the doctors did not come about. But if we are to make ethical judgments, they have to be ethical at the time the decision is made, not ethical by retrospect ten years later.

858    Is it the case that it is never in the best interests of the patient for doctors to go on strike? (Keep in mind that all of us are patients at one time or another.) Suppose that at some time in the future a violently anti-doctor government is elected, and passes a law that every doctor must have in his office a government-appointed committee of three consumer representatives, who will watch whatever he does and intercede at any time they feel the need. The staunchest supporters of national health insurance and consumerism among the medical profession would probably object that they could not practice medicine in that situation, and that giving no service at all would be preferable. However, if the public had by that time become so disenchanted with doctors and had so little trust in the profession, good medical practice would probably have been impossible already. The point is that a strike has to be viewed as a very extreme measure, and resorted to only on the basis of defensible predictions, not emotional upsets. Unless, of course, doctors are just bakers.

859    As a sidelight, we might note that Badgley and Wolfe state in their account of the Saskatchewan strike that the situation could have been averted if both sides had showed some more political awareness. The liberal government, in particular, seemed to feel that they were going to win, and that they did not have to consult with the medical organization or grant any concessions. Each side was sure that the other would back down before the time to strike arrived, as often happens in labor disputes. This further points out the need for realistic data in planning the strategy for social change.

860    The problem of gathering accurate data on which to base policy decisions is a major one, and is well illustrated in Case 57 in the dispute over the consequences of socialization of medicine. Since the U.S. is now debating the advantages of a national health insurance program, and trying to decide which of a dozen alternative proposals to accept, attention is being focused on Britain, which has had national health insurance since the late 1940's. Those who favor national financing go to Britain and report that their system is far superior to ours in every conceivable respect.

An example of this is Kaplan, quoting an unpublished Ph.D. thesis study:
"A study conducted among American physicians and British physicians employed
by the National Health Service revealed a higher degree of patient-centered
service orientation among the British practitioners. The British doctors evinced
satisfaction with many aspects of their system including the freedom they had
to dispense the care their patients needed without having to worry about their
financial means, and the freedom of patients to seek treatment irrespective
of cost. They also expressed satisfaction with the removal of billing responsibilities, which they had considered...essentially unrelated to their professional
tasks. Their American counterparts stressed the freedom they enjoyed under
the capitalist system and the competitive aspects of working in a free market.
The investigator concluded that British physicians manifested higher degrees
of professionalism, particularly with respect to the service norm."

In contrast, spokesmen for the American Medical Association have also
visited Britain and have come back painting a dismal picture of lowered quality
of care, monstrous inefficiencies and waste, and physicians leaving the country
in droves to escape oppressive restrictions.

One apparently has two possible conclusions. Either Britain has two
different systems of medical care and American visitors are shown one or the
other but not both; or else these "data" are highly colored by the political
biases of the observers.

## CASE 58

You are sitting on a government policy board which is considering regulations for health maintenance organizations, or HMO's. Since the regulations
will have an important impact on the structure of care delivery in the HMO's,
you are hearing testimony on the optimal form for that structure. Testifying
today are two experts in medical economics.

Dr. R.J. paints a rather grim picture of how the industry of medical
care compares to other major industries in the U.S., and states that medicine's
unfavorable comparison in terms of efficiency is a prime reason for the high
cost of medical care, and therefore in turn for the exclusion of the poor from
the system of care. Instead of small, isolated medical offices dispensing services
on an itemized fee basis, says Dr. J., medicine should be moving toward sys-
tematic organization and centralization, which has worked so well for other
industries. He concludes by suggesting a model of HMO's as large community
health centers, with financing somewhat similar to that of a public utility.

Your other expert, Dr. M.H., turns the tables by demanding decentraliza-
tion and smaller unit size for HMO's, even if the cost is some loss in efficiency
as measured in strictly economic terms. From an economic analysis, he says,
it can be shown that in a field in which much of the professional's effectiveness
stems from a direct personal contact with the "consumer," the economies of
scale (i.e., increased efficiency with increased size) will disappear very early
in the game, while this is not true of production industries. Far from allowing
more poor to enter the system due to increased efficiency, Dr. H. states, de-
personalized monster facilities may well discourage the poor from coming at all.

How do you weigh these two testimonies in making your final decisions?

(Adapted from arguments summarized by Halberstam)

864       The two experts in Case 58 are taking positions about as diametrically opposed as the opposite views on socialized medicine; however, they have fleshed out their positions with some statements about how they reached their conclusions, so that you have a bit more to work with. Your analysis should include:

      1)   Does the expert state the basic assumptions from which his conclusions are drawn? If so, are these supported (or supportable) by evidence?

      2)   Do the conclusions follow from the basic assumptions?

      3)   Especially important in Case 58: Do the data cited by the expert actually measure the variable you are interested in? That is, if you think emotional encouragement is an important part of the doctor's "output," trying to measure this in strictly economic terms might be like trying to measure land area in degrees Centigrade.

865       Notice in Case 58 that the ethical values claimed by the two opposing experts are identical—the idea of opening the medical care system to people who are presently being denied services, which fits into the category of distributive justice we discussed in Chapter 12. Therefore the debate is not at the core an ethical one. The disagreement is one of which consequences would actually follow from a given action. This is common in socio-politico-economic debates; the ethical assumptions are agreed upon, and the sources of disagreement are of the type which could, at least in theory, be settled by empirical observation or experimentation.

      (Since the ethical values or "scales of preference" are often agreed upon, are these the types of questions to which the model of rational decision-making by Bayesian theory described in Chapter 2 may be applicable? Or do you think there are too many variables or too much uncertainty over probability?)

REVIEW
BAYESIAN THEORY     86–97

866       If the points of dispute are empirical rather than ethical questions, why have we included this material instead of banishing this topic to the realm of medical sociology? Clearly medical sociology plays an extremely important role here. However, what we want to focus upon here, for the purposes of this book, are the ethical consequences of social actions.

867       Just what is meant by ethical consequences? On a very simple level, this is just a repetition of what was discussed in Chapter 2. Consequences have to be weighed against values, once the probabilities are taken into account, and if the consequence is found to contradict the values, then we could call it an unethical consequence.

But for these issues we are interested particularly in a more complex meaning of ethical consequences. *The consequence of any social change is a new social environment, which may differ only a little or may differ greatly from the present one. We know that human behavior is shaped to a great extent by environmental factors, and that the environmental shaping may tend toward behavior that is contrary to what rational ethical decision-making would support. We conclude from this that there are certain environments in which it is harder to act ethically than in others, and we know that people are less likely to do hard things. Therefore, the general level of ethical behavior may go up or down within the health professions as a result of a particular social change, and the challenge is to be able to predict this.*

868

An example of such a prediction was that made by Sade in the quotations earlier in this chapter—that increased governmental control of medicine will create an atmosphere in which the personal values underlying ethical behavior will be lessened.

869

Another prediction was the one we made in Chapter 4 when we recommended the "Contractual Model" of the doctor-patient relationship. The idea was that with that sort of distribution of decision-making responsibilities, along with the acknowledgment of the potential conflicts of interest that we just alluded to, ethical behavior was more likely to result than would be the case if either the "Priestly Model" or the "Engineering Model" were accepted instead.

REVIEW
MODELS     106—110

To go into this business of ethical prediction in a bit more detail, as well as to give the opponents of Sade equal time, we can turn to an essay by Kaplan on the fee-for-service system of financing medical care. Kaplan's contentions are that the present system of financing medicine in the U.S. leads to more ethical problems than would be the case under alternative systems. He quotes another author on the proper role of financing in the medical profession: "The professional man, it has been said, does not work in order to be paid; he is paid in order that he may work." On this somewhat idealistic note Kaplan distinguishes his doctor from the baker in Sade's analysis.

870

Why should it necessarily be the case that the goal of service to the patient—the ethical goal upon which both Kaplan and Sade would agree—is in conflict with fee-for-service? Kaplan states that a lack of mercenary interest on the physician's part is an essential ingredient in establishing trust between doctor and patient; and the patient must trust, since (along the lines of the "Contractual Model") the technical details of the treatment are left to the doctor's discretion. If the doctor says that an $800 surgical procedure will cure the disease while a $10 bottle of pills won't, the patient must have faith that this is a true medical opinion and not one colored by profit motives.

871

872        On the other hand, says Kaplan, we all know the basic value espoused by mercantile enterprise: "caveat emptor" or "let the buyer beware." Since it would seem that the buyer who is spending all his time being beware has little chance left over to trust, Kaplan concludes that the "caveat emptor" philosophy is directly contradictory to the goals of the medical profession as far as the service orientation goes, and that doctors who think they can be private merchants without this leading to a conflict with their patient's welfare are, given the standard amount of human frailty, kidding themselves.

873        As an example of ways in which the mercantile ethic can either over-shadow or overturn the professional ethic, Kaplan offers into evidence the titles of articles that appeared in the periodical Medical Economics in 1969, such as:

"The Fine Art of Heading Off House Calls"
"Writing Out the Fee Isn't Enough"
"How to Tell if You Need a Business Manager"
"A Tax Free Haven for Your Cash Reserves"

874        Presumably the justification for offering this type of evidence (which is more for illustration than for proof of the argument) is that figures are available to show that a significant number of doctors do read that periodical, and that therefore it is safe to assume that the editors, in their choice of material, are speaking to the true interests of the medical profession, or at least a large segment thereof. This illustrates the problems in getting adequate data on social issues; while we might want to criticize an author who based his entire argument on such data, it might well be that the data which would really prove the case one way or the other are nonexistent.

875        Another important fact to remember is that, while a social change taken alone will produce a new social environment, we are never going to have one change alone; and the new environment which will actually come about, not the hypothetical one that we are basing our predictions on, will result from the interactions of all the social changes. Kaplan takes this into account by noting that the fee-for-service system would work better than it does (although there are still inherent problems) if we had an environment of equal distribution and accessibility of medical care personnel and facilities, both geographically and socio-economically. However, since we have unequal distribution, the problems of the fee-for-service system are worsened. In rebuttal, a fee-for-service advocate might argue that all the problems of fee-for-service arise from maldistribution, and so our efforts should be directed against the maldistribution instead of against the financing. (Kaplan could still have the last word by then contending that fee-for-service stands in the way of achieving equal distribution.)

It is important to note some of the things that are NOT being said, to be fair to the real and hypothetical disputants in this case. No one is saying that in either a fee-for-service or in a nationally financed system, all the doctors would be unethical; or likewise that under the opposite system all doctors would be ethical. And, if you were to get his back against the wall, each disputant would acknowledge that there are SOME ethical problems with the system he is recommending. The actual contention in each case is that the ethical problems would be fewer, and those that arise would be more easily solved, under the recommended system.

876

877

At the beginning of the chapter we emphasized the medical-social problems that require action on the professional or governmental level, and it is now time to get back to the actions of the individual. It is perfectly true that if each soldier decided on his own to throw down his rifle and go home, there could be no wars—even though pacifists who based their policy decisions on the possibility of this occurring might be disappointed. By the same token, any social action is an aggregate of individual actions. In some cases, the best way to institute change is to address yourself to the group-level problem, but in other cases the actions of the individuals are more open to leverage. Case 59 illustrates a situation which seems of little social import when taken alone, but which has broad social consequences when we remember that similar decisions are being made in thousands of doctors' offices.

## CASE 59

878

You are a busy practitioner on the west side of Lansing, and you have just been complaining to your receptionist about your case load. In addition to long hours at the office, you are making hospital rounds either between 7 and 8 in the morning or 7 and 8 in the evening. You have been unsuccessful in four years of effort to attract a partner to your practice.

Over the years you have watched the neighborhood in which you practice becoming increasingly black and poor in its socioeconomic makeup, and you have had to hire a special billing clerk just to fill out Medicaid and Medicare forms so that you can be reimbursed at a level just above costs. You are somewhat proud that you have not joined the exodus of some of your colleagues to the middle-class neighborhoods. Yet you are envious when you realize that their patients come in regularly, follow directions, and have a positive attitude toward medical care, while your own patients often go to the emergency room so that you have no good records of their histories, and often miss appointments and fail to fill prescriptions. You are not going to complain about the extra income you could have in another neighborhood, but this inability to practice what you consider good medicine is particularly frustrating. At this point you reach a resolution and tell the receptionist that as of now you are accepting no new patients.

878 cont. As if on cue, the phone rings and Mrs. M.N. calls asking for an appointment, saying she was your patient 10 years ago. The receptionist learns that in the interim Mrs. M.N. has utilized emergency rooms and was being seen by Dr. R.Q., but since he has now refused to take Medicaid patients, she can't go to him, and she is not feeling well. When the receptionist says that given the 10-year interval Mrs. M.N. would have to be considered a new patient, and you are not taking any, Mrs. M.N. replies that she has called six doctors and none will take her. She says she has constipation and headache as well as having been deserted again by her alcoholic husband, and her kids are in trouble again, and she feels run down, and if you could just give her something for the constipation and headaches she would feel better.

The receptionist is firm and says again that you are taking no new patients, and she should call the county medical society to be referred to a doctor. At this time Mrs. M.N. volunteers the information that in addition to her constipation, she is having blood in her stools occasionally.

The receptionist puts Mrs. M.N. on hold and tells you what has transpired.

What do you do now?  What do you think the doctor did do?

---

879 To take the second question first, we can say almost with certainty what a real doctor under those circumstances would do. The idea of limiting patient load is one of those ideas which sounds great in the abstract, but putting it into practice requires drawing the line. When you draw the line, the person on the other side of the line is not "some patient," but a real person with specific problems, whom the doctor is bound to have sympathy for. At least, if he did not have sympathy, he would have moved to the rich suburbs long ago. So it is a safe bet that the real doctor did agree to see Mrs. M.N., and that he also agreed to see the next patient that called, until his resolution was forgotten.

880 The other question is what the doctor should ethically have done. By agreeing to take each new patient without regard to his total case load, he is acting somewhat similar to the nurse back in Case 27, who was going to adopt the retarded baby rather than allow the rest of the staff to turn off the respirator. We agreed then that it is simply not practical for her to adopt each baby that comes along in that state. Neither is it practical for this doctor to treat every patient on the west side of Lansing. From a strictly ethical and rational standpoint—from the standpoint of consistency of behavior—either the doctor is committing himself to treating all these patients, or else he must draw the line somewhere. And drawing the line means drawing the line on Mrs. M.N. or someone like her.

REVIEW
CASE 27 : 350

As this argument indicates, it is hard for a physician to act consistently    881
on this matter. So physicians as a rule act inconsistently; or rather they solve
the problem in their own ways according to their own life styles. It is possible
to hear practitioners complaining about "nine-to-five doctors" who limit their
practices severely in order to have plenty of leisure time, and also about the
doctors who are "breaking their backs" under such a large case load that they
cannot give adequate care. If you then ask the doctor to define his terms, you
get a variance. If the doctor sees about 30 patients a day, then a nine-to-five
doctor is one who sees 20, while breaking your back means seeing 40; if he
sees 50 patients a day, the nine-to-five doctor is defined as one who sees 40,
and so on up the line.

Despite the realities of large patient loads and 14-to-16 hour work days,    882
most doctors agree that they could give better quality care if they saw fewer
patients, although most would indignantly deny that what they are giving right
now is actually bad care. Therefore one might argue that it is unethical to
one's patients to allow the case load to increase to these levels, and that one
ought to cut it down. Furthermore, if all doctors did limit their case loads,
there would be more people without doctors, and this would lead to public
pressure to build more medical schools and turn out more doctors, which is
what we need anyway.

This argument may look attractive until it is defined in terms of what
it actually is—doctors going on strike in order to gain a certain political end.
If you were opposed to the Saskatchewan strike described in Case 57, how
might you go about defending this proposal? (Presumably an essential ingredient
of a justification of this partial strike would be that there is no other alternative,
short of denying care, to get society to commit itself to the necessary steps.)

In leaving Case 59, it should be noted that, while the individual question    883
may be the rights of the doctor's patients and whether or not the doctor
will have a coronary before age 55, the societal question is that of equitable
and effective distribution of a scarce resource, namely physician man-hours.
Therefore, any attempt to approach this problem on the social level with
an eye toward defining policy would have to begin from the allocation of
resources viewpoint, as outlined in Chapter 12.

Also in this chapter we ought to take note of two problems which are    884
very much on physicians' minds as this is written: professional standards
review organizations (PSRO's) and malpractice suits and insurance. We might
ask whether these are strictly political issues, or whether significant ethical
implications are involved.

885    PSRO's constitute an attempt by the government to force physicians to form groups for the purpose of overseeing the quality of care given by their peers. The PSRO idea is more or less a social dimension of the physician accountability we have already postulated under the notion of the doctor-patient contract and informed consent. The argument might say that while doctors owe individual patients an explanation of the care that they propose to render, in most cases the patient himself lacks the knowledge to judge the technical aspects. Therefore, the community of doctors owes it to the community of patients to set up peer-review mechanisms, to insure that at least no doctor gives treatment that is grossly out of line with accepted scientific practice. Furthermore, since every doctor wants to insure that he gives the best care possible, and that his inevitable human mistakes will be corrected, he should welcome the PSRO concept.

886    Naturally the idealistic approach just given takes a lot for granted. While a few of the most conservative groups pushing for repeal of PSRO legislation disagree with the basic assumption that the physician is accountable to anyone else, most of the anti-PSRO argument alleges instead the unworkability of any such bureaucracy in practice. Certainly there is the potential of miring physicians down in additional forms and red tape, and of setting such rigid standards of care that individual patient needs are lost sight of. Unfortunately there is little data to prove the truth of such claims; the PSRO experience that is just beginning to accumulate tends to suggest that such a bleak fate is not inevitable.

887    The malpractice problem is another hotly debated issue, and often seems to boil down to a dispute between the physicians and the lawyers. The doctors state with justification that  the number of frivolous malpractice suits has been increasing; even where real malpractice exists, the amount of damages awarded by juries is often unrealistically high; because of this, malpractice insurance rates for doctors have risen astronomically, and in some states new doctors or doctors in high-risk types of practice such as surgery cannot get insurance at all; the rates must be passed along to patients in the form of higher medical bills; and finally, the patient suffers when the doctor feels forced to practice "defensive medicine" by ordering unnecessary tests and X-rays in fear of a possible later suit.

888    With somewhat less justification, the doctors charge that all of the above is mainly caused by the cupidity of lawyers. The lawyers retort that under law, everyone is entitled to his day in court and to repayment of damages suffered through negligence; that true malpractice does indeed exist and that with the absence of strong peer review, malpractice suits are the only way to hound an incompetent doctor out of practice.

We have also had occasion to see that the progress of medical ethics is not divorced from malpractice actions in the courts. In Chapter 5, we saw much to suggest that the present concern of doctors over informed consent arose not from a new ethical enlightenment among the profession, but rather from a rash of lawsuits.

889

The problem obviously is to retain right of redress for the patient who really has suffered damages, while eliminating the abuses in the present system. While for many doctors and lawyers the debate has not progressed beyond the name-calling stage, cooler heads see that any lasting solution (such as some form of binding arbitration, for instance) depends upon cooperation between the two professions.

890

This is just another reminder that medicine is and must be practiced in a social context, and that physicians cannot enjoy the luxury of "doing their thing" without coming up against other social groups and institutions that must be dealt with. It is also of passing interest that progress in PSRO's may play a role in the eventual solution of the malpractice problem.

891

This concludes our overview of some issues in medical economics and organized medicine. In a more comprehensive presentation, this subject would have been divided into a number of sub-categories to be explored in depth. To aid in further reading, some of these sub-categories are listed:

892

Legal implications of the "right to health care"
Present health "crisis" in U.S.—real or imaginary?
History of medical societies and their roles as government lobbies
Alternative forms of financing medical care—e.g., health maintenance organizations, foundations of medical care
Alternative forms of delivering care—solo vs. group practice
Institutions involved in care—hospital, clinic, home care
Organized medicine as professional society and as trade union
Relationship of medical profession to the drug industry
Physicians in positions of limited options, with threat to doctor-patient relationship: prison doctors, military doctors
National health insurance and "socialized medicine"
Medical care systems in other countries—communist and Western European nations
Diseases of poverty, and problems of access into care system
Diseases of affluence—environmental pollution, socio-cultural factors of obesity and overconsumption
Social responsibility of medical-education system
Means of selecting and training medical students, as ways of solving or perpetuating socio-political-economic problems

The last discussion case we will have in this unit, provided for your thought without the distraction of our commentary, has to do with one of the areas listed above—the responsibility of the military doctor. As an added attraction, the case also leads nicely into the key topic of the next chapter—the problem of the concept of disease and what sorts of hidden value judgments play a role in describing disease.

---

## CASE 60

The following news item regarding an event during the Vietnam War appeared in an Air Force military surgeons' newsletter of December, 1966.

"Fear of Flying: A 26-year-old SSgt AC 47 gunner with 7 months active duty in RVN (Republic of Vietnam), presented with frank admission of fear of flying. He had flown over 100 missions, and loss of several aircraft and loss of several crews who were well known to the patient, precipitated his visit. He stated he would give up flight pay, promotion, medals, etc., just to stop flying. Psychiatric consultation to USAF Hospital, Cam Ranh Bay, resulted in 36 days hospitalization with use of psychotherapy and tranquilizers. Diagnosis was Gross Stress Reaction, manifest by anxiety, tenseness, a fear of death expressed in the form of rationalizations, and inability to function. His problem was "worked through" and insight to his problem was gained to the extent that he was returned to full flying duty in less than 6 weeks. This is a fine tribute to the psychiatrists at Cam Ranh Bay."

1.  Were the Air Force psychiatrists serving the best interests of the patient? What was the nature of their "contract"?

2.  What do you think of the diagnosis reached in this case? Do you think that a "disease" was indeed present? If the sergeant displayed diseased behavior, what would have constituted "normal" behavior under the circumstances?

3.  Are anxiety, tenseness, fear of death, and inability to function symptoms of disease whenever they appear, or only in some circumstances? What sorts of value judgments play a role in determining these circumstances?

4.  If you were the psychiatrist at Cam Ranh Bay in charge of this case, what would you have done?

(Case brought to our attention courtesy of Robert G. Newman, M.D., and H. Tristram Engelhardt, Jr., M.D., Ph.D.)

# 17. Defining Health and Disease

In the previous eight chapters, we have gone over some of the specific issues in medical ethics which are of interest today, and have tried to deal with them both by developing general principles and by making reference to specific cases. In the course of doing this, we were often led to a more abstract level of discussion, in order to see what the underlying source of the problem was. In the final two chapters of this book, we shall go back and deal with some of these more abstract questions, which we have postponed considering until now. These chapters will be restricted to discussion without the use of illustrative cases.

895

The present chapter deals with definitions of health and disease. The point we are trying to illustrate here goes back to Chapter 1, when we pointed out that all medical decisions have ethical components, and thus include value judgments as well as purely clinical or scientific decisions. That is, whenever the doctor acts, he must make value judgments. This formed the basis of the need to study medical ethics, but it still left open the possibility that medicine, as a purely research-oriented or speculative endeavor, might engage in the study of health and disease without the need of making value judgments. So now we shall illustrate a more radical thesis—that the very definitions of "health" and "disease" are based on value judgments, and are bound to be no matter which definitions we choose.

896

This thesis may be upsetting to anyone who would like to think that medicine is, or can become, an exact science, since it is usually assumed that in the objective pursuit of scientific truth, value judgments are an obstacle and a prime source of error. It may (or may not) be of consolation to such a reader that an analysis of the basic assumptions of any of the "exact" sciences, such as physics, reveals that they are based on value judgments as well, even though the practicing physicist may find it convenient to forget about this (if he knows it at all). For instance, there is no empirical proof for the proposition that nature is orderly and that we can discover the laws of this order, yet all of science is based on that proposition. And since medicine is a science of human beings, we should not be surprised to find relatively more room for value judgments there than would be the case in a science of atoms or molecules.

897

Let's start out by considering some alternative definitions of "health" and "disease." Recently, in reform-minded circles, it has been suggested that we ought to be concentrating on the concept of health, and that many of the problems with medicine today can be traced to an emphasis on disease, while allowing health to be defined by default as the absence of disease. These people argue that the best role of medicine ought to be that of preserving health rather than that of treating disease. However, in order to get a better idea of where we are now, as opposed to where we ought to be, we'll start by concentrating on the idea of disease.

898

**899** It is extremely useful to compare the concept of disease in different cultures—cultures separated by time, and cultures separated by geography. It is a loss that present-day medical schools, in their attempts to streamline the curriculum, have been forced to a large extent to neglect these cross-cultural comparisons. When one learns only one concept of disease, there is a strong unconscious tendency to assume that it is the only correct one. When one learns many different concepts, and sees the defects in them, one tends to turn a more critical eye on present-day concepts as well. This is important because, as we shall see, a number of practical weaknesses in medicine arise almost directly from the definition of disease that one employs.

**900** Remember as we go along that all concepts of disease (as well as, indeed, all scientific explanation) are simply ways of trying to make sense of the complex and often confusing array of sense-data that the world throws at us. It is sometimes useful to think of such concepts as metaphors or mythologies—their utility lies in how well they hang together and how much of the world they allow us to make sense of, although even the best will leave some loose ends.

**901** The many different concepts of disease can be nicely divided into two categories. The first concentrates on disease as a distinct entity. In this approach, there is a set of individuals, $(A_1, A_2, A_3, ...A_n)$ and a set of diseases having some kind of independent existence, $(B_1, B_2, B_3,....B_n)$. A healthy individual A becomes sick when one of those disease entities is visited upon him, and he becomes A+B. The problem of diagnosis is then deciding whether this B is $B_1$ or $B_2$ or whatever.

This approach to defining disease has a number of names attached to it, most common of which is the ontological approach. Not to be stuffy about it, we shall refer to the "A+B view" instead.

**902** The second major approach deals with disease as deviation from the normal. In this view, a well person, A, undergoes a series of physiological changes, with the end result being a deviation from the normal state. We then can call the individual A' to signify that he is sick, but still emphasizing that he is the same individual and that no new entity has been added.

A quick way of spotting this approach is to observe that under it diseases often (but not always) come in pairs. Thus, if we are interested in a physiological function or substance x, we can have either hyper-x disease or hypo-x disease, depending on whether there is an excess or a deficit of x.

This view is commonly labeled the physiological approach, and we shall abbreviate this as the "A' view."

Note that any hard and fast distinction between these two views is bound to break down. When we say that normal persons may become diseased through hyperfunction of the thyroid, we are working strictly within the A' view. When we start to see that certain symptoms are characteristic of this condition and start to diagnose "hyperthyroidism" by the presence of the symptom complex, we are adding in some of the A+B view. And if someone catches us saying "the disease hyperthyroidism is present in this patient," he will accuse us of selling out to the A+B model completely.

903

↓

It is not hard to see that modern medical practice depends on a combination of these two views. The A+B view is very strong in textbooks of medicine, where diseases are described with typical manifestations for each. The A' view comes on strongest in the use of screening tests such as for blood pressure or hemoglobin, where we take a deviation outside normal limits as the indication for a more extensive diagnostic workup.

904

↓

A major point about concepts of disease is that they are very closely tied up with ideas of proper therapy. The ancient Greeks may have been content to speculate about the nature of the universe, with no thought to exercising any control over it; but when it came to speculations about disease, they wanted practical results when they were sick. A quick historical tour illustrates how the changing concepts of disease each pointed to a certain therapy. It also shows how the changes in concepts of disease reflected a "borrowing" by medicine of the philosophic or scientific ideas which were in vogue at the time.

905

↓

One of the earliest (and still prevalent) concepts of disease grew up in magic-oriented cultures, and formed the concept of possession by a spirit or a demon. Clearly the treatment for disease was then removal of the demon. If this was strictly a bad spirit, it might be exorcised by the appropriate incantation or potion. If the spirit was suspected to have been sent by a god, who might become angry if a lack of hospitality were shown, the spirit was allowed to remain, but sacrifices or prayers were offered to the god in hopes of changing his malevolent purpose to a friendlier one.

906

↓

↓

Ancient Greek rational thought developed the theory of the four humors of the body—blood, phlegm, yellow bile, and black bile—which was essentially a biological application of the then-current notion of the four elements—earth, air, fire, water. Disease could arise from an excess or deficit of one of the humors, or from a humor arising outside of its proper location in the body. Health, then, was a sort of harmony in which all the humors were in equilibrium. Treatment could be directed at the restoration of this balance.

907

The idea of health as a harmony of elements was taken up from the Greeks by Arabic medicine, and similar views prevailed in the traditional medicines of India and China. In all three of those cultures, the traditional medicine is practiced today alongside Western medicine; in fact, some of current Chinese medical research is directed toward developing an integration between imported Western medicine and traditional therapies, such as acupuncture and herbal remedies.

↓

908     A later development of Greek medicine (about the 2nd century B.C.) was termed Methodism, and was based on the atomistic philosophy of the structure of matter. Diseases were classed as being due either to abnormal opening of the pores or to abnormal constriction of them; and the corresponding therapy consisted of either cold or hot baths and similar measures. This may represent an extreme of simplicity in disease-and-therapy concepts, at the expense, of course, of precision and effectiveness.

909     In Europe in the 1600's, one of the most talked-about new developments was Linnaeus' scientific classification of plants by families, genera, species, etc. The great English physician Sydenham developed a similar classification of diseases—thereby establishing the ascendency of the A+B view after centuries of the A' view in the form of the four humors. Since all these diseases were separate entities, it was useless to seek any general theory of therapy; rather one had to discover a specific therapy for each disease entity. Partly as a result of this approach, there was a tendency within some schools of European medicine into the 1800's for the science of therapy to take second place to the science of diagnosis.

910     The A+B view became even more firmly established with the advent of the germ theory of disease in the mid-1800's. In an ironic way, this represented a sort of return to the possession-by-spirit concept; treatment consisted of exorcising the spirit (through antibiotics) or placating it to soothe its evil effects (through symptomatic therapy) or else preventing its entry by charms or amulets (vaccination). Another similarity between the germ theory and the demon theory was the tendency to concentrate on B and ignore A. In the modern form of the germ theory, we realize that not all people who are exposed to a germ will get the disease, and that the host responses are as important as the microbe in determining the manifestations of the disease. However, the simplistic form of the A+B view still (unconsciously) pervades much of medical thinking today.

911     As we noted that crosscultural comparisons are useful in highlighting disease concepts, it is worth looking at concepts of disease present in various folk subcultures within the U.S., such as the lower-class black, Spanish-American, and southern white communities. Some folk beliefs, especially in Spanish speaking areas, are holdovers from the humoral theories of medieval medicine and reflect an A' approach. Such diseases will be ascribed to natural causes, and natural remedies such as foods and herbs will be prescribed. Often side by side with these diseases is another set of diseases ascribed to magic or witchcraft, in the oldest A+B tradition; here a "healer" with special powers might be called in.

Snow points out that while any isolated folk belief (such as putting a knife under the bed of a woman in labor to "cut" her pains) seems silly, the entire system of folk beliefs and folk remedies functions as an integrated whole for that subculture. In short, it provides for them an alternate metaphor or mythology where the scientific world view is either not understood or is unattractive for cultural reasons.

912

We mentioned that modern medicine represents a mixture of the A+B and the A' views. The reason for this is simple—either view, taken alone, is unable to explain all the facts that we now know. Each view is prone to particular types of errors. The A+B view suggests that one diagnoses an unknown by comparing it with a catalog of knowns—as one author said, "the method of recognizing an elephant by having seen one before." It also encourages a penny-in-the-slot approach to diagnosis, with lab tests providing handy short cuts, thereby tending to reduce the amount of thinking required. It works well when the case before one closely resembles the textbook description, but leads to mistaken diagnosis when the case has several unique features. In sum, it has all the defects associated with the practice of sticking labels on reality instead of trying to understand it.

913

Engelhardt and Fabrega have also suggested that there is at least some tendency for the A+B view to lead to episodic, crisis-oriented health care. If the emphasis is on the B, which is present only temporarily and then departs, and not on the conditions within the A that allow the B to gain a foothold, there is little motivation for a continuity of health care or for much effort devoted to prevention.

914

The A' view has its own set of difficulties. Since everyone deviates from normal to some extent, this view does not tell us how much deviation constitutes disease. While it is nice to say "two standard deviations above and below the mean," many measures do not fit a mathematical, normal distribution; and even when they do, 5% of all "normal" cases will be diagnosed as disease if those statistical limits are rigidly applied. This may lead to the diagnosis of "nondisease" through overuse of lab tests, again reducing thought to a minimum. In the extreme cases, we might be led to conclude that people with obvious symptoms are not "really" sick, or else that everyone is sick, depending on where we draw the line.

915

916     In addition to historical comparisons, it is enlightening to compare concepts of disease in different cultures today, with most marked differences being found between technological and pre-literate societies. In order to make these comparisons, it helps to bring in a third concept of disease—disease as different behavior. Since each society recognizes some kind of sickness, each society has a "sick role" which is a set of behaviors people adopt when sick and cease when restored to health. To an anthropologist, who is sick in a given society can be determined by how that person acts and also by how others act towards him. The "sick role" has implications beyond the question of medical care and treatment; for instance, it has an economic side in that the sick person is excused from work responsibilities.

917     The question we want to ask is whether certain objective biological events are considered criteria for the sickness label in all cultures, or in some but not in others. On a very superficial level, we would assume correctly that diseases which we detect by special tests or lab methods, such as mild anemia, borderline diabetes, etc., would not be viewed as sickness in cultures which did not have the means to do the tests. But in addition there are more basic variations. Some have to do with the flaw of the A' view of where to draw the line. For example, in some tribes that inhabit very humid jungle climates, essentially everyone has a condition that we would classify as a skin disease in our culture. In that tribe, however, a person with that condition is considered normal.

918     Another basic variance has to do with the traits that a certain culture has selected as essential—that is, the value judgments of that culture. A good example is moderate mental retardation. This is a severe handicap in our culture and is considered a disease, worthy of being prevented by prenatal diagnosis and abortion where possible. In a hunting or a simple agricultural society, such an individual might well be considered normal.

919     Based on this sort of analysis, Fabrega compiled a table of diseases showing "cultural masking" and "cultural invariance." In the latter category he included items such as stroke, acute asthma, seizure, severe vision loss, hip fracture, and acute shortness of breath as conditions which would be considered "sick" in almost any culture. The other category included such things as nutritional deficiencies, chronic bronchitis, early stages of cancer, mild anemia, and senility as examples of conditions which are subject to wide variation in the way they are treated by different cultures.

920     However, we do not have to go to other cultures to see how the same condition may have different labels attached to it; we can look at the changing concepts in our own culture of conditions such as alcoholism. It has always been agreed that alcoholism is deviant behavior, but just what type of deviant behavior has never been settled. Until recently it was universally thought that alcoholism was a problem of moral weakness and depravity. For a decade or so, the U.S. toyed with the idea that alcohol consumption was a criminal deviancy, but this created more problems than it solved. More recently we have had alcoholism redefined as an illness, and medical-type therapies have been applied. We could say that alcoholism really is an illness and that this change in definition represents our growing understanding of the root causes. We could say just as plausibly that we still do not understand the problem any better, and the changing definitions simply represent the failure of each social institution, in turn, to make a dent in the problem.

So far in this historical and anthropological discourse we have not made    921
any major reference to values, but the line of thought is probably clear by
now. When we note the arbitrary and "non-scientific" features of definitions
of disease in other cultures, we are bound to wonder whether the problem
is that the others are stupid and we are smart, or whether *in fact some degree
of arbitrariness is bound to occur in any definition of disease. If the latter,
then it seems clear that our values will play a major role in defining disease.
However, since in most cases almost all people in our society will share the
same value judgment—say, that it is bad to have a heart attack—we will probably
not be aware that we are making these value judgments.*

A corollary to the argument that the concept of disease contains a value    922
judgment is that, if disease actually were a biologically objective fact, we
should see disease in the animal and plant worlds. Several authors argue that
we do not—until we subject those worlds to interpretation in social terms.
For instance, Sedgwick writes, "Plant-diseases may strike at tulips, turnips, or
such prized features of the natural landscape as elm trees; but if some plant
species in which man had no interest (a desert grass, let us say) were to be
attacked by a fungus or parasite, we should speak not of a disease, but merely
of the competition between two species."*

Where do the values come in to the different concepts of disease? In the    923
A' view, we have already noted that the major value judgment is where to
draw the line. Another value judgment concerns what factors or qualities to
measure. For instance, we could conceivably measure rate of hair growth,
plot a normal curve for a population, and say that if your hair grows at a
rate two standard deviations above or below the mean, you are diseased. In
fact we don't do that, because no one has yet related rate of hair growth to
a state which we consider undesirable; concern about rate of hair growth is
a low-priority value in our society.

Still another value judgment in the A' view occurs when we look at    924
deviation in only one direction from the norm. We can plot a normal distribution curve for hemoglobin concentration in the blood, and we have defined
two diseases: one for low hemoglobin (anemia) and one for high hemoglobin
(polycythemia). Similarly, we can plot I.Q. on a normal curve, and we define
the disease of mental retardation when an I.Q. falls below a certain limit—
since normal I.Q. is about 100, the highest limit of mental retardation might
be given as 70. By consistent reasoning, we should also say that anyone who
has an I.Q. above 130 is diseased; they deviate as much but in the opposite
direction. In fact, we are not consistent, and we do not consider high I.Q. to
be a disease.

*Reprinted from the Hastings Center Studies, Vol. 1, No. 3, 1973, with the permission
of the Institute of Society, Ethics and the Life Sciences, Hastings-on-Hudson, N.Y. 10706.

**925**  The role of value judgments in the A+B view is analogous to the role of value judgments in any descriptive science (which is not surprising because, as we saw, the A+B view is largely patterned after botany). There are, in the world out there, an infinite number of things that can be observed, or if you will, an infinite number of data that can be plotted. In practice, we select some of those data as being of significance and some as being immaterial. This is a value judgment, based on which data we judge, subjectively, as being most likely to lead us to the "laws of the universe" which we assume (without any conclusive evidence) to exist.

**926**  In the A+B view, we consider certain observables, and when a particular set of them occur together we deduce the presence of the B, the disease or syndrome. For instance, when we see an A with the collection of observables including joint pain, elevated blood uric acid, etc., we declare that he has the disease gout. Now, any enterprising medical scientist could find a person with another set of observables, for example, thick eyebrows, low blood strontium, birthmark on the left arm, etc., and declare that this individual has the disease glarf. There is no objective way in which gout differs from glarf in its right to be called a disease entity. The real difference is a subjective one—I don't care if I have glarf; but if I have gout, I don't like it one bit, and I will put myself to a considerable amount of trouble to get rid of it, and if someone tells me I am in the process of developing gout, I will likewise go to some trouble to head it off if possible.

**927**  We also mentioned a third concept of disease, a behavioral concept. If anything, the value judgments here are even more obvious than with the other two views, because there is more disagreement about what constitutes good and bad physical sensations and life span. (Many people in this country would consider going to see an X-rated movie evidence of sick behavior, while probably few readers of this book would agree.) This is the same problem which we referred to in Chapter 9 in discussing the problems of defining mental illness and mental health.

REVIEW
"MENTAL ILLNESS" ↑ 451—454

**928**  A striking example of value judgments in the behavioral concept of disease is found in the census figures for the city of Baltimore. Between 1933 and 1936 the number of individuals with "psychopathic personality" dropped sharply. There was no increase in the cure rate, or mass influx of psychiatrists into the city, during this period. What happened was simply that the census takers, in 1933, had included unemployment as a sign of psychopathic personality; by 1936 they had revised their definition.

270

*In saying that value judgments play an important role in defining disease, we do not mean to suggest that empirical data and scientific evidence play no role, any more than the ethical method of Chapter 2 excluded factual knowledge as an ingredient in ethical decisions. The facts and the value judgments interact.*

For instance, if I have high blood pressure, I will probably have no symptoms that I can be aware of, so I will have no reason to ascribe any negative value judgment to my present status. But if someone tells me that my life expectancy is twenty years less than it would be if the condition were treated, this new data might lead me to revise my valuation.

However, we will insist that, even though facts may play a large role, value judgments are essential to defining disease. Even if the value judgment is a trivial one, like it is bad to die at age 20, it still must be there or else the definition of disease is incomplete.

However, we might note in passing that while value judgment is essential for the presence of disease, the existence of a negative value judgment based on biologically observable factors is not always a guarantee that the label of disease will be applied. A good example is the trait of having black skin, which is a biological objective fact and which carries a negative value connotation in many societies. While black individuals are discriminated against in those societies, however, they are not regarded as being sick. This relates to the sociological concept of "deviancy," as illness is only one of several possible forms that deviancy may take. We observed this classification problem earlier with alcoholism.

At the beginning of this chapter we mentioned that it might be more desirable to define health instead of disease. We can choose two ways to do this. If we choose to say that health is simply the absence of disease, then we have to define disease, and all the same value judgments we have been discussing enter in. If we take the more positive route and wish to define health as some state with its own characteristics, then we are implying that some individuals might be neither diseased nor healthy. With this extra distinction to make, we have allowed room for even more value judgments.

One approach to defining health is the ecological-evolutionary one that considers health as fitness to the environment. Disease is then defined in terms of absence of health rather than the other way around. Fabrega, paraphrasing Dubos, accordingly describes disease in this view as "temporary setbacks in the perpetual struggle between man and the forces of nature," although a strict ecologist would probably prefer "interaction" to "struggle." This would allow an objective measure of the absence or presence of health—if we had a mathematical measure of "fitness" which was applicable to biological systems. As noted in Chapter 15, we have no such measure; therefore we must fall back on value judgments in defining "fitness" also.

REVIEW
"GENETIC HEALTH" | 811–818

933    Another often-cited definition of health is that of the World Health Organization, "Health is a state of complete physical, mental, and social well-being and not merely the absence of disease or infirmity." This definition has the advantage of being positive (visionary, in fact) and of relating health to the totality of the human condition, instead of treating man as a collection of organs. It does, however, present serious problems, not the least of which is the fact that the definition of "health" is, for all practical purposes, identical to the definition of "happiness." If we assume that the role of the medical profession is to preserve health, it follows that anyone who is unhappy for whatever reason ought to be able to go to a doctor with reasonable expectation of being helped. This would require either a major reorganization of medical practice and medical training, or else a rejection of that concept of health.

934    If the concepts of disease that we have gone over all fall short of being "objective," one's first response might be to ask how they could be modified or replaced to achieve greater objectivity. However, is this really at the top of our priorities? Recall in the historical discussion the way in which concepts of disease have been closely tied to therapy. Necessity being the mother of invention, treatment in the past has often been discovered in spite of the prevailing disease concept, but from a scientific standpoint we would consider this inefficient. We would prefer to have a concept of disease that is fruitful in suggesting new treatments and new openings for medical research. If treatment is our goal, then our definition of a good concept of disease is a pragmatic one. If the new disease concept also turns out to be more "objective" in some ways, that is very nice, but of secondary importance.

935    Since it may be too much to expect that cures for all sorts of diseases will immediately fall out of the sky, a more modest hope is that a new concept of disease might allow us at least to avoid some of the errors produced by other concepts, which we have already listed. We mentioned that modern medical thought consists largely of a mix of the A+B and the A' views of disease (with the behavioral concept thrown in on the psychiatric side). However, this is not a well-integrated mix, but often an uneasy coexistence. Instead of the strengths of one view counteracting the weaknesses of the other, it too often happens that the errors are simply reinforced and compounded.

936    An integration of these different concepts would lead us to some sort of unified concept of disease. A unified concept would allow us to point out certain properties that are present in all diseases, which would serve as a base for us to go on to consider the differences between diseases. The problem is that in order to achieve the degree of generality needed to do this, a unified concept loses on the side of practical application. This has led some medical authorities to deny the existence of any useful unified concept of disease. However, if a concept could highlight some new approaches to medical research and the understanding of disease processes, new practical applications might result ten or twenty years down the road; so the long-term payoffs might be there even if the concept looked impractical at first glance.

It so happens that we have a unified concept of health and disease to offer, which at this point does not have many obvious direct applications, but which may serve to clarify thinking and which may serve as a model for the strengths and weaknesses of the unified approach. In addition, it will serve as a basis for our discussion of the nature of man when we come to Chapter 18.

937

Our concept of health and disease is related to the ecological-evolutionary view mentioned earlier, with some important additions. It is based on a medical application of some concepts of systems theory and information theory, which so far have been disciplines mainly associated with computer technology. To start, we have to be clear on some terms, including "system," "information," and "hierarchy." The essence of this concept is the nature of man as a biological system. A "system" is an organized set of subcomponents; it is made up of a number of subsystems, and each subsystem could be considered a system with its own subsystems, and so on down the line. These systems, as we rank them in order of complexity, form a hierarchy. In biology, we are familiar with the idea of a hierarchical system with the individual at the highest level. At the next lowest level are the organ systems, and each of them in turn has the organs as their subsystems. Each organ has a variety of tissues as its subcomponents. We can carry this down through cells to molecules or atoms.

938

We can imagine a collection of organs, tissues, cells, etc., all lying in a heap on the floor of an anatomy laboratory. What distinguishes a biological system from this heap of the different subcomponents? We already mentioned the orderly nature of a system, but of what does this order consist? The order is maintained by information flow within the system, and between the system and its environment ("information" here is being defined in a very broad sense, as something which has the potential to change the activities of a component of the system). Very commonly the information flow pattern takes the form of "feedback loops," in which component A influences component B, and the new state of B in turn acts upon A, so that it is possible to maintain a balance. In this way a system can maintain its orderly structure; if one subsystem starts to get out of line, the other subsystems act on it to set things right. If your cardiovascular system starts to pump blood too fast, it activates neural and hormonal feedback mechanisms which work to restore the normal state. Thus, each subsystem has the freedom to do what it chooses within certain limits, but once it crosses those limits, feedback loops are activated to return it to its proper place.

939

What we have just described is no more than the physiological concept of homeostasis. However, we want to go beyond the levels of the hierarchy that are usually considered in purely physiological terms. Why stop with the individual organism? First we might want to include some allowances for behavior. We can say that simple motor behavior is at a lower hierarchical level than behavior which requires the use of language; and that sophisticated problem-solving behavior is at a still higher level, and so on. So we might want to subdivide the individual or "person" into these different levels of behavior and experience. Further, we note that "persons" are not content to remain isolated, but form themselves as the subcomponents of still higher-level systems such as families, communities, nations, etc. If we are going to have a really comprehensive view of man, it would seem that our systems view would have to include all these hierarchical levels.

940

941    Clearly, the exact nature of the information flow is going to be different at different levels of the hierarchy. Atoms in a molecule keep each other in line by means of electrostatic attractions and repulsions; family members keep each other in line mainly by language behavior; and cultures keep their individual members in line mainly by transmitting values. However, if we are willing to regard all of these examples as information flow (and information theory provides a basis to do this), then the basic characteristics, such as the nature of the feedback loop, should be applicable to each level of the hierarchy.

942    Figure 4 summarizes what we have just described; it shows the levels of the hierarchy and describes some of the types of information flow that occurs between two adjacent hierarchical levels. There are also information-flow circuits between levels more widely spaced, as when the nation feeds back directly to the "person," say, to order him to produce his income tax. Also do not forget that each level of the hierarchy has information circuits to connect it with the environment. Since it takes energy to move all this information around it is characteristic of biological systems that they must take in energy from the environment to maintain themselves.

943    Now, take a look at the picture just drawn of this biological system we call man. It is maintaining itself as an orderly array of subcomponents. It is taking energy in from the environment, and it is interacting with the environment in other ways to maintain the "fitness" we mentioned earlier. Each of its subcomponents at all the different levels is "doing its own thing" within the limits allowed, while the various feedback circuits are standing ready to be activated once those limits are crossed and the subcomponent embarks on a course that could threaten the stability of the whole system. It would be reasonable to identify this state of overall equilibrium as what we mean by a "healthy" system.

944    However, this idyllic state of affairs does not always prevail. Every once in a while a subcomponent oversteps its bounds (often as a response to some disruption originating in the environment, which the usual feedback loops were unable to prevent). Or in some cases, the limits imposed by the feedback circuits might become too rigid, so as not to allow the subcomponent any "breathing room," and thus hampering its function. In either way, the particular level of the hierarchy has its equilibrium disrupted, and we could say that a "disease" has occurred.

945

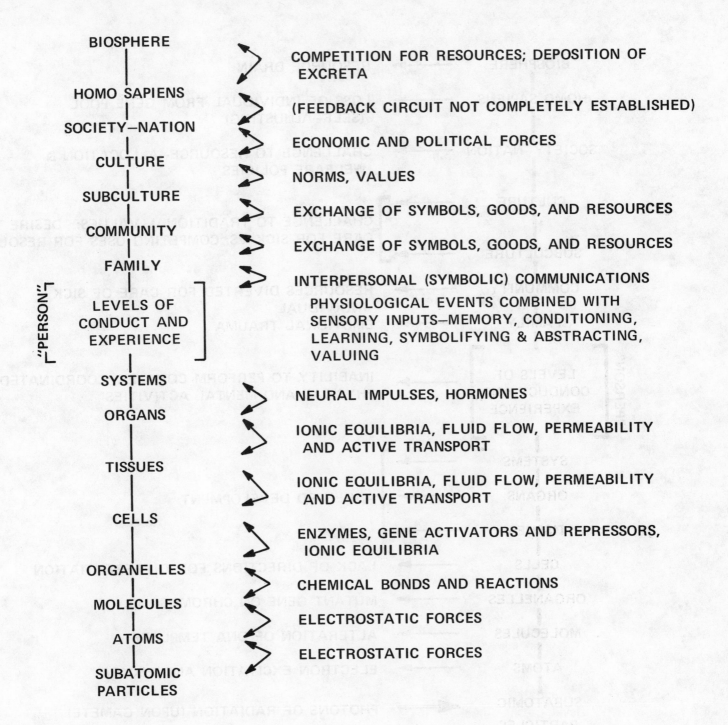

BIOSPHERE
⟶ COMPETITION FOR RESOURCES; DEPOSITION OF EXCRETA

HOMO SAPIENS
SOCIETY–NATION
⟶ (FEEDBACK CIRCUIT NOT COMPLETELY ESTABLISHED)
⟶ ECONOMIC AND POLITICAL FORCES

CULTURE
⟶ NORMS, VALUES

SUBCULTURE
⟶ EXCHANGE OF SYMBOLS, GOODS, AND RESOURCES

COMMUNITY
⟶ EXCHANGE OF SYMBOLS, GOODS, AND RESOURCES

FAMILY
⟶ INTERPERSONAL (SYMBOLIC) COMMUNICATIONS

"PERSON" — LEVELS OF CONDUCT AND EXPERIENCE
PHYSIOLOGICAL EVENTS COMBINED WITH SENSORY INPUTS—MEMORY, CONDITIONING, LEARNING, SYMBOLIZING & ABSTRACTING, VALUING

SYSTEMS
⟶ NEURAL IMPULSES, HORMONES

ORGANS
⟶ IONIC EQUILIBRIA, FLUID FLOW, PERMEABILITY AND ACTIVE TRANSPORT

TISSUES
⟶ IONIC EQUILIBRIA, FLUID FLOW, PERMEABILITY AND ACTIVE TRANSPORT

CELLS
⟶ ENZYMES, GENE ACTIVATORS AND REPRESSORS, IONIC EQUILIBRIA

ORGANELLES
⟶ CHEMICAL BONDS AND REACTIONS

MOLECULES
⟶ ELECTROSTATIC FORCES

ATOMS
⟶ ELECTROSTATIC FORCES

SUBATOMIC PARTICLES

Figure 4. Systems approach to the nature of "man," showing levels of the hierarchy on the left and the nature of the information flow between different levels on the right.

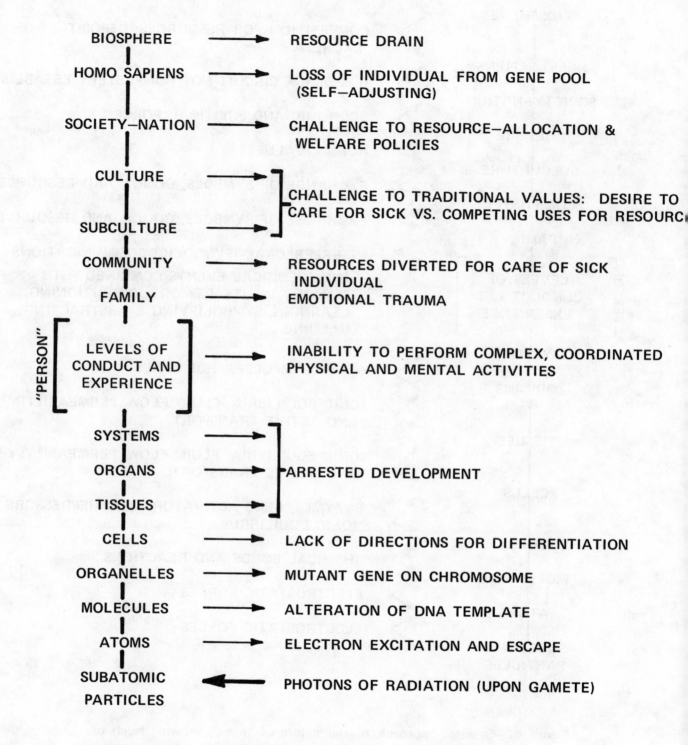

BIOSPHERE → RESOURCE DRAIN

HOMO SAPIENS → LOSS OF INDIVIDUAL FROM GENE POOL (SELF—ADJUSTING)

SOCIETY—NATION → CHALLENGE TO RESOURCE—ALLOCATION & WELFARE POLICIES

CULTURE →

SUBCULTURE → CHALLENGE TO TRADITIONAL VALUES: DESIRE TO CARE FOR SICK VS. COMPETING USES FOR RESOURC

COMMUNITY → RESOURCES DIVERTED FOR CARE OF SICK INDIVIDUAL

FAMILY → EMOTIONAL TRAUMA

"PERSON" [LEVELS OF CONDUCT AND EXPERIENCE] → INABILITY TO PERFORM COMPLEX, COORDINATED PHYSICAL AND MENTAL ACTIVITIES

SYSTEMS →

ORGANS → ARRESTED DEVELOPMENT

TISSUES →

CELLS → LACK OF DIRECTIONS FOR DIFFERENTIATION

ORGANELLES → MUTANT GENE ON CHROMOSOME

MOLECULES → ALTERATION OF DNA TEMPLATE

ATOMS → ELECTRON EXCITATION AND ESCAPE

SUBATOMIC PARTICLES ← PHOTONS OF RADIATION (UPON GAMETE)

Figure 5. Disease example. Severe physical and mental retardation caused by a radiation—induced mutation in the gamete: example of spread of disruption upwards through the hierarchy.

Key:

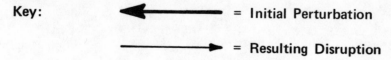

← = Initial Perturbation

→ = Resulting Disruption

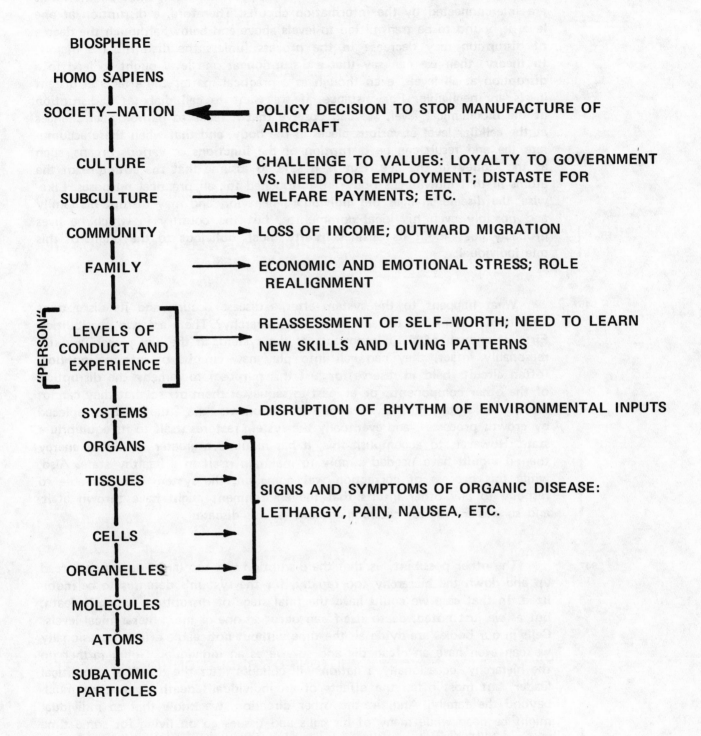

BIOSPHERE

HOMO SAPIENS

SOCIETY—NATION ← **POLICY DECISION TO STOP MANUFACTURE OF AIRCRAFT**

CULTURE → **CHALLENGE TO VALUES: LOYALTY TO GOVERNMENT VS. NEED FOR EMPLOYMENT; DISTASTE FOR**

SUBCULTURE → **WELFARE PAYMENTS; ETC.**

COMMUNITY → **LOSS OF INCOME; OUTWARD MIGRATION**

FAMILY → **ECONOMIC AND EMOTIONAL STRESS; ROLE REALIGNMENT**

"PERSON" { LEVELS OF CONDUCT AND EXPERIENCE } → **REASSESSMENT OF SELF—WORTH; NEED TO LEARN NEW SKILLS AND LIVING PATTERNS**

SYSTEMS → **DISRUPTION OF RHYTHM OF ENVIRONMENTAL INPUTS**

ORGANS →

TISSUES → **SIGNS AND SYMPTOMS OF ORGANIC DISEASE: LETHARGY, PAIN, NAUSEA, ETC.**

CELLS →

ORGANELLES →

MOLECULES

ATOMS

SUBATOMIC PARTICLES

Figure 6.   Disease example. Stress-related psychosomatic illness in an unemployed aerospace engineer: example of spread of disruption downward through the hierarchy.

Key:   ← = **Initial Perturbation**

→ = **Resulting Disruption**

945    But as a rule, the disease does not stop at one level, since all the levels are interconnected by the information circuits. Therefore, a disruption at one level is bound to be transmitted to levels above and below, although the degree of disruption may decrease in the process (unless the disruption is major). In theory, then we can say that a disruption at one level ought to lead to a disruption at all levels, even though as a practical matter the effects at distant levels are negligible. For instance, if we want to call diabetes a disruption at the biochemical level, we can observe that it leads to pathological changes at the cellular level at various places in the body, and that when these accumulate the end result can be disruption of the functions of various organs, such as the kidney or the eye. But it is safe to assume that the structure of the atoms in that individual's body are untouched for all practical purposes. Likewise, the disease changes the individual's behavior, and may disrupt his family and possibly even his local community, but the country in which he lives probably goes about its business pretty much oblivious to the plight of this one individual.

946    What happens to the system after a disease occurs, and its disruptions have been transmitted up and down the hierarchy? There are two possibilities. First, if enough of the components of the system, in the key places, are still reasonably intact, they can call into play new circuits of information flow (often circuits held in reserve for just this purpose) to remedy the disruption of the other components, or at least to sequester them off so that they cannot disrupt the system further. If some subcomponents "die," they can be replaced by growth processes; and eventually the system restores itself to its equilibrium state. However, to accomplish this, it has required a greater supply of energy than it would have needed simply to maintain itself in a healthy state. Also, while this process of correction was going on, the system was less able to respond to any other insults that the environment might have thrown at it, and so was at risk for catching a more serious disease.

947    The other possibility is that the disruption was too large, or that it spread up and down the hierarchy too rapidly, for the system's defenses to be mobilized. In that case we could have the final stage of disruption, which is death; but as we just noted, death itself can occur at one or more hierarchical levels. Cells in our bodies are dying all the time without noticeable effect; occasionally we can even have an organ die and survive as an individual. Going farther up the hierarchy, occasionally a nation will collapse after the death of a political leader, but most often the effects of an individual's death do not go much beyond the family. And, in the other direction, we know that an individual might be dead while many of his cells and tissues go on living for some time afterward. (Does a hierarchical view of death help us clarify the problem of defining death that was raised in Chapter 6?)

REVIEW
DEATH          285

948    Because most of the information circuits in the system are in the form of feedback loops—bi-directional instead of unidirectional—we can conclude that the disruptions associated with disease can move down the hierarchical levels as well as up. The differences between different disease "entities" (as described by the A+B view) may be related to such factors as where the initial disruption arises, which hierarchical levels are most affected, and so on. It should also be noted that often what we take to be signs of disease may be the efforts of the system to restore order—fever is a common example.

For further illustration, Figures 5 and 6 explain two disease processes in systems terms. In Figure 5, a case of genetic disease resulting in physical and mental retardation is shown; the initial disruption is presumed to be radiation from the environment that produces a mutation in the reproductive cells of one parent, and the resulting spread of disruption is up the hierarchical levels. In Figure 6, a case is shown of so-called psychosomatic disease resulting from emotional stress on an individual—here, an airplane engineer thrown out of work by budget cuts. The initial disruption is at the national level, and the spread of disruption is downward.

Since the idea of therapy is closely tied up with the idea of disease, how does therapy fit into this model? We would have to say that a therapy is a disruption from the environment which is intended to counteract the disease-disruption and aid the system in returning to equilibrium. If diseases and therapies are both disruptions from the environment, what is the difference between them? None—other than the value judgment placed on the final results, or the predicted final results, of the disruption. (We have noted repeatedly that the cure is often worse than the disease. We also gave, in Case 37, an example of deliberately injecting live virus. While we would generally expect this to result in "disease," the virus was actually being introduced in hopes of "therapy.")

Now, the disadvantages of this systems concept of health and disease are obvious. Not only are the practical applications hard to imagine; but in addition we seem to have been deliberately obscure by redefining a number of familiar concepts in unfamiliar terms. On the other side of the ledger, what are some of the advantages of this system?

First, it does represent an increase in unification. It takes into account the A' view of disease, since the physiological processes of homeostasis and deviation from normal limits are already being explained in terms of feedback loops. By showing the possibilities of differences between diseases in terms of what kind of disruption may cause them, on what levels their primary manifestations are located, etc., the systems view indicates that there is utility in adopting at least some of the classifications of the A+B view, even if we want to deny the theoretical validity of the "separate entity" concept. Furthermore, since the various levels are all interconnected, we expect that diseases involving organ and tissue disruptions also to have associated disruptions on the behavioral levels; so the behavioral concept of disease is explained as a view that focuses on the particular aspect of the total picture.

This leads us into the second advantage, that of eliminating the sharp distinction between organic and mental diseases which has been plaguing medical thought recently, and which has been adhered to despite accumulating evidence that it is dysfunctional. If disruptions can move equally well up and down the hierarchical levels, as was illustrated in Figures 5 and 6, there is no reason why psychosocial disruptions cannot cause tissue or biochemical manifestations, and vice versa. Under the old concepts, medicine has tended to act surprised when it was discovered that such interconnections existed—for instance, when it was discovered that persons with certain personality traits were more likely to develop certain types of organic disease such as ulcer, or that a procedure such as kidney dialysis could lead to severe psychiatric problems. Applying the systems model, we should be surprised if these interconnections DID NOT exist.

949

950

951

952

953

954    In abolishing this sharp distinction between types of disease, we also abolish the sharp distinction between the biological and the behavioral and social sciences. We drew an analogy between things like social values and things like hormones—they are both parts of the system's information circuitry, but they occur at different levels. We know that it is easier to measure and quantify hormones than values, but it seems erroneous to extend that and say that a science which tries to observe information flow at one level of the hierarchy is "less scientific" in any way than a science which addresses itself to another level.

955    A third advantage is particularly useful in ethical discussions, which, as we saw, often come to grief by looking only at the anticipated results and not at possible undesirable side effects. If we start from the idea that all levels are interconnected, we are not only reminded that side effects are bound to occur; we also have a handy check list as to where to look for them. All we have to do is follow each of the feedback loops—we have to look at other levels; a other subsystems in the same level, and at the environment. Of course, there are actually an infinite number (almost) of these feedback circuits, so that explains why we can never exhaustively explore all the possible consequences before making a decision.

956    Here a caveat is appropriate: remember how the A+B view comes to grief when the "disease entities" are viewed as real things and not as concepts. Similarly, the levels of the hierarchy should be seen as ways of guiding us in our search for interrelations among real-world phenomena, not as real-world phenomena in themselves, although they agree well with some of our intuitive views. Thus Engelhardt agrees in saying that disease-concepts must be seen as complex relations among many different factors, but he avoids any specific hierarchical or other model of these factors.

957    This search for side effects is especially important when applied to therapy. Again, the medical field tends to act surprised, even when it should know better, when a drug turns out to have a side effect. This surprise can be traced to the A+B or the A' views which tend to label a drug as doing one thing— either removing the B in the A+B view, or pushing the variant physiological factor back within normal limits in the A' view. On the other hand, since "man" in the systems view of disease is an ecosystem, we are reminded to apply the sayings that have become popular with ecologists—"You can't do just one thing" (or, "There is no such thing as a free lunch").

958    As a matter of fact, from the systems perspective, it is little short of a miracle that there are any therapies at all whose benefits outweigh all the possible side effects. This alone serves to remind us that modest attempts to aid the natural restorative reactions of the system are often to be preferred to heroic intervention. This also reminds us that longer-range changes in the system which make it more adaptable and better able to cope with stresses are to be preferred to one-shot interventions after the disease has occurred. Thus, while antibiotics have to be regarded as one of the greatest medical advances of this century, their effect on the infant mortality statistics in the U.S. was only a fraction of the effects of chlorinating city water supplies and pasteurizing milk.

A fourth advantage comes from the fact that disruption at one level leads to disruptions at many other levels, and the level of primary manifestation (if there is one) is not necessarily the level of the initial insult. Likewise, while "ideally" we might want to direct therapy at the "primary cause" of a disease, this "primary cause" may not exist if the disease was caused by a constellation of factors. (For example, psychiatric depression is probably a complex response to psychological stress, genetic predisposition, and biochemical state of the brain, among other factors.) Even where there is an identifiable primary cause, it may be better from a practical standpoint to direct the therapy-disruption at a different level.

If these are kept in mind, we can avoid the simplistic notions that hamper much of medical understanding, such as those of confusing the level of intervention with the level of "disease." From the fact that the complex constellation of interactions which we call "depression" can be treated with certain drugs, we cannot deduce that therefore depression is "just" a disease of the biochemical level and nothing else. Similarly, if an illness gets better because of the "placebo effect" (which is intervention on the language-behavior level), we cannot conclude that the person was not "really" sick and that it was "all in his mind." (The symptoms of incurable cancer have been shown to respond to placebos.)

However, in the process of including so many hierarchical levels in the "man" system, we have blundered into the same problem presented by the WHO definition of health. There is no way that the doctor, or even an interdisciplinary health care team, as presently constituted, can address itself to preserving health across all these levels. For instance, we look to politicians to handle disruptions that occur at the society-nation level; are politicians then to become members of the health care team?

On the other hand, we cannot deny that the various hierarchical levels are interconnected, and that events at the social level have major implications for the health or sickness of individuals. If we try arbitrarily to confine the concept of health to only a few levels of the hierarchy, we run the risk of speaking nonsense; also we are putting ourselves in a bad position to go on to discuss bioethics in the next chapter.

These arguments lead us to the conclusion that, if we accept the systems concept of health, it cannot be the task exclusively of the medical profession to preserve health. The medical profession must be very much concerned with health, because ethical behavior demands reasonable attempts to predict the various consequences of one's actions, including consequences at other levels. But since the techniques by which one can intervene to change the system vary greatly among levels, we may decide to respect the tradition which decrees that certain sorts of intervenors confine their activities to one level, and others to others. If we have to choose between an arbitrary definition of health on one hand and an arbitrary definition of the medical role on the other, we might as well be arbitrary about roles and try to be theoretically consistent about the concept of health.

964    If the medical profession is not supposed to preserve health, in this view, what does it do? First we have to note that an intervenor, at any level, becomes a part of the environment interacting with the "man-patient" system, and does so by setting up information-flow circuits between the "patient-person" and the "doctor-person." We would like the major intervention of the doctor to be at the "person" level; this is what is meant by "treating the whole person" instead of regarding the patient as a collection of organs. We would, in addition, allow the doctor to intervene at lower levels of physiology and biochemistry, and at the next higher level of the family, depending on the skills he has acquired in his training.

965    While our model has not specified what "self-awareness" is, it seems intuitively clear that whatever it is, it takes place at the "person" level. (Societies can have values and act in accordance with them, but only individuals can specifically claim values for themselves.) We have already noted the high risks involved in attempting to intervene in a complex set of systems; and any intervenor who directs his attentions to the "person" level would want to have the powerful resource of self-awareness working for him, so that it can point out related factors to him that he might otherwise miss.

966    Thus this model suggests the key importance for the doctor-patient relationship of the sort of communication we have been stressing all along, in the "contract" and in informed consent. (The justification just given is a pragmatic one; but if we assume that self-respect and dignity follow naturally from self-awareness, we can derive sound ethical justification as well.) This is a feature of our model that is not shared by either the A+B or the A' models, since they concern themselves with what is going wrong at the level of cells and organs. But the organs, from the point of view of the "person," are not ends in themselves; their function is to allow him to carry out his chosen goals that arise from his self-awareness.

967    *The foregoing is essentially a repetition of the role of the doctor as we have defined it elsewhere in this unit—his tasks are  1) to relieve suffering where possible; and  2) to implement, where possible, the decisions of the patient with regard to control over his own body and behavior. The first task is a minimal condition and gets high priority. The second task is more open to question, and should be looked at in terms of resource allocation and of possible conflicts of interests with the desires of others before making the decision that a particular practice should be used medically.*

968    Rather than continue discussing aspects of the health-disease concept, we will focus on one aspect of the systems view of "man" that we have described— namely, the role that such a model can play in explicating just what we mean by "human nature" or the nature of man. This concept will play a key role in the development of bioethics, a subject to which we shall now proceed.

# 18. Bioethics

At long last we are prepared to go back and pick up a major problem that we put on the back burner in Chapter 2. We described an ethical method in which consequences of ethical statements were compared with values, but we did not say, other than in a general way, how to determine the validity of those values. Thus, up till now, we have essentially been operating with an ethical method into which the values of a saint or the values of a Hitler could fit equally well. Is this as far as we can go, or can we do better? Of the various proposals for doing better, we believe that the most promising is a relatively new line of thought which Potter has christened "bioethics." In this final chapter we will have room to give only a brief and somewhat superficial exposition of it.

969

To avoid confusion, we must note that the term "bioethics" is being used in two ways at present. Most commonly it is used as an abbreviation for "ethical problems that arise in biology and medicine," which seems to be the case with the Kennedy Bioethics Institute of Georgetown University and the "Encyclopedia of Bioethics" which they are presently compiling, to name one example. But Potter, in naming his first book <u>Bioethics</u>, had in mind rather a unifying plan in which ethics and science interact to complement each other in specified ways. Our use of "bioethics" in this chapter follows Potter's.

970

Where do our values come from? Basically, we get our values from our indoctrination into the culture into which we are born, usually at an early age and continuing through our schooling and social interactions. Cultures, in turn, get their values as a part of the process of cultural evolution, analogous to Darwinian biological evolution. Values arise in response to the society's needs, often related to changes in the environment which the society must cope with. Then, by a process of selection, those values which have survival value for the culture are maintained, and strengthened by being associated with social institutions; while useless values are dropped along the way.

971

There are a couple of reasons why we might want to improve upon this process. By analogy with Darwinian evolution, it would appear that a culture with non-adaptive values will die out and be replaced by new, better fitted cultures. But if we are a member of the condemned culture, we cannot be expected simply to sit back and let this happen; we will want to make modifications in our values to head off this fate. In effect, the only alternative to letting evolution take its course is for us to take our evolution into our own hands.

972

973     The other reason for avoiding a laissez-faire approach to values comes about because of the present rapid rate of change in our society due to the exponential increase in technology. Today we can change the environment as much in one decade as would have taken thousands of years in the pre-historic times when man was evolving as a biological creature. Man is still evolving biologically, but biology alone cannot keep pace any more. In older times, up until a few centuries ago, the chance that values would become obsolete due to sudden changes was less than the chance that useful values might be lost due to failure to transmit them from one generation to the next. Therefore, it made good sense from the cultural-evolution standpoint to "rigidify" good values in self-perpetuating social institutions, such as the church, which could transmit them to succeeding generations with a minimum of distortion.

974     The result is that now, when maintaining static values is no longer necessarily in our best interests, we are prevented from making progress by these same institutions which resist change; social institutions, by their design, are made to transmit values and not to re-examine them. This problem is not just one of social policy. All of us have gone through the same cultural indoctrination, and all of us have come to identify emotionally with our social values and institutions; so we are all hard-pressed to reject these values and institutions, even when our reason tells us that failure to do so may have dire consequences. The job of personal reform is as hard or harder than the job of social reform.

975     Given this common cultural indoctrination, we presently go about testing the validity of our values by the means described in Chapter 2. As we saw there, we can simply turn the ethical decision-making method around; instead of deciding on the validity of an action or an ethical principle by weighing its consequences against our values, we can weigh the validity of our values by seeing what sorts of actions they would permit and what they prohibit. If we find the values consistently leading us toward actions that others in our society disparage, and leading us away from actions which others encourage, then we will either accept the role of a social deviant, or else go shopping for some different values. But this just boils down to basing our ethics on current popular opinion or "common sense." Since, in the scientific world, we have been given ample proof of how deficient these are as a basis for reasoning, we might well seek a better method.

976     A handy way out of this bind is to select a set of values which have some attractive authority. These may be principles revealed by a suitable religion, or they may be the basic principles of a philosophy of life, such as Western humanistic thought. In any case, we choose an authority which is sufficient to dispel any desire to raise questions about the validity of these principles. Since we then have "given" principles, the validity of which is not open to question, we can deduce what is right in a particular case along the fashion of a proof of geometry, reasoning from general principles to specific cases. We described this as the method of deontological ethics in Appendix I.

We have been giving examples all through this book of the flaws in this approach. If the values are very general, such as "primum non nocere," they are bound to be almost totally devoid of useful meaning. If they are meaningful, as with "absolute sanctity of life" which does give us a specific guide to behavior, they are likely to come into conflict with other basic principles. Since we cannot question the basic principles, and we are usually given little guidance as to how to assign them a priority ranking, the deontological approach leaves us in a bind when such a conflict of principles occurs. (If these basic conflicts did not arise with increasing frequency in medical practice, we would probably still be muddling through with our traditionally established values, and we would have felt no need to study medical ethics.)

977

978

Another approach we might try is to bring science into the picture in determining our basic principles. Here we have two different strategies. First, we can try to deduce basic principles directly from scientific facts. But in doing so we run into an elementary philosophical tangle. Recall our discussion of different types of statements in Chapter 2. Science deals with empirical statements, and we saw that these had basically different characteristics from ethical statements. As far back as the 1700's the philosopher Hume pointed out the conceptual error in trying to deduce "ought" statements logically from "is" statements. The transition from "ought" to "is" invariably signals the insertion of a value judgment independent of scientific facts, which the author is slipping by us (and usually himself) without stating it explicitly.

REVIEW EMPIRICAL  
VS. ETHICAL      18—20

From this view, we can conclude that trying to deduce ethical principles directly from science is like trying to make applesauce by chopping up oranges. But through the years many writers have concluded that they could do it, if only they chopped the oranges up fine enough, or took out all the seeds, or whatever. The results have been a mixed bag. At the crude level, we have had ethics based on supposed "natural law" which concluded that certain sexual practices were immoral in humans from observing animal behavior (and usually observing it erroneously at that); and the "social Darwinism" which concluded that capitalists would be immoral not to exploit the masses. In very sophisticated treatments, such as the recent "beyondism" of R.B. Cattell, the resulting ethic hangs together consistently and can be used to guide practical policy. But in all cases we can see that value judgments have been slipped in under the guise of science.

979

The other possible strategy, which avoids the philosophical hangup entirely, is to use scientific knowledge as a means of weighing values, as a more structured and developed form of the consequentialist ethical method such as we described in Chapter 2. This leads us to bioethics.

980

What are some of the basic kinds of scientific knowledge that bioethics will put to use? Recall two points that were made in Chapter 2. One was that the very possibility of making any sort of ethical judgment depends on actual possibilities in the real world. It makes no sense to tell someone he ought to do something which he either must do or which he cannot do. Traditionally our views of human capabilities have depended on the way we envisioned "human nature," and traditionally that view has contained a mixture of folklore and a priori beliefs derived from religion and philosophy. We are now gradually getting to the point where the science of man can give us some coherent information about human nature to compete with these traditional sources.

981

982    The idea of "Man" as a biological system with hierarchical levels and maintained by information flow within itself and with the environment, which we put forth in the last chapter, is an attempt to integrate the various things that science has been telling us about the nature of man. It is an attempt to avoid previous approaches which were based on empirical evidence, but which provide only piecemeal views. For instance, we can criticize certain abstract religious notions of human nature, which concentrate on one hierarchical level of behavior—abstracting or spiritual behavior—and neglect other levels. Similarly, we find that the views of many early psychologists, that man is basically an animal whose behavior is at the mercy of "drives" and "instincts," looks at man as if the hierarchy was chopped off at the level of motor behavior; all higher-level behavior as well as the levels of social organization are ignored.

983    *In summary, we can say that any adequate ethical framework must take into account three broad aspects of human nature: 1) man's biological dependence, which emphasizes that the individual is the result of continuing, reciprocal interaction between his heredity and his environment, and that these interactions follow the laws of physics and chemistry like other biological phenomena; 2) man's social dependence, which requires that the individual participate in a complex set of social interactions; and 3) the uniqueness of the individual when viewed at the individual level, no matter how homogeneous he might look in the aggregate.*

984    Another point that was made in Chapter 2 and elsewhere is that any ethical decision is a bet on the future, or a prediction that certain future worlds will come about if we take certain actions, and that we will value those possible future worlds in certain ways. Such a prediction of the future involves many features that are aided by judicious application of empirical data, and science today is giving us some reasonably clear signals that certain future states will result from certain present actions.

985    In this regard we want to pay particular attention to the various danger signals that we are getting from scientific thought. If certain catastrophes are in the offing, we might want to put our first attention toward avoiding those before we get too occupied in planning Utopias. According to modern biological and social science, a number of such catastrophes are waiting to be visited upon us if we do not change certain behaviors, although no one can predict how soon they might occur and just how preventable they are. The most obvious of these are the threat of major thermonuclear war, continued over-population with the corresponding decrease in resources, and massive pollution of the physical environment. While it is going too far to say that any of these would lead to man's biological extinction as a species, it is fairly likely that any one of these would put an end to anything resembling our present idea of the human culture.

Now that we have in mind the basic problem of deciding the validity of values, and the contributions that we have available from science, we can begin to define bioethics. But before doing this, you might have an objection. Why is the emphasis on something as abstract as values? After all, if we want to change society or head off possible disaster, we have to work on practical things, while values are obviously abstractions without substance and which have no ability to move events. If this view is true, and values are static instead of dynamic entities, it seems a waste of time to pay all that much attention to them when there is important work to be done.

986

↓

In the last chapter, we already stated the basis for the denial of this view when we pointed out that values are one of the types of information that participates in the biocybernetic feedback circuits that form the basis for the structure of the system. We also defined "information" in the broad sense as that which has the potential to bring about change in various parts of the system. Information is very dynamic as an entity, and appears even more so when one gets into some concepts of information theory and cybernetics, and begins to explore the relationships between information and energy.

987

↓

While we cannot go deeply into information theory here, we can give added credence to this view by outlining some of the biocybernetic feedback circuits in which values play an important part. One such circuit is that which connects some important fields of human activity, science and technology, with man's valuing behavior. This is diagrammed in Figure 7.

988

↓

Figure 7 shows what we already noted, that values come into being out of an interaction between our view of the world and concerns or anxieties, which are often precipitated by changes in the environment. These values then go on to become embodied in social institutions and transmitted by symbols. These institutions and symbols then go on, as we are indoctrinated into the ways of our culture, to determine our behavior at many levels, from simple biological-sustenance behavior all the way up to abstract and symbolic thought.

989

↓

The sum of the resulting behaviors could be termed our "life style." Our life style, of course, must take place within the physical-biological world, and because of the feedback loops between the "person" and the environment, our life style will have an environmental impact—as the ecology movement has taken pains to show us in recent years. The impact may change the environment to the extent that the environment no longer fits in with our existing world-view. This creates an anxiety and the cycle starts over again.

990

↓ 991

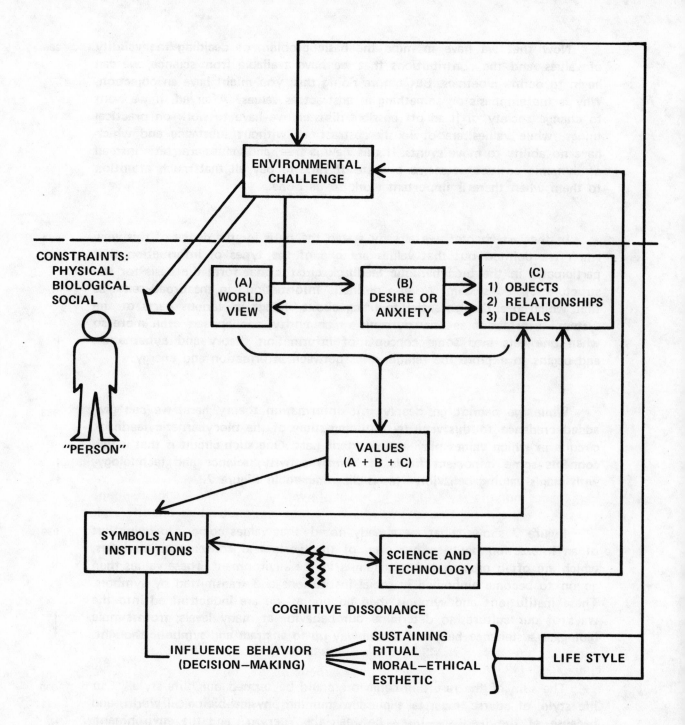

Figure 7.  Feedback circuits of information flow connecting science and values within the realm of human activity. Arrows beneath the horizontal broken line represent information circuits within the "man" hierarchy; arrows crossing broken line represent flow between "man" and external environment.

What we just described can be, in cybernetic terms, either a positive or negative feedback system. If it is a negative feedback system, the lifestyle will change the environment in a way that reverses the original environmental challenge. For example, suppose the original challenge which creates anxiety is the observation that our environment is littered with tin cans. If we then change our life style so that we recycle all cans instead of throwing them away, this is negative feedback and the problem is corrected. But there is no guarantee that this will be the case; our new lifestyle may make the matter worse instead of better. This is positive feedback or the proverbial vicious circle, which is an inherently self-destructive situation.

991

To make the circuit a little more complicated, Figure 7 shows science and technology as a separate social institution. It has interrelations with other social institutions, and we have already seen that these interrelations have significant potential for "cognitive dissonance." That is, the messages we get from science about the nature of the world may conflict with the messages we are getting from other social institutions. This can lead (following the arrows backwards) directly to an alteration in our values.

992

Through its direct applications, technology also acts directly on the environment to produce change. This sets up the opportunity for some additional instances of positive and negative feedback. Technology A can counteract technology B's effects, such as the use of catalytic converters to control auto emissions. When a technology produces undesirable environmental changes, we can change our life style, possibly in such a way as to require less of the commodity produced by the technology. Or, where some aspect of our life style other than technology is responsible for a change, technology can be called into play to correct the situation. But in all these circuits, note that values are important intermediate steps in the process.

993

Having thus shown the importance of values, and the nature of their interactions with science and technology, we are prepared to go on to define bioethics. We shall do so by making several points about it.

994

1) Bioethics endorses the consequentialist method of ethical decision-making. It supports an ethical method such as that used in this book, where an action or a principle is to be judged according to its consequences.

995

996    2)    Bioethics demands that human values be examined in light of our biological knowledge. We must investigate the practical consequences of holding certain values, making predictions based on scientifically sound principles, so that these predictions can be made:

    a)    with more precision,

    b)    with more breadth—that is, with all the ecological relationships taken into account,

    c)    farther into the future, so that long-range as well as short-range effects will be included.

997    3)    Following the analysis of No. 2, bioethics demands that we stand ready to change our values. *As we saw, we cannot derive new values directly from scientific facts. We can, however, call for the rejection of values whose consequences contradict scientific accounts of human nature and of man's future.* We can also choose certain basic values as the primary ones, and then emphasize those secondary values which, on scientific analysis, seem most likely to lead to a future world most consistent with the primary values.

998    4)    Since, as we saw, science tells us that if we change nothing in our present world we are heading for catastrophe, and if we change things the wrong way we may only accelerate the catastrophe, it follows that all of us have an interest in other people being "bioethical" as well as ourselves. In the same way, bioethics cannot be thought of as supporting any narrowly defined self-interest to the exclusion of broader considerations.

999    5)    Since the view of human nature we developed has included, as a major point, the uniqueness of the individual, bioethics requires us to design a morality that permits and encourages cultural and individual diversity, so long as society as a whole is not jeopardized by this, and human uniqueness is balanced against the equally important human trait of social dependence.

1000    6)    To accomplish these ends, bioethics should place a high priority on the development of scientific ways to distinguish biological, psychological, and social <u>needs</u> (without which the hierarchy of systems would be in danger of disintegration) rather than catering to arbitrary <u>wants</u> (even when those wants are erroneously labeled "rights"). This injunction is essentially the same as distinguishing the different categories of needs, as cited in Chapter 12.

REVIEW
NEEDS     613

Remember again that while science can predict possible future worlds, science alone cannot tell us if these worlds will be good or bad. Therefore, to apply bioethics, we need at least one value which we decide, on a priori grounds, to consider as a primary value against which all others can be weighed. A reasonable choice for this, since we have seen that survival of our present-day human culture is in danger, is the continued survival of a human culture (as opposed to mere survival of homo sapiens on a strictly biological level). This choice, which Potter has called the "survival imperative," serves to focus our attention on the crucial problems that need to be tackled at once. Our first order of business is to distinguish and eliminate those courses of action which would lead to our cultural destruction. Many courses will still remain, and we will then have time to choose which among those are preferable to others.

We can restate the "survival imperative" in terms of the systems hierarchy. The systems levels are not static; they can be seen as stages of evolutionary growth. We assume that there had to evolve one-celled creatures before multi-celled creatures could develop; we assume that a child has to learn to move his arms in a co-ordinated fashion before he can write the alphabet, and so on. These jumps of "hierarchical growth" often take place in response to challenges from the environment, which present problems that cannot be solved at the old level of organization. But hierarchical regression is also possible, in which a short-range security is gained at the expense of the longer-range adaptability. For example, if the nations of the world created an international authority to oversee equitable distribution of scarce resources, that would be an indication of hierarchical growth. If the nations responded to the problem by fighting wars with each other to get possession of the resources they wanted—as a result of which all the resources were used up in fighting—we would call this hierarchical regression.

*We can therefore state a bioethical injunction consistent with the survival imperative: whenever possible, seek to solve a problem by hierarchical growth rather than hierarchical regression. In this way, adaptability for future crises will best be preserved.*

The survival imperative also gives additional weight to point No. 5 in our definition of bioethics, maintaining diversity. In Chapter 15, we saw the arguments in favor of genetic diversity as the best way to "keep options open" for the future of the species. Our best guess now is that cultural evolution is analogous in this regard, and that any measures which restrict diversity within too narrow limits may severely decrease cultural adaptability and survivability. This further suggests that the social and psychological sciences should place particular priority on determining the optimal levels of diversity at different levels of the hierarchy.

1005     Now suppose that at some time in the future, we have gotten to the point where we can say that the demands of the survival imperative have been met. We have analyzed the different social policies and courses of action open to us and determined the consequences of each, and we have ruled out those policies which would lead to the destruction of human culture. We are left with a number of alternative policies. Now that we have, in this optimistic hypothesis, effectively headed off the threat of outright catastrophe, has bioethics completed its task?

1006     At this point in the future, we would still have choices to make among the remaining alternatives, and we will have the luxury of some more time to make them, knowing that the culture will still be there when we wake up the next morning (which is something we cannot be sure of now). A logical next step is to continue to weigh the alternatives according to bioethical considerations, but we will need some more basic principles, in addition to the survival imperative, to do this. Presumably, those other basic principles will serve to accomplish what we have been talking about all through this book—setting up practical and specific criteria for "quality of life," and seeing how they can best be applied to the largest number of people in the world.

1007     You have seen that within the confines of this book we have not had much luck in designing a set of specific, practical quality-of-life criteria, although we have continually seen the potential benefits of such a set. However, if we make a determined and consistent attempt to apply the bioethical method of integrating science and values, and as we gain more practice in the method through our attempts to apply it to meet the survival imperative, the solution to the task begins to seem less impossible than it does now.

1008     All along we have been saying that the primary goal ought to be the survival of human culture, while at the same time we have stated that our present Western culture, as it is now shaped, is what is leading us down the road to certain catastrophe. This is not a self-contradiction; *it simply means that we must build a new culture, which will be a "human" culture in the sense that the essential humanistic values are preserved, but which will still differ in many significant ways from our present society.*

1009     Obviously what we are asking for is no easy task. Until now, only the Hitlers of history have had the arrogance to try to design a totally new world culture. Furthermore, we have been arguing that a person's values and attitudes are shaped by the culture into which he was born. This is an advantage once the bioethical culture is established; people will then act bioethically in large part all by themselves. But it is a very sticky problem when the new culture has yet to be set up, since people indoctrinated to the attitudes of the present culture are much less likely to accept kindly any moves that would lead to the replacement of one culture by another.

It would seem that we have argued ourselves into a vicious circle: we have to set up the new culture in order to get people to act bioethically, and we have to get people to act bioethically in order to set up the culture. But we know this is not impossible to accomplish, because such social changes (albeit unplanned) have occurred many times before, by the same process of hierarchical growth we mentioned earlier. (In fact such social revolutions are excellent examples of hierarchical growth—up until a very short time before the change occurs, it looks as if no change is possible, and the old order of things appears firmly entrenched. But once the right conditions come about, many previously independent components all fall into their places in the new pattern, and the change occurs with surprising rapidity. The French Revolution in politics and the relativity revolution in physics are often cited as examples.)

1010

While the bioethicist is not shy about his goals of creating a new culture, he is desirous of doing it in a more reasonable (and more effective) way than Hitler set about doing it. This immediately leads him to reject any use of coercion to get people to accept the new attitudes he is proposing, and to accept the fact that the bioethical message must be transmitted by some sort of educational process. There is good reason to believe that the speed at which this educational process can take place, more than any other factor, will determine whether or not we will be successful in avoiding cultural catastrophe.

1011

Our mention of Hitler may raise another question: granted that we reconstruct a culture based on bioethical values, whatever they turn out to be: would this be a just society? (Note that the bioethical emphasis on individual diversity already seems to have made specters of 1984 and Brave New World less likely.)

1012

In Chapter 12 we called upon John Rawls' theory of justice to supply the notion of self-respect, as a way of ordering human needs. What would Rawls have to say about bioethics? Rawls' theory, which he calls "justice as fairness," resembles Potter's notions in that one is supposed to figure out alternative ways of structuring society and then choose the best of these. Rawls' rule for choosing is: select the social scheme in which the basic social rights and goods are distributed as equally as possible, unless an unequal distribution would be to the advantage of the least-well-off class of individuals.

1013

A crude way of saying what Rawls has in mind might be to ask whether the president of General Motors ought to get a raise of $100,000 per year. The test is to look at the black mother on ADC in the Detroit inner city. If she benefits, say because the raise stimulates the economy, the raise is just; if not, the raise is unjust. Whether the president has "earned" it in any sense is irrelevant to Rawls' theory.

1014

1015    Now, set up a row of alternative schemes for structuring society, and set the bioethicist and a Rawlsian hypothetical decisionmaker on them——would they pick the same scheme? The bioethicist is looking to eliminate schemes which would lead to the destruction of the human culture, and after that, schemes which fail to maximize his idea of quality of life. Based on what we know about societies in general, we may well expect that in such schemes, the least-well-off class of individuals will be most affected. Thus the Rawlsian and the bioethicist may well choose the same scheme.

1016    In concluding this chapter, we ought to go back and remember that this was supposed to be an introductory book in medical ethics. How does all this grand talk about inventing new cultures relate to medical ethics? Other than the obvious fact that if the cultural catastrophe occurred, we would have no more medical practice, what is the relevance?

1017    We have answered this question by proposing the systems view of "Man," and making explicit the interconnections between the different levels of the hierarchy. At the beginning of this book, we stated that in ethical decision-making, it is crucial to give as much consideration to the long-range as well as the short-range consequences. We have now filled this in by showing what kinds of long-range consequences there can be and where to look for them. In fact, all the bioethical concerns can be viewed as the long-range consequences of medical ethics. Therefore there is no sharp dividing line between medical ethics and what we have described as bioethics; one merges into the other.

1018    Furthermore, the educational process that is the necessary first step toward bioethical attitudes is the same process that we have been stressing all through this book. *In simplest terms, it is nothing more than the assumption that we will act better, in the long run, if we get into the habit of making our values explicit and of being ready to examine our values critically.* In many cases, once we do this, we are nearly home. In other cases, even after we make our values explicit and examine them, there is still some hard decision-making that remains to be done. But it must be made very clear that that is the place to start.

END

# Appendix I. Alternative Ethical Methods

The ethical decision-making method proposed in Chapter 2 and then used as the basis for further discussion in this book is definitely not the only ethical method that has been proposed by ethical philosophers, nor is it a particularly popular position. In this Appendix we will list a few of the most common alternatives; we will have to restrict ourselves to Western philosophy in doing so.

First, some terms which describe different ethical theories:

Consequentialist ethics refers to a method in which an action is judged to be morally right or wrong by judging the consequences of the action.

Utilitarian ethics is a special kind of consequentialist ethics. It specifies that the ultimate principle against which consequences are to be judged is the general happiness of all people concerned, or the greatest net balance of good over evil. Rule-utilitarians select rules of conduct which are judged to promote the general happiness, and then act in accordance with those rules. Act-utilitarians judge each action individually according to whether it will promote the general happiness.

Deontological ethics maintains that there are rules or principles of action which have moral validity independent of the consequences of individual actions, and that one must act in accordance with these rules or principles. (Act-deontologists take an extreme position that each action must be judged solely on its own merits without recourse either to general rules or to the consequences. We need not consider it further, and will take deontological and rule-deontological to be equivalent terms.)

(Ethical philosophers distinguish deontological from consequentialist, or teleological, theories by noting that in teleological ethics, one first defines what is "good" and then defines as "right" whatever promotes the "good." In deontological ethics, one defines the "right" independently of the "good" and insists on an obligation to do what is "right" even where the "good" is not served by it.)

From this list, you can see that our ethical method is a sort of rule-consequentialist ethics, which, unlike utilitarianism, refers one to a set of personal values instead of to the general happiness as the final criteria. No method for testing the validity of the set of values was given in Chapter 2, but this deficiency was corrected in Chapter 18.

We shall come across deontological theories in several places in this book, such as the sanctity-of-life principle in Chapter 6. The deontological approach is particularly common in religious and theological circles, since God or the Bible can then be turned to as the source of authority for one's rules or principles.

Figure 8 shows how the deontologist would go about making an ethical decision. After listing the alternative courses of action, he compares them to his set of rules or principles. He need not make a choice now; however, if he is passing judgment on someone else's choice, he would compare just that choice to the rules. If this comparison shows that one alternative is in accordance with the rules, he is home free. If several alternatives are in accordance with the rules, any of them would be ethically correct, and he can choose among them according to preference, or by which promotes the greatest happiness, or whatever subordinate criteria he wishes. If one alternative is in accordance with some rules and in conflict with others (or if none of the choices are consistent with the rules), he has a problem. In a case of rule conflict, he might be able to appeal to a higher-level rule to settle it; otherwise he is stuck. (However, the method in Chapter 2 is not superior to this method on that ground alone; don't forget that our method also may give us more than one answer, or no answer.) Notice that there is no feedback loop in the deontological method as there is in Figure 1. If the deontologist finds that his rules are contradictory in one case, he cannot go back and modify his rules, since they have validity independent of their practical consequences. He can, however, sometimes rearrange the priority of his rules, and get out of a fix that way.

Figure 9 follows the decision-making of an act-utilitarian. Once he has listed his alternatives, he calculates the consequences of each, and then assigns a value depending on how much each consequence will increase or decrease the general happiness. He then selects as ethically correct whichever alternative has the greatest positive value, or the least negative one if all the choices are negative. The act-utilitarian can also get into trouble if several alternatives turn up with equal values, or if he is unable to predict the consequences, or if he is unable to estimate how much happiness or unhappiness would follow a particular consequence.

Fletcher's "Situation Ethics" resembles act-utilitarianism except that the central principle is not general happiness, but a quantity which Fletcher labels with the Greek word "agape", which can be translated as "love for humanity" or "general goodwill." Fletcher has as much trouble defining his "agape" as the utilitarians do in defining "happiness"; as a practical matter they end up amounting to pretty much the same thing. However, Fletcher is more condemnatory of rules and of "rights" than many other act-utilitarians.

The rule-utilitarian follows a procedure roughly similar to that of our own method in Figure 1, with some modifications. He need not make a choice at the beginning, and he usually will not have to frame a new ethical statement, since he can select a rule from his existing stock which applies to the case at hand. Once he chooses the appropriate rule, he can proceed just like the deontologist.

# Figure 8

## Deontological Ethical Method

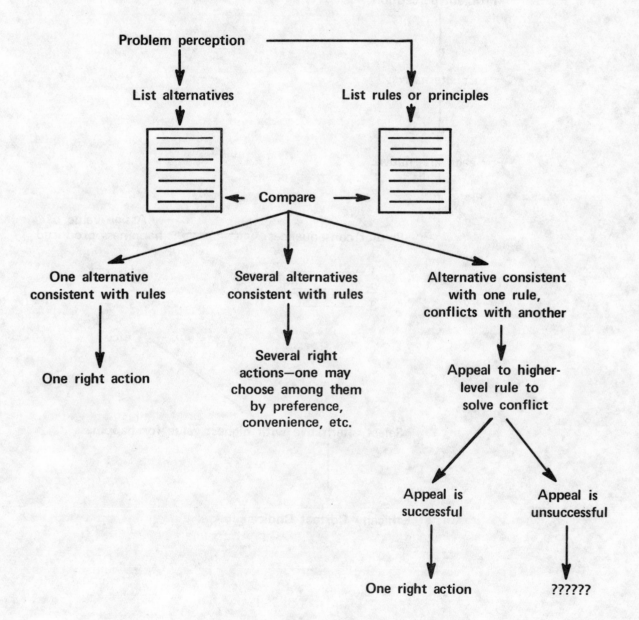

## Figure 9

## Act—Utilitarian Ethical Method

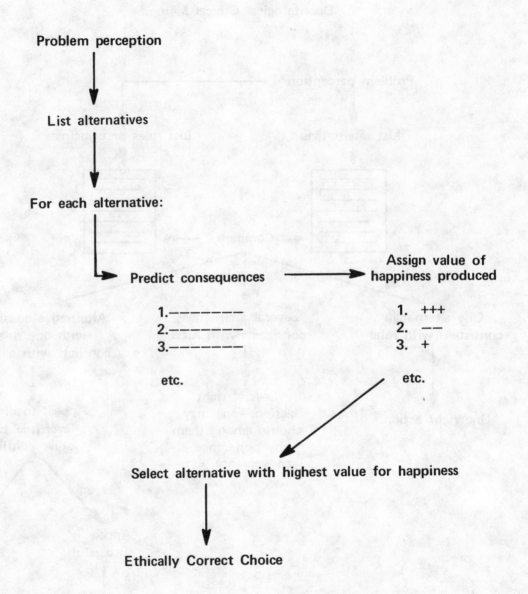

**Problem perception**

**List alternatives**

**For each alternative:**

**Predict consequences** → **Assign value of happiness produced**

1.———————
2.———————
3.———————

etc.

1. +++
2. ——
3. +

etc.

**Select alternative with highest value for happiness**

**Ethically Correct Choice**

Method fails if:
1) Unable to predict consequences accurately
2) Unable to estimate accurate happiness values

But in a problematic case he will do the same thing with his rule as we did with our ethical statement——list consequences, and compare them with values, although his values will not be a personal set, but rather the primary value of the greatest general happiness. (Since this is such a vague concept, however, he might well need a set of more specific values by which to apply it, and thus his method might come more and more to resemble our own.) If the rule-utilitarian finds that his rule is not conducive to the general happiness to the extent that he expects, he can revise it and go through the process again until it comes out to his satisfaction.

While we have talked about deontological ethics in general, we might add a specific note on one very famous deontologist, Immanuel Kant. Many people take to be of primary ethical importance Kant's principle, "Act always so as to treat people as ends and not merely as means only." (Note the language: we always are treating others and indeed ourselves as means; what is prohibited is treating them as means only without regard to their dignity as persons, that is, as free moral agents.) There is some question as to whether one can apply this principle in practice without confusion; and there is some evidence that Kant intended it to give added persuasive weight to his other formulations of the basic ethical principle, rather than to provide a means of testing ethical judgments. An example of a case in which Kant's principle might be illuminating is the question of removing an organ from a "brain-dead" person on a respirator for transplantation (see Case 21). By the notion that brain function is necessary for "personhood," the body is not a person and we are free to use it as a means toward some other value: saving someone else's life. But we are similarly not free to remove an organ from a living person without his consent to save another's life; that would be using the person as a means and not as an end in himself. Under strict utilitarian guidelines, we could do so if the general happiness would be increased——say the person needing the organ was a great scientist and the involuntary donor was a depraved criminal. Here the Kantian deontologist would claim his method to be superior to utilitarianism, because it attributes to the individual not just value, which is relative, but the dignity of being regarded as an end in himself.

A number of subjects usually regarded as being parts of ethics have been ignored in this book. We have left out the view of morality seen in Plato and Aristotle, that morality is dependent on virtue or good character, since our emphasis has been on decision-making. We have left out the whole ethical question of how to define and achieve the "good life," since our focus has been on how to act well as a physician and not on how to be a good person. We have also neglected the question of the relation between religion and ethics and the role of faith, if any, in ethical behavior; but do not forget that our decision-making method, into which one injects one's own values, in no way rejects religious values.

For a more complete but still very concise description of these ethical methods, see Ethics by Frankena (cited in references). The ethical method in Chapter 2 is based to a large extent on the ethics proposed by R.M. Hare in Freedom and Reason (see references).

# Appendix II. Patient's Bill of Rights

(American Hospital Association, November, 1972)

1. The patient has the right to considerate and respectful care.

2. The patient has the right to obtain from his physician complete current information concerning his diagnosis, treatment, and prognosis in terms the patient can be reasonably expected to understand. When it is not medically advisable to give such information to the patient, the information should be made available to an appropriate person in his behalf. He has the right to know by name, the physician responsible for coordinating his care.

3. The patient has the right to receive from his physician information necessary to give informed consent prior to the start of any procedure and/or treatment. Except in emergencies, such information for informed consent should include but not necessarily be limited to the specific procedure and/or treatment, the medically significant risks involved, and the probable duration of incapacitation. Where medically significant alternatives for care or treatment exist, or when the patient requests information concerning medical alternatives, the patient has the right to such information. The patient also has the right to know the name of the person responsible for the procedures and/or treatment.

4. The patient has the right to refuse treatment to the extent permitted by law, and to be informed of the medical consequences of his action.

5. The patient has the right to every consideration of his privacy concerning his own medical care program. Case discussion, consultation, examination, and treatment are confidential and should be conducted discreetly. Those not directly involved in his care must have the permission of the patient to be present.

6. The patient has the right to expect that all communications and records pertaining to his care should be treated as confidential.

7. The patient has the right to expect that within its capacity a hospital must make reasonable response to the request of a patient for services. The hospital must provide evaluation, service, and/or referral as indicated by the urgency of the case. When medically permissible a patient may be transferred to another facility only after he has received complete information and explanation concerning the needs for and alternatives to such a transfer. The institution to which the patient is to be transferred must first have accepted the patient for transfer.

8.  The patient has the right to obtain information as to any relationship of his hospital to other health care and educational institutions insofar as his care is concerned. The patient has the right to obtain information as to the existence of any professional relationships among individuals, by name, who are treating him.

9.  The patient has the right to be advised if the hospital proposes to engage in or perform human experimentation affecting his care or treatment. The patient has the right to refuse to participate in such research projects.

10. The patient has the right to expect reasonable continuity of care. He has the right to know in advance what appointment times and physicians are available and where. The patient has the right to expect that the hospital will provide a mechanism whereby he is informed by his physician or delegate of the physician of the patient's continuing health care requirements following discharge.

11. The patient has the right to examine and receive an explanation of his bill regardless of source of payment.

12. The patient has the right to know what hospital rules and regulations apply to his conduct as a patient.

No catalogue of rights can guarantee for the patient the kind of treatment he has a right to expect. A hospital has many functions to perform, including the prevention and treatment of disease, the education of both health professionals and patients, and the conduct of clinical research. All these activities must be conducted with an overriding concern for the patient, and above all, the recognition of his dignity as a human being. Success in achieving this recognition assures success in the defense of the rights of the patient.

# Appendix III. Criteria for Determining Quality of Life*

A. "Tentative Profile of Man" by Joseph Fletcher: Fletcher, a theologian and professor of medical ethics, has proposed a set of "positive human criteria" specifically designed to serve as indicators of "personhood" in decisions regarding abortion, allowing to die, etc. With brief explanation, his list consists of:

1. MINIMAL INTELLIGENCE: Below 40 on Stanford-Binet or similar I.Q. test is questionably a person; below 20, not a person

2. SELF—AWARENESS

3. SELF—CONTROL: if condition cannot be rectified medically, individual without self-control is not a person

4. A SENSE OF TIME: a sense of the passage of time and of the need to allocate time

5. A SENSE OF FUTURITY: a sense of time to come; looking forward and planning

6. A SENSE OF THE PAST: a sense of time gone by; memory

7. CAPABILITY TO RELATE TO OTHERS: includes both inter-individual and diffuse social relationships

8. CONCERN FOR OTHERS: while role this trait actually plays is debatable, its absence is indicator of psychopathology

9. COMMUNICATION: completely isolated individual who cannot communicate, as opposed to being disinclined to communicate, is not a person

10. CONTROL OF EXISTENCE: when absent leads to state of irresponsibility [compare No. 3]

11. CURIOSITY: "Man is a learner and knower as well as a tool maker and user"

12. CHANGE AND CHANGEABILITY of one's mind and conduct

13. BALANCE OF RATIONALITY AND FEELING: person can be neither coldly rational nor given over completely to feelings

14. IDIOSYNCRASY: must have recognizable identity

15. NEO—CORTICAL FUNCTION: all other traits hinge upon this; offers legitimacy of brain-function approach to defining death

*Adapted from the Hastings Center Report, Vol. 2, November 1972, with the permission of the Institute of Society, Ethics and the Life Sciences, Hastings-on-Hudson, N.Y. 10706.

For purposes of clarification, Fletcher also lists a five-point list of negative human criteria, which he deems not essential to personhood. Man is not non- or anti-artificial (i.e., technology is a normal part of human existence); man is not essentially parental, and can be fully a person without reproducing; man is not essentially sexual; man is not a "bundle of rights"; and man is not a worshipper ("Faith in supernatural realities. . .is a choice some human beings make and others do not.")

Fletcher acknowledged many problems with his list and proposed it as a start for discussion rather than a final product. He noted that some items may be essential for human existence where others might merely promote optimal existence. He was unable to suggest how to rank-order the criteria. While he did state that the potential cannot be treated equivalently to the actual, he did not state how to regard precisely such "potential" persons as normal fetuses. He did not say just how many indicators, or which ones, had to be absent before the individual is no longer worthy of medical protection.

As noted in the text, in 1974 Fletcher had revised his notions to the extent that he acknowledged the primary importance of No. 15, cerebral function, and was willing to make life-and-death decisions based on that criterion alone.

B. Other "personhood" criteria: Other authors have developed lists of traits which they consider essential for humanhood, but which were developed for other purposes and so are not directly applicable to medical-ethical decisions without clarification.

G.G. Simpson has listed the activities which he considers as the biological basis of human nature:
1) Abstracting
2) Communicating
3) Tool-making
4) Ethicizing or valuing

These, of course, are stated in the most abstract form, and thus are of limited practical use in deciding specific cases.

T.S. Clements, in an attempt to explicate the philosophy of scientific humanism, lists a number of "personality atoms" which are part of what he calls the "good life." These include:
1) Desire to be loved
2) Desire to be excited
3) Desire to satisfy curiosity and exercise intelligence
4) Desire for order
5) Desire to feel healthy and unified
6) Desire to feel meaningfully related to world and to others
7) Desire to share experiences socially

Again, the "good life" label suggests that these are criteria for optimal existence, rather than the minimal criteria needed for making quality-of-life decisions in a medical-ethical context.

References for this appendix are included in the references to Chapter 6.

# Appendix IV. Declaration of Helsinki

(Recommendations Guiding Doctors in Clinical Research)

Resolution adopted at the 18th World Medical Assembly, June, 1964, by the World Medical Association, of which the American Medical Association is a member.

INTRODUCTION: It is the mission of the doctor to safeguard the health of the people. His knowledge and conscience are dedicated to the fulfillment of this mission.

The Declaration of Geneva of the World Medical Association binds the doctor with the words: "The health of my patient will be my first consideration" and the International Code of Medical Ethics which declares that "Any act or advice which could weaken physical or mental resistance of a human being may be used only in his interest."

Because it is essential that the results of laboratory experiments be applied to human beings to further scientific knowledge and to help suffering humanity, the World Medical Association has prepared the following recommendations as a guide to each doctor in clinical research. It must be stressed that the standards as drafted are only a guide to physicians all over the world. Doctors are not relieved from criminal, civil and ethical responsibilities under the laws of their own countries.

In the field of clinical research a fundamental distinction must be recognized between clinical research in which the aim is essentially therapeutic for a patient, and the clinical research, the essential object of which is purely scientific and without therapeutic value to the person subjected to the research.

## I.   BASIC PRINCIPLES

1.   Clinical research must conform to the moral and scientific principles that justify medical research and should be based on laboratory and animal experiments or other scientifically established facts.

2.   Clinical research should be conducted only by scientifically qualified persons and under the supervision of a qualified medical man.

3.   Clinical research cannot be legitimately carried out unless the importance of the objectives is in proportion to the inherent risk to the subject.

4.   Every clinical research project should be preceded by careful assessment of the inherent risks in comparison to forseeable benefits to the subject or to others.

5.   Special caution should be exercised by the doctor in performing clinical research in which the personality of the subject is liable to be altered by drugs or experimental procedure.

## II. CLINICAL RESEARCH COMBINED WITH PROFESSIONAL CARE

1. In the treatment of the sick person, the doctor must be free to use a new therapeutic measure, if in his judgment it offers hope of saving life, reestablishing health, or alleviating suffering.

If at all possible, consistent with patient psychology, the doctor should obtain the patient's freely given consent after the patient has been given a full explanation. In case of legal incapacity, consent should also be procured from the legal guardian; in case of physical incapacity the permission of the legal guardian replaces that of the patient.

2. The doctor can combine clinical research with professional care, the objective being the acquisition of new medical knowledge, only to the extent that clinical research is justified by its therapeutic value for the patient.

## III. NON—THERAPEUTIC CLINICAL RESEARCH

1. In the purely scientific application of clinical research carried out on a human being, it is the duty of the doctor to remain the protector of the life and health of that person on whom clinical research is being carried out.

2. The nature, the purpose and the risk of clinical research must be explained to the subject by the doctor.

3a. Clinical research on a human being cannot be undertaken without his free consent after he has been informed; if he is legally incompetent, the consent of the legal guardian should be procured.

3b. The subject of the clinical research should be in such a mental, physical, and legal state as to be able to exercise fully his power of choice.

3c. Consent should, as a rule, be obtained in writing. However, the responsibility for clinical research always remains with the research worker; it never falls on the subject even after consent is obtained.

4a. The investigator must respect the right of each individual to safeguard his personal integrity, especially if the subject is in a dependent relationship to the investigator.

4b. At any time during the course of the clinical research the subject or his guardian should be free to withdraw permission for research to be continued.

The investigator or the investigating team should discontinue the research if in his or their judgment, it may, if continued, be harmful to the individual.

# Appendix V.  A Living Will

(Prepared and distributed by the Euthanasia Educational Council, 250 West 57th Street, New York  10019; has also been used as a model for "death with dignity" bills introduced into state legislatures.)

To my family, my physician, my clergyman, my lawyer—

If the time comes when I can no longer take part in decisions for my own future, let this statement stand as the testament of my wishes:

If there is no reasonable expectation of my recovery from physical or mental disability, I,_____, request that I be allowed to die and not be kept alive by artificial means or heroic measures. Death is as much a reality as birth, growth, maturity and old age—it is the one certainty. I do not fear death as much as I fear the indignity of deterioration, dependence and hopeless pain. I ask that medication be mercifully administered to me for terminal suffering even if it hastens the moment of death.

This request is made after careful consideration. Although this document is not legally binding, you who care for me will, I hope, feel morally bound to follow its mandate. I recognize that it places a heavy burden of responsibility upon you, and it is with the intention of sharing that responsibility and of mitigating any feelings of guilt that this statement is made.

Signed_____

Date_____

Witnessed By:_____

_____

_____

For an example of an individualized "living will" drawn up by a patient for personal use, see the article by Modell listed in the references for Chapter 13.

# References and Suggested Readings

Annotations are provided where the discussion in the text does not indicate the nature of the book or article. The following journal abbreviations are used: NEJM—New England Journal of Medicine; JAMA—Journal of the American Medical Association; HCR—Hastings Center Report; HCS—Hastings Center Studies; AIM—Annals of Internal Medicine; PBM—Perspectives in Biology and Medicine.

## Ethics: General

Aiken, H.D. Reason and Conduct: New Bearings in Moral Philosophy. New York, Knopf, 1962. See especially Chapter 4, "Levels of Ethical Discourse."

Dworkin, G. "Paternalism." In: Morality and the Law, ed. R.A. Wasserstrom. Belmont, Calif., Wadsworth (n.d.). A discussion of paternalism and the circumstances in which it is justified.

Fletcher, Joseph. Situation Ethics. Philadelphia, Westminster, 1966. See Appendix I for description.

Frankena, W.K. Ethics. Englewood Cliffs, N.J., Prentice-Hall, 1973. An excellent overview on an introductory level.

Gewirth, A. "Positive 'Ethics' and Normative 'Science.'" Philosophical Review 69:311, 1960. An examination of the fallacy that the scientific method yields firm answers while ethics is only vague and subjective.

Gewirth, A. "Categorical Consistency in Ethics." Philosophical Quarterly 17:289, 1967. An analysis of ethical methods.

Hare, R.M. Freedom and Reason. New York, Oxford University Press, 1965. An exploration of ethics emphasizing the notion of universalizability; much of Chapter 2 here is derived from Hare's treatment.

Kant, I. Foundations of the Metaphysics of Morals, trans. L.W. Beck. New York, Bobbs-Merrill, 1959.

Rawls, J. A Theory of Justice. Cambridge, Mass., Belknap Press, 1971. A difficult book, considered a modern classic on the subject of social justice.

Stevenson, C.L. "Ethical Fallibility." In: Ethics and Society, ed. R.T. de George. New York, Anchor. Comparison of ethics and scientific methodology.

## Medical Ethics: General

Bibliography of Society, Ethics and the Life Sciences. Issued yearly to members of the Institute of Society, Ethics and the Life Sciences, 623 Warburton Avenue, Hastings-on-Hudson, New York 10706. Annual student membership fee is $10. This bibliography is presently the most extensive on the medical-ethical literature. Like the Hastings Center Report, it is essential for anyone seriously interested in the field.

Clouser, K.D. "What is Medical Ethics?" <u>AIM</u> 80:657, 1974.

_____. "Medical Ethics: Some Uses, Abuses and Limitations." <u>NEJM</u> 293:384, 1975. Clouser gives an excellent brief overview of medical ethics in its practical applications.

Fletcher, Joseph. <u>Morals</u> <u>and</u> <u>Medicine</u>. Boston, Beacon Press, 1960. A classic book by a liberal Protestant theologian.

Greenberg, D.S. "Medicine and Public Affairs: Ethics and Nonsense." <u>NEJM</u> 290:977, 1974. Greenberg views current ethical debates and sorts out substantive issues from polemics.

Ingle, D.J. "The Ethics of Biomedical Interventions." <u>PBM</u> 13:364, 1970. Ingle places medical ethics within the context of all the ways in which biological applications impinge on human life; compare with the systems model of health and disease in Chapter 17.

Kass, L.R. "The New Biology: What Price Relieving Man's Estate?" <u>Science</u> 174:779, 1971. Kass gives an overview of recent biological advances giving rise to a range of ethical questions.

Nelson, J.B. <u>Human</u> <u>Medicine</u>. Minneapolis, Augsburg, 1973. An overview of issues in medical ethics from the viewpoint of a Protestant minister.

Torrey, E.F., ed. <u>Ethical</u> <u>Issues</u> <u>in</u> <u>Medicine</u>. Boston, Little, Brown, 1968. A collection of essays on ethical issues; some are cited individually by topic.

Vaux, K. <u>Biomedical</u> <u>Ethics</u>. New York, Harper & Row, 1974. Overview by a Protestant theologian.

Wertz, R.W., ed. <u>Readings</u> <u>on</u> <u>Ethical</u> <u>and</u> <u>Social</u> <u>Issues</u> <u>in</u> <u>Biomedicine</u>. Englewood Cliffs, N.J., Prentice-Hall, 1973. A collection of readings from other sources.

### Chapter 2.  A Method of Ethical Reasoning

Jeffrey, R.C. <u>The</u> <u>Logic</u> <u>of</u> <u>Decision</u>. New York, McGraw-Hill, 1965. Includes a discussion of Bayesian decision theory.

## Chapter 4.  The Doctor-Patient Relationship

Davidson, H.A. "Professional Secrecy." In: Ethical Issues in Medicine, ed. E.F. Torrey. Boston, Little, Brown, 1968. Davidson discusses confidentiality problems, giving several examples.

Dworkin, G. "Paternalism." In: Morality and the Law, ed. R.A. Wasserstrom. Belmont, California, Wadsworth. See "Ethics—General".

Guttentag, O.E. "The Meaning of Death in Medical Theory." Stanford Medical Bulletin 17:165, 1959. Guttentag begins with the doctor-patient relationship as one involving two human beings, and develops the notion of "finite freedom."

"How Well Are Patients' Rights Observed?" Hospital Practice, March, 1973, p. 31. Summarizes the Patient's Bill of Rights and surveys evidence for the need of such a statement.

Meyer, B.C. "Truth and the Physician." In: Ethical Issues in Medicine, ed. E.F. Torrey. Boston, Little, Brown, 1968. Meyer shows the flaws in various arguments supporting a general policy of non-disclosure toward patients.

Pemberton, L.B. "A Comprehensive Understanding of the Doctor-Patient Relationship." Journal of Religion and Health 11:252, 1972. Pemberton, starting from a theological groundwork of human relations, ends up with a position close to Veatch's.

Veatch, R.M. "Models for Ethical Medicine in a Revolutionary Age." HCR, Vol. 2, June 1972, p. 5. Veatch outlines the models of the doctor-patient relationship given in the text.

## Chapter 5.  Informed Consent

Alfidi, R.J. "Informed Consent: A Study of Patient Reaction." JAMA 216:1325, 1971. "Controversy, Alternatives, and Decisions in Complying with the Legal Doctrine of Informed Consent." Radiology 114:231, 1975. Alfidi here expands his earlier study and concisely summarizes the doctor's legal responsibility.

Curran, W.J. "The Patient's Bill of Rights Becomes Law." NEJM 290: 32, 1974. Summary of actions by state legislatures based on the hospital patient's Bill of Rights (Appendix II).

Fletcher, John. "Human Experimentation: Ethics in the Consent Situation." Law and Contemporary Problems 32:620, 1967. Discussion of the moral rules of informed consent.

"How Well Are Patients' Rights Observed?" Hospital Practice, March 1973, p. 31. Review of the adoption of the patient's Bill of Rights and its implications in the hospital setting.

Ingelfinger, F.J. "Informed (but Uneducated) Consent." <u>NEJM</u> 287:465, 1972. Brief editorial on problems in informing patients adequately.

Katz, J., with A.M. Capron and E.S. Glass. <u>Experimentation with Human Beings</u>. New York, Russell Sage Foundation, 1972. One section of this reference work is devoted to informed consent and lists many relevant court cases with discussion.

Romano, J. "Reflections on Informed Consent." <u>Archives of General Psychiatry</u> 30:129, 1974. A physician reflects on informed-consent problems from his experience as clinician and researcher.

Rubsamen, D.S. "What Every Doctor Needs to Know About Changes in Informed Consent." <u>Medical World News</u>, February 9, 1973, p. 66. A concise summary by a physician-attorney with recommendations.

## Chapter 6. Determination of the Quality of Life

Bennett, J. "Whatever the Consequences." In: <u>Moral Problems</u>, ed. J. Rachels, New York, Harper and Row, 1971.

Capron, A.M., and L.R. Kass. "A Statutory Definition of the Standards for Determining Human Death: An Appraisal and a Proposal." <u>University of Pennsylvania Law Review</u> 121:87, 1972. Discussion of ambiguities in present "brain death" laws and a recommended model statute.

Clements, T.S. <u>Science and Man: The Philosophy of Scientific Humanism</u>. Springfield, Ill., Charles Thomas, 1968. See Chapter 4 for the quality-of-life criteria listed in Appendix III.

Clouser, K.D. " 'The Sanctity of Life': An Analysis of a Concept." <u>AIM</u> 78:119, 1973.

Dinello, D. "On Killing and Letting Die." <u>Analysis</u> 31:83, 1971.

Fletcher, John. "Attitudes Toward Defective Newborns." <u>HCS</u>, Vol. 2, No. 1, 1974, p. 21. Fletcher traces the roles of social values and new scientific awareness in shaping attitudes toward life-death decisions in newborns.

_____. "Abortion, Euthanasia, and the Care of Defective Newborns." <u>NEJM</u> 292:75, 1975. Argues that the decision to abort a fetus with a diagnosed genetic defect is logically separate from the approval of infanticide on such an infant after birth.

Fletcher, Joseph. "Elective Death." In: Ethical Issues in Medicine, ed. E.F. Torrey. Boston, Little, Brown, 1968. Joseph Fletcher argues for quality-of-life approaches and rejects the sanctity notion.

____. "Indicators of Humanhood: A Tentative Profile of Man." HCR, Vol. 2, November 1972, p. 1. See Appendix III. See also Fletcher's subsequent revision of his criteria to cerebral function, in HCR, Vol. 4, December 1974.

Kass, L.R. "Death as an Event: A Commentary on Robert Morison." Science 173:698, 1971. In objecting to the views of Morison (see below) Kass notes that Morison has confused the questions of when life is no longer worth living with when a person is actually dead.

McCormick, R.A. "To Save or Let Die: The Dilemma of Modern Medicine." JAMA 229:172, 1974. A Jesuit priest says that decisions to allow to die are appropriate when the individual has no chance to develop any meaningful interpersonal relationships.

Morison, R.S. "Death: Process or Event?" Science 173:694, 1971. Morison argues that death takes place over time; see also reply by Kass (see above).

Rachels, J. "Active and Passive Euthanasia." NEJM 292:78, 1975.

Simpson, G.G. Biology and Man. New York, Harcourt, Brace, and World, 1969. See Appendix III.

Smith, D.H. "On Letting Some Babies Die." HCS, Vol. 2, No. 2, 1974, p. 37. Smith applies quality-of-life notions to decision-making on defective infants.

Task Force in Death and Dying of the Institute of Society, Ethics, and the Life Sciences. "Refinements in the Criteria for the Determination of Death: An Appraisal." JAMA 221:48, 1972. Lists the Harvard brain-death criteria and discusses their implications. (Harvard criteria originally appeared in JAMA 205:337, 1968.)

Veatch, R.M. "Brain Death: Welcome Definition or Dangerous Judgment?" HCR, Vol. 2, November, 1972, p. 10. Veatch reviews a court case in which brain death was introduced as an issue in removing organs for transplant without consent of relatives.

## Chapter 7. Determination of Ethical Participation

Hook, E.B. "Behavioral Implications of the Human XYY Genotype." Science 179:139, 1973.

Valentine, G.H., M.A. McClelland, and F.R. Sergovich. "The Growth and Development of Four XYY Infants." Pediatrics 48:583, 1971. This and the above paper review the data on the connection between XYY and behavior disorders (see Case 28).

## Chapter 9. Behavior Control

Breggin, P.R. "Psychotherapy as Applied Ethics." Psychiatry 34:59, 1971. Breggin, a psychiatrist, is an outspoken opponent of psychosurgery.

____. "The Return of Lobotomy and Psychosurgery." Congressional Record, 118, February 24, 1972. Breggin traces the history of psychosurgery techniques and concludes that even new "refined" types are unacceptable.

Chorover, S.L. "Big Brother and Psychotherapy II: The Pacification of the Brain." Psychology Today, May 1974, p. 59. A review of the anti-psychosurgery position for the general audience.

Delgado, J. Physical Control of the Mind. New York, Harper and Row, 1969. Delgado is a leading advocate of psychosurgery and electrode implantation for both medical and social-control purposes.

Fish, B. "The 'One Child, One Drug' Myth of Stimulants in Hyperkinesis." Archives of General Psychiatry 25:193, 1971. Fish reviews questionable basic assumptions in the use of drugs in behavior control.

Holden, C. "Psychosurgery: Legitimate Therapy or Laundered Lobotomy?" Science 179:1109, 1973. Good short summary of the pro and con positions, the weight being toward the con.

Klerman, G.L., R.M. Veatch, L.J. West, and P.H. Wender. "Controlling Behavior Through Drugs" (special section of four articles). HCS, Vol. 2, No. 1, 1974, p. 65. See the Veatch article for classifications of justifications for drug use.

Mark, V.H., and F.R. Ervin. Violence and the Brain. New York, Harper and Row, 1970. Good monograph on the use of psychosurgery to control violent behavior, arguing its superiority to environmental means in specific cases.

Mark, V.H. "Brain Surgery in Aggressive Epileptics." HCR, Vol. 3, February 1973, p. 1. Mark argues for an organic basis for some violence and so justifies psychosurgery.

_____. "A Psychosurgeon's Case for Psychosurgery." Psychology Today, July 1974, p. 28. A reply to Chorover (see above).

Platt, J. "Beyond Freedom and Dignity: A Revolutionary Manifesto." Center Magazine, Vol. 5, March-April 1972, p. 34. Platt reviews Skinner's book and reformulates some of the features he finds oversimplified in it.

Rhinelander, P. Is Man Incomprehensible to Man? San Francisco, Freeman, 1974. Rhinelander surveys various philosophical views of human nature, including Skinnerian behaviorism, which he finds flawed on several counts.

Rosenhan, D.L. "On Being Sane in Insane Places." Science 179:250, 1973. Widely quoted study in which normal volunteers were admitted to mental institutions with nonexistent symptoms.

Skinner, B.F. Beyond Freedom and Dignity. New York, Knopf, 1972.

Sweet, W.H. "Treatment of Medically Intractable Mental Disease by Limited Frontal Leucotomy: Justifiable?" NEJM 289:1117, 1973.

Szasz, T.S. The Myth of Mental Illness. New York, Hoeber, 1961. Classic presentation of the view that so-called "illness" is really "problems in living," and that medical treatment does more harm than good.

_____. "Problems Facing Psychiatry: The Psychiatrist as Party to Conflict." In: Ethical Issues in Medicine, ed. E.F. Torrey. Boston, Little, Brown, 1968. Discussion of conflicts of interest between therapeutic and societal motives.

Bok, S. "Ethical Problems in Abortion." HCS, Vol. 2, No. 1, 1974, p. 33.

Callahan, D. Abortion: Law, Choice, and Morality. New York, Macmillan, 1970. A detailed discussion of social and moral issues drawing upon abortion experience in other nations; however was published prior to 1973 Supreme Court decision.

Curran, W.J. "Birth of a Healthy Child Due to Negligent Failure of 'Pill': Benefit or Loss?" NEJM 285:1063, 1971. Good case for discussion.

———. "Legal Abortion: The Continuing Battle." NEJM 290:1301, 1974. The evolving legal issues since the Supreme Court decision, and reaction to it by anti-abortion forces.

Dyck, A.J. "Perplexities of the Would-Be Liberal in Abortion." Journal of Reproductive Medicine 8:351, 1972. Dyck finds that so-called "liberal" values conflict in the abortion issue.

———. "Procreative Rights and Population Policy." HCS, Vol. 1, No. 1, 1973, p. 74. Dyck discusses the dangers in coercive population control policies which are favored by some experts.

Engelhardt, H.T. "Viability, Abortion, and the Difference Between a Fetus and an Infant." American Journal of Obstetrics and Gynecology 116:429, 1973.

Fost, N. "Our Curious Attitude Toward the Fetus." HCR, February 1974, p. 4. Fost notes some internal contradictions in views on abortion and fetal research.

Guttmacher, A.F. "Contraception." In: Ethical Issues in Medicine, ed. E.F. Torrey. Boston, Little, Brown, 1968. An overview of techniques and a defense of contraception against moral objections.

Hall, R.E. "Abortion: A Non-Catholic View." In: Ethical Issues in Medicine, ed. E.F. Torrey. Boston, Little, Brown, 1968. A brief coverage of common pro and con arguments.

Ingram, I.M. "Abortion Games: An Inquiry into the Working of the Act." Lancet ii:969, 1971. A "games doctors play" discussion of how the abortion act has been promoted and thwarted in England.

McGarrah, R.E. "Voluntary Female Sterilization: Abuses, Risks, and Guidelines." HCR, Vol. 4, June 1974, p. 5. Problems in insuring truly voluntary consent.

Moore, E.C., H. Edgar, K.A. Lebacqz, and D. Callahan. "Abortion: the New Ruling." HCR, Vol. 3, April 1973, p. 4. Brief comments in the aftermath of the Supreme Court rulings.

Nelson, J.B. Human Medicine. Minneapolis, Augsburg, 1973. Chapter 3 offers a clergyman's view of artificial insemination.

Peck, S. "Voluntary Female Sterilization: Attitudes and Legislation." HCR, Vol. 4, June 1974, p. 6. A survey of current practices.

Ramsey, P. "Abortion: A Review Article." The Thomist 37:174, 1973.

Taylor, H.C. "The Ethics of the Physician in Human Reproduction." In: Humanistic Perspectives in Medical Ethics, ed. M.B. Visscher. Buffalo, Prometheus Books, 1972. A brief overview of the topic.

Tooley, M. "Abortion and Infanticide." Philosophy and Public Affairs 2:37, Fall 1972. Tooley concludes from his use of personhood criteria that judgments on abortion imply similar judgments about infanticide.

Viola, M.V. "Abortion: A Catholic View." In: Ethical Issues in Medicine, ed. E.F. Torrey. Boston, Little, Brown, 1968. Viola sketches a liberal Catholic approach to the issue.

Wood, H.C. "Sterilization." In: Ethical Issues in Medicine, ed. E.F. Torrey. Boston, Little, Brown, 1968. A brief introduction.

## Chapter 11. Human Experimentation

Altman, L.K. "Auto-experimentation: An Unappreciated Tradition in Medical Science." NEJM 286:346, 1972. Historical examples of researchers who used themselves as subjects.

American Medical Association Judicial Council. Opinions and Reports. Chicago, 1971. Includes "Principles of Medical Ethics," with statement on human experimentation.

Barber, B., et al. Research on Human Subjects. New York, Russell Sage Foundation, 1973. Emphasis on social implications; includes Sullivan's study of risk-benefit ratios in experiments involving subjects of different social status.

Beecher, H.K. "Ethics and Clinical Research." NEJM 274:1354, 1966.

_____. Experimentation in Man. Springfield, Ill., Charles Thomas, 1959. A pioneering book by an experimenter.

Capron, A.M. "Medical Research in Prisons: Should a Moratorium be Called?" HCR, Vol. 3, June 1973, P. 4. Reviews the problem of voluntary consent for research in prisons.

Curran, W.J. "Experimentation Becomes a Crime." NEJM 292:300, 1975. Criticism of a 1974 Massachusetts law prohibiting research in fetuses.

Department of Health, Education, and Welfare, National Institutes of Health. "Protection of Human Subjects: Policies and Procedures." (Draft Form) Federal Register, Vol. 38, No. 221 (November 16, 1973). Proposed NIH regulations of research on children, prisoners, mentally ill, and fetuses, which attempt to safeguard rights while still permitting useful research to continue.

Freund, P.A., ed. Experimentation with Human Subjects. New York, George Braziller, 1970. A collection of several important essays covering both ethics and law.

Guttentag, O.E. "Ethical Problems in Human Experimentation." In: Ethical Issues in Medicine, ed. E.F. Torrey. Boston, Little, Brown, 1968. Includes as appendices the Nuremburg Code, Declaration of Helsinki, and U.S. Public Health Service Code.

Katz, J., with A.M. Capron and E.S. Glass. Experimentation with Human Beings. New York, Russell Sage Foundation, 1972. A large reference work, including notes on ethics and especially legal cases of relevance to experimentation and consent.

Lasagna, L. "Human Experimentation." In: Humanistic Perspectives in Medical Ethics, ed. M.B. Visscher. Buffalo, Prometheus Books, 1972. An introductory overview.

Lowe, C.U., D. Alexander, and B. Mishkin. "Nontherapeutic Research in Children: An Ethical Dilemma." Journal of Pediatrics 84:468, 1974. Seeks a compromise between the problem of consent in minors and the benefits of experimentation on children.

Murton, T. "Prison Doctors." In: Humanistic Perspectives in Medical Ethics, ed. M.B. Visscher. Buffalo, Prometheus Books, 1972. The account includes some "horror stories" of exploitative research on prisoners.

Schwartz, A.H. "Children's Concepts of Research Hospitalization." NEJM 287: 589, 1972. Data on the extent to which children are informed about their status as subjects; has implications for children having "veto power" over experimentation on them (see NIH proposed guidelines, above).

Veterans Administration Cooperative Study Group on Antihypertensive Agents. "Effects of Treatment on Morbidity in Hypertension." JAMA 202:1028, 1967. The basis for Case 35.

Weinstein, M.C. "Allocation of Subjects in Medical Experiments." NEJM 291: 1278, 1974.

## Chapter 12.   Allocation of Scarce Resources

Childress, J.F. "Who Shall Live When Not All Can Live?"; and F.B. Westerveldt, "A Reply to Childress: The Selection Process as Viewed from Within," in: Readings on Ethical and Social Issues in Biomedicine, ed. R.W. Wertz. Englewood Cliffs, N.J., Prentice-Hall, 1973.

Dukeminier, J., and D. Sanders. "Organ Transplantation: A Proposal for Routine Salvaging of Cadaver Organs." NEJM 279:413, 1968. Ideal methods to insure supplies of transplantable organs conflict with prevalent societal notions about death.

Kass, L.R. "The New Biology: What Price Relieving Man's Estate?" Science 174:779, 1971. Kass sketches the levels from the individual to the global on which resource allocation decisions must be made.

Rawls, J. A Theory of Justice. Cambridge, Mass., Belknap Press, 1971.

"Scarce Medical Resources." Columbia Law Review 69:620, 1969. Considered to be an excellent review article on legal and policy questions, with recommendations for legislative solutions.

See also references to Chapter 6, especially Bennett, Dinello, and Rachels on active and passive euthanasia.

Brill, H.W. "Death with Dignity: A Recommendation for Statutory Change." University of Florida Law Review 12:368, 1970. Discussion of legal implementation of "living wills."

Duff, R.S., and A.G.M. Campbell. "Moral and Ethical Dilemmas in the Special-Care Nursery." NEJM 289:890, 1973. A review of a number of decisions to allow diseased newborns to die, reached jointly by physicians and parents.

Fletcher, Joseph. "Elective Death." In: Ethical Issues in Medicine, ed. E.F. Torrey. Boston, Little, Brown, 1968. A defense of the individual's right to choose his own death.

Freeman, J.M. "Is There a Right to Die—Quickly?"; and R.E. Cooke, "Whose Suffering?" Journal of Pediatrics 80:904, 1972. A debate on active euthanasia for children with severe meningomyelocele (see Case 45).

Jaretzki, A., III. "The Doctor's Dilemma." In: Dilemmas of Euthanasia, excerpts from the Fourth Euthanasia Conference, 1971. Available from the Euthanasia Educational Council (see Appendix V for address).

Kass, L.R. "Death as an Event: A Commentary on Robert Morison." Science 173:698, 1971.

Kubler-Ross, E. On Death and Dying. New York, Macmillan, 1970. The classic study of psychological reaction to death and the need of the dying patient for communication with physician and family.

Modell, W. "A 'Will' to Live." NEJM 290:907, 1974.

Morgan, L.G. "On Drinking the Hemlock." HCR, Vol. 1, December 1971, p. 4. A personal account of the indignity of protracted terminal illness.

Poe, W.D. "Marantology: A Needed Specialty." NEJM 286:102, 1972. Poe argues that success-oriented physicians cannot humanely treat hopelessly ill patients because they wish to deny any evidence of "failure." A new type of physician who can accept failure is needed to treat such patients with empathy and compassion.

Ramsey, P. "The Indignity of 'Death with Dignity.'" <u>HCS</u>, Vol. 2, No. 2, 1974, p. 47. A dissection of the notion of "death with dignity" from a religious perspective. See also commentaries by R.S. Morison and L.R. Kass in the same issue.

Shaw, A. "Dilemmas of 'Informed Consent' in Children." <u>NEJM</u> 289:885, 1973. Shaw takes up the fact that "informed consent" implies the right to refuse treatment, and that if parents are competent to consent for children they are also competent to refuse. He includes a number of case illustrations.

## Chapter 14. Mass Screening Programs

Culliton, B.J. "Sickle Cell Anemia." <u>Science</u> 178:138, 178:283, 1972.

Fraser, F.C. "Genetic Counseling." <u>Hospital Practice</u>, January 1971, p. 49. Description of types of data that might be presented to patients in a counseling situation.

Hemphill, M. "Pretesting for Huntington's Disease." <u>HCR</u>, Vol. 3, June 1973, p. 12.

Institute of Society, Ethics, and the Life Sciences, Research Group on Ethical, Social, and Legal Issues in Genetic Counseling and Genetic Engineering. "Ethical and Social Issues in Screening for Genetic Disease." <u>NEJM</u> 286: 1129, 1972. Cites important issues and offers guidelines for setting up a community screening program. See also editorial by Gaylin, "Genetic Screening: The Ethics of Knowing," same volume, p. 1361.

Leonard, C.O., et al. "Genetic Counseling: A Consumer's View." <u>NEJM</u> 287: 433, 1972. An important study of the results of genetic counseling, showing that many patients do not understand the information or reach decisions based on other factors.

Ramsey, P. "Screening: An Ethicist's View." In: <u>Ethical Issues in Human Genetics</u>, ed. B. Hilton and D. Callahan. New York, Plenum, 1973.

Whitten, C.F. "Sickle-Cell Programming: An Imperiled Promise." <u>NEJM</u> 288: 318, 1973; related correspondence in <u>NEJM</u> 288:971, 1973. Whitten puts forth the need to weigh the beneficial results of knowing one's carrier status against the psychological burden.

## Chapter 15. Genetic Engineering

Berg, P., et al. "Potential Biohazards of Recombinant DNA Molecules." Science 185:303, 1974.

Crow, J.F. "Rates of Genetic Change Under Selection." Proceedings of the National Academy of Sciences 59:655, 1968.

_____. "The Effects of a Changing Environment on Man's Genetic Future." Bioscience 21:107, 1971. This and the preceding article discuss the idea of genetic deterioration through treatment of disease from the standpoint of technical genetics.

Edwards, R.G., and R.E. Fowler. "Human Embryos in the Laboratory." Scientific American 233:45, December 1970. Discusses the technical aspects of in vitro fertilization.

Fletcher, Joseph. The Ethics of Genetic Control. Garden City, N.Y., Anchor, 1974. A defense of the use of genetic engineering as a reflection of man's rationality.

Friedmann, T., and R. Roblin. "Gene Therapy for Human Genetic Disease?" Science 175:949, 1972.

"Genetic Engineering in Man: Ethical Considerations." JAMA 220:721, 1972. A call for a moratorium on attempts at in vitro fertilization because of the ethical issues involved.

"Genetics and the Quality of Life." World Council of Churches, Study Encounter 53, Vol. X, No. 1, 1974. Report of a symposium among theologians, physicians, and scientists.

Gottesman, I.I., and L. Erlenmeyer-Kimling. "Prologue: A Foundation for Informed Eugenics." Social Biology 18, Supplement S1-S8, 1971. A defense of positive eugenics.

"Human Genetic Engineering: No Brave New World but Brand New Medical Potentials." Medical World News, May 11, 1973, p. 45. Sympathetic discussion of real potentials of various techniques in the near future.

Kass, L.R. "Babies by Means of In Vitro Fertilization: Unethical Experiments on the Newborn?" NEJM 285:1174, 1971. Kass feels such techniques are unethical because of possible undetected harm to the child-to-be.

Lappe, M. "Moral Obligation and the Fallacies of 'Genetic Control.'" Theological Studies 33:411, 1972. A geneticist shows how some moral arguments on the topic misconstrue biological facts.

_____. "Genetic Knowledge and the Concept of Health." HCR, Vol. 3, September 1973, p.1.

_____, and Steinfels, P. "Choosing the Sex of Our Children." HCR, Vol. 4, February 1974, p. 1. A discussion on values to be used in genetic engineering and the social and ethical consequences.

Ramsey, P. "Shall We 'Reproduce?'" JAMA 220:1346, 220:1480, 1972.

Twiss, S.B. "Parental Responsibility for Genetic Health." HCR, Vol. 4, February 1974, p. 9. A discussion of procreation rights versus responsibility when parents are known to carry deleterious genes.

## Chapter 16. Organized Medicine and Medical Economics

American Medical Association Judicial Council. "Opinions and Reports" (includes "Principles of Medical Ethics.") Chicago, 1971.

Badgley, R.F., and S. Wolfe. "The Doctor's Right to Strike." In: Ethical Issues in Medicine, ed. E.F. Torrey. Boston, Little, Brown, 1968.

Bay Area Chapter, Medical Committee for Human Rights. Billions for Band-aids: An Analysis of the U.S. Health Care System and of Proposals for its Solutions. P.O. Box 7677, San Francisco, California 94119. A statement of the "radical" position on health care reform.

Bean, W.B. "The Medical Profession and the Drug Industry." In: Ethical Issues in Medicine, ed. E.F. Torrey. Boston, Little, Brown, 1968. Includes government hearings on the regulation of the drug industry.

Brian, E.W. "Government Control of Hospital Utilization: A California Experience." NEJM 286:1340, 1972. Provides some data suggestive of some possible results of PSRO's.

Bruhn, J.G., and D.C. Smith. "Social Ethics for Medical Educators." In: Humanistic Perspectives in Medical Ethics, ed. M.B. Visscher. Buffalo, Prometheus Books, 1972. Short essay on the importance of social responsiveness in medical education.

Chapman, C.B., and J.M. Talmadge. "The Evolution of the Right-to-Health Concept in the U.S." In: Humanistic Perspectives in Medical Ethics, ed. M.B. Visscher. Buffalo, Prometheus Books, 1972. A detailed historical review emphasizing legislative action and the reaction from organized medicine.

Curran, W.J. "The Right to Health in National and International Law." NEJM 284:1258, 1971.

____. "The 'Class-Action' Approach to Protecting Health Care Consumers——The Right to Psychiatric Treatment." NEJM 286:26, 1972. A good case for discussion as well as an example of court protection of rights.

Enterline, P.E., et al. "Effects of 'Free' Medical Care on Medical Practice——the Quebec Experience." NEJM 288:1152, 1973. Detailed analysis of a transition to "socialized" medicine.

Friedman, E.A., and S.L. Kountz. "Impact of HR-1 on the Therapy of End-Stage Uremia." NEJM 288:1286, 1973. Practical implications of the decision to provide federal funds for anyone needing an artificial kidney.

Greenberg, D.S. "Medicine and Public Affairs——Kennedy Urges Further Pharmaceutical Regulation." NEJM 290:1211, 1974. Strong testimony against the pharmaceutical industry from Senate hearings.

Halberstam, M.J. "Liberal Thought, Radical Theory, and Medical Practice." NEJM 284:1180, 1971. See Case 58.

"Health Radicals: Crusade to Shift Medical Power to the People." Science 173:506, 1971. Review of the activities of the "radical" health movement.

Kaplan, H.R. "The Fee-for-Service System." In: Humanistic Perspectives in Medical Ethics, ed. M.B. Visscher. Buffalo, Prometheus Books, 1972.

Kennedy, E.M. In Critical Condition: The Crisis in America's Health Care. New York, Simon and Schuster, 1972. Statement by the leading proponent of national health insurance in the Senate.

Kline, N.S., and M. Gordon. "Amphetamine Quotas and Medical Freedom." HCR, Vol. 3, December 1973, p. 8. Case study of conflict between physician's freedom to prescribe vs. desirability of regulating abusable drugs.

Lifton, R.J. "Beyond Atrocity." In: Humanistic Perspectives in Medical Ethics, ed. M.B. Visscher. Buffalo, Prometheus Books, 1972. What can psychiatry as a profession say about Hiroshima and My Lai?

Livingston, G. "Medicine and the Military." In: Humanistic Perspectives in Medical Ethics, ed. M.B. Visscher. Buffalo, Prometheus Books, 1972. Conflicts between the military doctor's obligations to his patient and to the military system.

MacLeod, G.K., and J.A. Prussin. "The Continuing Evolution of Health Maintenance Organizations." NEJM 288:439, 1973. Discussion of ways of implementing group pre-paid care via HMO's. See Case 58.

McNamara, J.J. "The Revolutionary Physician—Change Agent or Social Theorist." NEJM 287:171, 1972. Paradoxes between theory and practice in health reform.

Murton, T. "Prison Doctors." In: Humanistic Perspectives in Medical Ethics, ed. M.B. Visscher. Buffalo, Prometheus Books, 1972. Focuses on the abuses of an especially corrupt prison system in Arkansas in the 1960's.

"National Health Insurance." The New Physician 19:986, 1970. A handy and extensive run-down on the issue.

Navarro, V. "Women in Health Care." NEJM 292:398, 1975. Navarro notes the scarcity of women in decision-making positions in the health care system and calls for increased institutional democracy.

Newhouse, J.P., C.E. Phelps, and W.B. Schwartz. "Policy Options and the Impact of National Health Insurance." NEJM 290:1345, 1974. A Rand Corp. analysis of the impact of national health insurance on demands for medical services. One may conclude either that national health insurance would swamp present facilities and be a disaster (as the AMA concluded), or that the data show the inadequacy of the present health care system.

"Our Doctor Shortage Exists only on Paper." Hospital Physician, October, 1970, p. 33. Criticism of the widely held idea that the U.S. needs to train an increasing number of physicians.

Sade, R.M. "Medical Care as a Right: A Refutation." NEJM 285:1288, 1971.

Schwartz, H. "Health Care in America: A Heretical Diagnosis." Saturday Review, August 14, 1971, p. 14. Attack on the "liberal" position that U.S. health care lags behind European countries and that basic changes in the health structure are needed.

Shenker, B.N., and D.C. Warren. "Giving the Patient His Medical Record: A Proposal to Improve the System." NEJM 289:688, 1973. Discussion of beneficial results of opening such information to scrutiny by "consumers."

Stevens, R. American Medicine and the Public Interest. New Haven, Yale University Press, 1971.

Wise, H.B. "Medicine and Poverty." In: Ethical Issues in Medicine, ed. E.F. Torrey. Boston, Little, Brown, 1968. Discussion of patient care requirements and social responsibility.

## Chapter 17. Defining Health and Disease

Akiskal, H.S., and W.T. McKinney. "Depressive Disorders: Toward a Unified Hypothesis." Science 182:20, 1973. The authors review recent research on depression and conclude that it can be understood only by a model that takes into account its biochemical, genetic, and social aspects.

Brody, H. "The Systems View of Man: Implications for Medicine, Science and Ethics." PBM 17:71, 1973.

Cohen, H. "The Evolution of the Concept of Disease." In: Concepts of Medicine, ed. B. Lush. New York, Pergamon Press, 1961. A historical overview.

Dubos, R. Man Adapting. New Haven, Yale University Press, 1965. Dubos is the most prominent of the authors using an evolutionary-ecological model of disease.

Engel, G.L. "A Unified Concept of Health and Disease." PBM 3:459, 1960. Engel notes the error in selecting a single "cause" for a disease, and stresses psychological as well as biological variables.

Engelhardt, H.T. "Explanatory Models in Medicine: Facts, Theories, and Values." Texas Reports on Biology and Medicine 32:225, 1974. Engelhardt emphasizes that all disease ascriptions include value judgments, and that we can look at disease causes from many viewpoints depending on our therapeutic intentions.

Fabrega, H. Jr. "Concepts of Disease: Logical Features and Social Implications." PBM 15:583, 1972. Fabrega calls for a unified or systems view of disease and sketches the implications of the view for health care delivery.

————. "The Study of Disease in Relation to Culture." Behavioral Science 17:183, 1972. Discusses cross-cultural variables in responses to various biological states.

HCS, Vol. 1, No. 3, 1973. This issue is devoted to five articles on the concept of health. See especially the article by Peter Sedgwick on values in disease concepts; and Daniel Callahan's discussion of the World Health Organization definition of health.

Laszlo, E. The Systems View of Nature. New York, George Braziller, 1972. Laszlo develops the systems-theoretical view of biological systems which is applied specifically to disease by Brody (see above).

Snow, L. "Folk Medical Beliefs and their Implications for the Care of Patients." AIM 81:82, 1974. Snow reviews systems of folk beliefs prevalent in the U.S.

Temkin. O. "The Scientific Approach to Disease: Specific Entity and Individual Sickness." In: Scientific Change, ed. A.C. Crombie. London, Heinemann, 1963. A historian reviews two themes in the development of disease concepts——disease as entity and concern for the individual patient.

Wolf, S. "Disease as a Way of Life: Neural Integration in Systemic Pathology." PBM 4:288, 1961. Wolf reviews the neurophysiological data to demonstrate the intimate way in which thoughts and feelings are tied in with bodily function.

## Chapter 18.   Bioethics

Callahan, D. "Living with the New Biology: Search for an Ethic." Center Magazine, Vol. 4, July-August 1972, p. 4. Callahan argues that changes at the cultural level are necessary to meet the challenges posed by new technologies.

Cattell, R.B. A New Morality From Science: Beyondism. New York, Pergamon, 1972. Cattell develops a system of ethical injunctions which he claims follow logically from evolutionary considerations.

Heilbroner, R. An Inquiry into the Human Prospect. New York, Norton, 1974. An economist views the long-range consequences of present human behavior and lists changes that will be necessary if the culture is to survive.

Potter, V.R. Bioethics: Bridge to the Future. Englewood Cliffs, N.J., Prentice-Hall, 1971. Potter lays the framework for "bioethics" as a way of analyzing the long-range consequences of holding values, and using scientific knowledge to make better value choices.

    . "Disorder as a Built-in Component of Biological Systems: The Survival Imperative." <u>Zygon</u> 6:135, 1971. Discusses the essential role of randomness and diversity in adaptation and survival.

    . "Probabilistic Aspects of the Human Cybernetic Machine." <u>PBM</u> 17:164, 1974. Develops the model of human beings as showing systems organization and interacting with the environment at all levels.

Trosko, J.E. <u>The Bioethics of Human Intervention</u> (in preparation). Trosko gives an overview of Potter's bioethics and applies it to problems in medical ethics as well as other types of intervention.

# Self-Evaluation

You may complete this self-test to see whether you have fulfilled the Objectives listed at the beginning of this book. Complete the test all the way through, and then compare your answers with the answers that follow.

The first group of questions refer to the case below.

## SELF-EVALUATION CASE

You are a pediatrician who gets a frantic call at 11:30 one night from the resident on duty at the local hospital, concerning your 11-month-old patient, L.K. The baby was diagnosed as having a congenital hernia which was successfully operated on four days ago. L.K. seems to have been making an uneventful recovery, although he has been mostly sedated by medication.

The resident tells you that about 16 hours ago, the hospital pharmacy erred and sent up a bottle of 50% glucose solution for the patient's IV, instead of the 5% you had ordered. The nurse on the floor failed to catch the error and the bottle was hung and the fluid administered. The patient is now comatose and shows signs of severe dehydration.

You rush to the hospital, where you find that the resident has also called in an expert in fluid therapy from a nearby medical school. He tells you that the child has an extremely high blood glucose level which is already producing severe damage to the kidneys. He will try to correct the situation, he says, but this must be done very delicately; the outlook right now for L.K. is very grim.

At this point Mr. and Mrs. K. approach you. They are very anxious and perceive from the activity that something has gone wrong; so far no one has told them anything. They urgently demand an explanation.

What do you tell Mr. and Mrs. K.?

1. How many alternative courses of action are open to you?

2. Which of these seems most acceptable to you? Write a formal ethical statement which expresses this choice.

Questions 3 through 9 refer to the following formal ethical statement:

"When an error in therapy that has significant consequences for the patient is made, the doctor ought to inform the patient or a responsible guardian as soon as possible of the true circumstances. He should decide for each case how and when this disclosure may best be made."

3. Make as extensive a list as you can of the consequences of this formal ethical statement. For each consequence, indicate by "high," "medium," or "low" the relative probability that you attribute to this consequence actually occurring.

4. Suppose one places a high value on the terms of the doctor-patient "contract" as we have described it in this book. Which of the consequences are consistent with this value, and which are not? Does the formal ethical statement serve this value well or poorly?

5. Suppose one places a high value also on the efficiency of the cooperation of all members of the health care "team." Which of the consequences are consistent, and which are inconsistent with this value? Is this value well or poorly served by the ethical statement?

6. If, in Question No. 5, you found significant inconsistencies between the formal ethical statement and the value of health care cooperation, how could you modify the formal statement to decrease them?

7. In this case, what effect does the course of action that you choose have upon L.K.?

8. Your answer to Question No. 6 above has some implications for how you determine the rights of ethical participation in this decision. What are your criteria for determination here?

9. Does your response to this case represent any basic modifications in the doctor-patient relationship, according to your answer to Question No. 6?

The remaining questions represent fragments of arguments in defense of various ethical propositions. For each one, indicate the ethical "error" that it contains, if any.

10. "It can't be ethical to deny me, as an expectant mother, the opportunity for a screening amniocentesis if I want it. Why, you're saying that I can't do everything possible to assure myself of having a normal child."

11. "You say that the man who came into the emergency room just now has a brain tumor causing increased intracranial pressure, and needs an immediate craniotomy to keep him alive long enough for us to do the tests to decide if the tumor is treatable or not, and now his wife won't give consent for the operation? How am I supposed to decide what to do? Sure, I'm the doctor in charge, but I don't have all the data. We need more data."

12. "Now, Mrs. Jenkins, after all, I am your doctor. So don't worry about little things like unlikely side effects. Just have the surgery as I recommend and everything will be all right."

13. "You can't allow infertile mothers to have 'test tube babies.' Sure, it would be nice for them, but pretty soon everyone would want a test tube baby instead of one born the regular way. What would become of the foundations of the sexual relationship?"

14. "How can you possibly be recommending brain surgery for that child? Have you forgotten that the doctor's first responsibility is to do no harm?"

15. "If we look at animals in the natural world, it is clear that sex is used only for purposes of procreation, and that it takes place only between members of opposite sexes. Therefore homosexuality is unnatural and clearly wrong, and deserves immediate and aggressive psychiatric treatment when detected."

16. "You say that the county medical society ought not take a stand on national health insurance because it ought to be free of political involvement. Yet in the past I have heard you encourage the society's lobbying efforts on behalf of publicly financed school vaccination programs, genetic screening, and improved sanitation. You can't accept some political involvement and reject another without giving a better reason than the one you just gave."

17. "Well, it's been five years now since I diagnosed that city bus driver's dangerous heart condition, and he hasn't had a heart attack. I guess that I was right in not violating confidentiality, as he requested, and in not notifying the bus company when he refused to quit his job."

18. "Abortion can't possibly be justified under any circumstances. Why, it's murder!"

19. "I make it a rule never to stop to give medical aid at the scene of an accident. I once knew a doctor who had a cousin who heard of one case where a physician stopped and gave first aid. The victim died and the poor jerk got sued for his shirt as a result."

# Self-Evaluation: Answers

Throughout this book we have avoided claiming to have any special access to "right answers," and the answers that follow should be interpreted in this light. They should be regarded as representing a minimal level of competence in fulfilling the objectives listed at the beginning of the book. If you have spent time in careful thought, you may well have come up with additional consequences, or you may possibly have thought of some more subtle distinctions, beyond what is given here.

If your answer differs significantly from the one given below, you will have to decide whether your own answer is "better" than ours according to the criteria for ethical validity used in this book or whether you have misunderstood part of the material. If the latter is the case, you may wish to reread the appropriate section which is given in parentheses at the end of each answer.

1. You have been cautioned against jumping to the conclusion that there are two and only two alternatives. As was noted in connection with Case 1, when the question is "What do you say?" there are as many alternatives as there are things that could be said, up to an infinite number. On a purely practical level, there are a large number of alternatives which are significantly different from each other. Compare the following:

"Don't worry, everything is all right with your child."

"Your child seems to have taken a sudden turn for the worse. We don't know what caused it but we're working hard to correct it."

"Your child is very sick now; this may be due to some of the medication he has been given."

"We just now discovered that an error was made in the type of IV fluid the child has been getting. He's very sick now but we shall do everything possible to correct the situation."

"We just now discovered that an error was made in the type of IV fluid. I'm afraid that the child is going to die."

"Well, right now the child is very sick, and it's all because the pharmacist sent up the wrong bottle of IV fluid and the nurses were too busy drinking coffee and gabbing to notice."

You can see that saying each of these would lead to a different set of consequences. With a little ingenuity you can make the list almost as long as you like, so we cannot give an exact number of alternatives. (Frames 32, 76)

2.    Since there are so many alternatives, we cannot phrase a formal ethical statement for each. In order to qualify as a formal statement, yours should have included what is to be done, who is to do it, and under what circumstances; the circumstances may have been as broadly or as narrowly defined as you saw fit. (Frames 16, 34)

3.    While the consequences of the ethical statement on the specific case of L.K. is a good place to start, don't forget that you are determining the consequences of the general (universalizable) ethical statement, not a specific statement about what the doctor should do in just this one case. Therefore, if your list of consequences pertains only to this one case and does not apply to possible similar cases, it is incomplete.

Your list of consequences should have included most of the following:

a)    The doctor maintains his duties under the doctor-patient "contract." (high probability)

b)    The doctor has told the truth, which we tend to view as a worthwhile exercise in general. (high probability)

c)    The parents will appreciate the frankness and candor of the doctor. (high probability)

d)    The parents will be made angry at someone, depending on exactly how the doctor phrased his account of what happened. (medium probability; doctor can help parents deal with anger)

e)    The parents may institute a lawsuit against the doctor. (medium probability, depending on circumstances)

f)    The parents may institute a lawsuit against the hospital or against other members of the health care team. (medium probability)

g)    If (e) occurs, the parents may win the suit. (low probability if the circumstances are like those of the case given)

h)    If (f) occurs, the parents may win the suit. (high probability under circumstances given)

i)    If the error was made by another member of the team, and the doctor tells the parents, the team members may feel "betrayed" by the doctor, and the team solidarity and efficiency may be weakened. (high probability)

j)    The doctor will avoid the consequences of not telling the parents the truth—i.e., they will probably determine that something had gone wrong, and will feel frustrated and left out if not told. (high probability)

k)   The doctor and the other team members, having suffered the embarrassment of exposure, will make fewer mistakes in the future. (low probability, since such errors are already uncommon, and since there are other forces acting to prevent them)

l)   People in general, hearing of these errors, may lose faith in the medical professions. (low, since it is probably known already that such mistakes can be made)

m)   If (l) occurs, people may demand and get more governmental regulation of medicine. (low probability; more regulation is likely, but for other reasons) (Frames 35-38)

4.   Consequences (a), (b), (c), and (j) would be viewed as positive from the viewpoint of the doctor-patient "contract" as we have defined it: i.e., giving significant information to the patient so that he can make his own ethical decisions. While instituting a lawsuit may in fact be a decision the patient may make upon receipt of the data, we would tend to regard that as indicating a breakdown of the "contract," albeit a justifiable one from the patient's viewpoint. So we might say that consequences (e) and (f) are contrary to a high value in the doctor-patient "contract." In all, however, the value of the "contract" would seem to be served well by the formal ethical statement as written. (Frames 110, 123, 129)

5.   The consequence which addresses itself most directly to this value is (i), which is contradictory to the state of affairs desired. Other consequences which might contradict the stated value are (d) and (f). Consequence (k) might further the value of team performance, but it is a low-probability consequence. In sum, if one places a high value on team cooperation and efficiency, one might decide that the formal ethical statement is in need of revision.

6.   The core of the problem with Consequence (i) appears to be the fact that the doctor is placing his "contract" with the patient above his responsibility to the other team members; the team has to shoulder the blame while the doctor has washed his hands of the matter. The team-patient "contract" may indeed require that the parents be told, but if so, the team, not just the doctor, ought to be in on the decision. Therefore, one might wish to alter the formal ethical statement to:
"When an error in therapy that has significant consequences for the patient is made by a member of the health care team, a team member, usually the doctor, ought to inform the patient or guardian as soon as possible. The health care team should decide among themselves how and when the disclosure ought best to be made, depending on the circumstances of the individual case."
Of course, having looked at Consequences (e) and (f) as well as (i), you might have decided that the entire ethical statement ought to be reversed, and that it would be better not to tell the parents the truth. If you do this, however, you would have to be ready to accept all the consequences of withholding important information. (Frames 43-47)

7. In the case described, which course of action you choose can have little effect on L.K. Even if L.K. were conscious, and a patient in the physiological state described would not be in all likelihood, he is too young to understand what is happening. One might speculate that if L.K. were conscious, and the parents were not told what was happening and were very anxious and confused as a result, L.K. might sense this emotional atmosphere and be adversely affected by it; but that is about all the effect that the ethical decision could possibly have on him directly. The therapy that you will give him does not depend on his parents knowing the true cause of the problem.

To digress a bit, the fact that L.K. cannot be harmed in any material way by not telling the truth, while the doctor or the hospital could be hit with a lawsuit if the truth is known, might lead an ethical utilitarian to the conclusion that the true cause of the accident ought to be concealed. In that way the "greatest good for the greatest number" would best be served. On the other hand, an ethicist who places high priority on some concept of "justice" might say that the parents ought definitely to be told, and if the responsible parties are sued, they are just getting what they deserve. If you are not clear on how these ethical decision-making methods differ from the one we have been using, see Appendix I.

8. If you answered No. 6 as we did, you were extending the original concept of the doctor-patient contract to that of a team-patient contract, and you decide that therefore the entire health care team, not just the doctor, ought to have a say in the matter. Or possibly you reasoned that while the main "contract" is still between patient and doctor, the pharmacist and nurses, who stood to suffer significant and deleterious consequences if the truth were told, had acquired rights of participation for that reason. (Frames 166, 346-349)

9. Again, if you were extending the "contract" to cover the rest of the team members as well as the doctor, this represents a basic modification in the doctor-patient relationship. (Frame 166)

10. The statement suggests that the speaker is regarding "doing everything possible to have a normal child" as something to which she is entitled by some higher authority, regardless of the consequences. Thus, she is claiming this as a "right." Since this is not a "right" as traditionally defined in the legal sense, the speaker is obligated to state 1) by what authority she has this right, and 2) exactly who is obligated to carry out the required actions (since this is a "right" requiring action instead of a right prohibiting action). She has failed to do both of these. (Frames 157-165)

11. Every ethical decision requires both data and a value judgment. The speaker here seems reluctant to make the needed value judgment, so, consciously or unconsciously, he is misstating the nature of the ethical question and confusing it with an empirical question, in order to get himself off the hook. In fact, the one-sentence case description provides nearly all the data needed to make the ethical judgment, with the exception of the psychological nature of the husband-wife relationship. (Frames 18-20)

12. The speaker here, by prefacing his remarks with "I am your doctor," seems to be assuming that because of his good motives in his role as physician, he is more competent than the patient to make the required ethical judgments. He is attributing ethical expertise to himself merely on the basis of 1) his socially "good" role and 2) his socially "good" motives—neither of which is adequate insurance that the best course of action will be chosen. These errors have led him into the "Priestly Model" of the doctor-patient relationship. (Frames 107-110, 847-853)

13. What is the actual likelihood that everyone will want to have a "manufactured" baby even when they could have a real one? On the face of it, the proposition seems highly unlikely, and the speaker has offered no evidence to the contrary. If the probability of this consequence is that low, it should be of very low weight in the ethical decision-making process, yet the speaker has based his entire argument on it. We have here the "domino theory" or "foot in the door" theory of ethics, which has the various flaws described in Frames 227-230.

14. Presumably the speaker is treating the injunction "do no harm" as if it settled the question definitively in favor of not doing surgery. But with the little data available, we cannot judge whether the "harm" done by surgery will be greater or lesser than the harm of not doing surgery. It makes a great deal of difference whether the child has a brain tumor or whether he has simply been showing signs of hyperactivity, but, by using "do no harm" as a "catch phrase" the speaker has avoided these issues entirely. (Frames 308-309)

15. From an empirical statement about what animals do in the natural world, the speaker has jumped to an ethical judgment that homosexuality is "wrong" and to an ethical statement about how homosexuality should be handled. Clearly he has made a value judgment in the process, but the form of his statement has served to obscure this. The speaker is engaging in another form of confusion between ethical and empirical statements, by deriving an ethical statement purely from empirical evidence—and erroneous evidence at that. (Frames 18-20)

16. No ethical error.

17. The speaker here is indulging in retrospective ethics. It is just as likely, indeed more likely from the data available at the time of the original decision, that the bus driver would have had a heart attack, and it is possible that he would have had it on the job. The ethical decision at the time should have been based on the consequences as best they could be judged then; the ethical decision does not become right in hindsight just because the doctor "lucked out." (Frame 155)

18.	The speaker here is making a moral judgment by definition of words, rather than by the consequences of actions. If it were true that 1) abortion is indeed the same as murder, and that 2) murder could be shown to have very bad consequences, which are not outweighed by good consequences, then it would indeed follow that abortion is immoral. But both these propositions require some supporting evidence, which the speaker has not provided. (Frame 269)

19.	Like the speaker using the "domino theory," this speaker is putting decisive weight on one possible consequence of very low probability, while ignoring relevant consequences which are much more likely to occur. In effect, this sort of person is making ethical decisions by anecdote rather than by weighing consequences according to values. This can never lead to any general agreement, since anyone can come up with an anecdote which "proves" the opposite side. (Frames 267-268)

# Index*

*Numbers refer to frames except for those with the prefix "A", which refer to pages.